Small Animal Arthroscopy

Small Animal Arthroscopy

BRIAN S. BEALE, DVM, DIPLOMATE ACVS
Gulf Coast Veterinary Specialists
Houston, Texas

DONALD A. HULSE, DVM, DIPLOMATE ACVS
College of Veterinary Medicine
Texas A&M University
College Station, Texas

KURT S. SCHULZ, DVM, MS, DIPLOMATE ACVS
Department of Surgical and Radiological Sciences
University of California, Davis, California

WAYNE O. WHITNEY, DVM, DIPLOMATE ACVS
Gulf Coast Veterinary Specialists
Houston, Texas

Illustrated by

JOHN H. DOVAL, BPA
Department of Surgical and Radiological Sciences
University of California, Davis, California

and

KURT S. SCHULZ

SAUNDERS
An Imprint of Elsevier Health Sciences

SAUNDERS
An Imprint of Elsevier Science
The Curtis Center
Independence Square West
Philadelphia, Pennsylvania 19106

NOTICE

Veterinary Medicine is an ever-changing field. Standard safety precautions must be followed, but as new research and clinical experience broaden our knowledge, changes in treatment and drug therapy may become necessary or appropriate. Readers are advised to check the most current product information provided by the manufacturer of each drug to be administered to verify the recommended dose, the method and duration of administration, and contraindications. It is the responsibility of the treating veterinarian, relying on experience and knowledge of the animal, to determine dosages and the best treatment for each individual animal. Neither the Publisher nor the editor assumes any liability for any injury and/or damage to animals or property arising from this publication.

The Publisher

Library of Congress Cataloging in Publication Data

Small animal arthroscopy / Brain S. Beale . . . [et al.].—1st ed.
   p. cm.
  Includes bibliographical references.
  ISBN 0-7216-8969-8
   1. Dogs—Surgery. 2. Cats—Surgery. 3. Joints—Endoscopic surgery. 4. Veterinary arthroscopy.
  I. Beale, Brian.
SF991.S585 2003
636.7′0897—dc21

2002066972

Acquisitions Editor: Raymond R. Kersey
Senior Developmental Editor: Denise LeMelledo

RT/QWK

Printed in the United Sates of America

Last digit is the print number: 9 8 7 6 5 4 3 2 1

This book is dedicated to our families for their understanding and support, our fellow arthroscopists for their inspiration and perseverance, and our clients for entrusting us with their canine companions.

Foreword

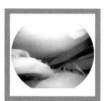

I t is a great pleasure to be asked to write a foreword to the text of *Small Animal Arthroscopy*. It is also pleasing to see the coming of age of arthroscopic surgery in the dog, and I am confident that this text will enable many small animal surgeons to achieve expertise in arthroscopy. When I wrote the first edition of *Diagnostic and Surgical Arthroscopy in the Horse* in 1984, I did so in response to numerous requests for the photos and diagrams from our courses. Budding arthroscopists need clarification of the exact locations for portals, knowledge of the unique arthroscopic anatomy, and the techniques available to them in real time. I am confident that *Small Animal Arthroscopy* will be used constantly in small animal surgery practices.

There are many challenges to the surgeon learning arthroscopic surgery, including exactly locating portals, relearning anatomy, developing the unique hand-eye coordination that goes with minimally invasive surgery, and operating off a video screen. The advantages of arthroscopy over arthrotomy include decreased surgical morbidity, greatly enhanced visualization and diagnostic evaluation of joints, and an enhanced success rate. However, there is a price to pay including the cost of the equipment and the time investment in learning and training. Ultimately, such challenges should not prevent surgeons from embracing this technique.

I predict that there will be resistance to acceptance of the technique in some quarters. There will be those who say, "I want to do an arthrotomy and really see the joint," when you actually see so much more with the arthroscope. Small animal arthroscopic surgeons will be accused of using the technique to get cases and to make money or of promoting a gimmick; I know because we heard these accusations when we started performing equine arthroscopy. The truth is that the naysayers have a fear of the new, do not want to learn new techniques, or do not want to change. Regardless of their age, surgeons should embrace this new—though difficult—technique for the welfare of the dog. Arthroscopy in the dog has arrived and will take its place as the only way to perform joint surgery in the dog, as it has in the horse. I congratulate the authors on achieving the skills, developing the techniques, and now writing the text.

Wayne McIlwraith

Preface

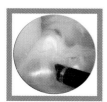

The last 15 years have been perhaps one of the most exciting periods in veterinary orthopedic medicine. During this period the profession has witnessed tremendous advances in techniques, including total joint replacement, TPLO, advanced musculoskeletal imaging, ring and interlocking nail fracture fixation, and limb spare procedures. Not the least of these advances has been the growth of the use of arthroscopy in the diagnosis and treatment of articular diseases in the dog.

The application of arthroscopy to the relatively small joints of the dog has been made possible through the development of small joint arthroscopy equipment and the perseverance of pioneers in the field such as George Seimering, Myron Person, Jean Francois Bardet, Henri Van Bree, and Bernadette Van Ryssen. The outcome of their work and that of others is a practical and invaluable method for the visual evaluation and treatment of diseases of the major joints of the dog.

Arthroscopy has become the modality of choice for the diagnosis and treatment of many diseases of the joint in dogs. Arthroscopic surgery is minimally invasive, thus reducing postoperative pain and accelerating recovery. Arthroscopy improves visualization by magnifying and intensely illuminating the joint within its natural fluid medium. Finally, because of its low morbidity, arthroscopy is an excellent choice when it becomes necessary to treat two or more joints at the same time.

The benefits of complete visualization and magnification of articular surfaces and structures cannot be overstated. In particular, arthroscopy gives the surgeon a new understanding of osteoarthritis. This condition is the most prevalent of all orthopedic diseases of the dog, and before the advent of arthroscopy, the presence and severity of osteoarthritis was judged almost exclusively on radiographs. Arthroscopy complements radiography as a means of evaluation and staging of osteoarthritis and may soon replace it as the gold standard in the assessment of canine osteoarthritis.

The use of arthroscopy has had a particularly significant impact in the diagnosis and treatment of lameness of the forelimb. In our practices, before the use of arthroscopy, a significant percentage of adult canine forelimb lameness went undiagnosed. The use of arthroscopy on the forelimb has enabled greater awareness of osteoarthritis of the elbow, diseases of the biceps tendon and bursa, and injuries of the supporting structures of the shoulder. While arthroscopy has greatly enhanced our ability to diagnose these problems, the challenge now is to develop effective therapies for these widespread conditions.

The goal of the authors was to produce a book that was easy to read, well-illustrated, and practical in nature. Chapters describing arthroscopy of the joints were organized in a uniform fashion and include sections on instrumentation, patient preparation, anesthesia and pain control, portal sites, surgical anatomy, and surgical treatment. The text is written with some duplication so that the reader rarely needs to refer to other sections of the book. A large number of illustrations are presented because arthroscopy is very visual in nature and is initially technically demanding. Computer-generated graphics, exterior photographs, and intra-articular photographs are used to guide the reader. Although we have attempted to provide a thorough written description of each technique, the illustrations in each chapter simplify the learning process and present information that words could never provide. Graphics and photographs were contributed by all the authors, but special recognition goes to John Doval for the many hours put into the development of these quality illustrations. A compact disc has been developed to complement the textbook with short video clips of topics addressed in the book.

The book contains chapters on the history of arthroscopy; equipment and instrumentation; shoulder, elbow, carpus, hip, stifle, and tarsus arthroscopy; clinical arthroscopic cases; and medical management of osteoarthritis. We are particularly pleased with Chapter 9, which discusses clinical arthroscopic cases. The content of this chapter meets our goal of providing clinically relevant material that can be used on a regular basis in the private practice setting. All authors contributed to all chapters, although each chapter was assigned to a primary author for initial organization and composition.

We have decided to use a format for references and further reading that has been popular in other recent veterinary textbooks. Specific pertinent references are included at the end of each chapter either as references (specific studies) or as suggested readings (important related publications). Reference numbers are not used in the body of the text.

Authors

Acknowledgments

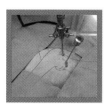

We would like to recognize the hard work, dedication, and patience of Denise LeMelledo of W. B. Saunders and Ray Kersey of W. B. Saunders for giving us the opportunity to produce this book. Thanks also to Peggy Gordon of P. M. Gordon Associates. We also thank all the veterinary arthroscopists around the world who collaborated with us over the years. Much of the information included in this textbook is the result of inspirational discussions with our colleagues, often late at night and in a multitude of venues. Lastly, we thank our families for the support and understanding they provided during the many hours required to complete this project.

About the Authors

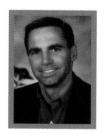

Brian S. Beale, DVM, Diplomate ACVS, Gulf Coast Veterinary Surgery, Houston, Texas. Brian joined Gulf Coast Veterinary Specialists in 1992 after completing his residency and serving on the faculty of the University of Florida's College of Veterinary Medicine. Brian has a special interest in arthroscopy, minimally invasive fracture management, medical management of osteoarthritis, and perioperative pain management. He has authored many publications and speaks internationally on these topics. Brian is an adjunct assistant professor at Texas A&M College of Veterinary Medicine. He is past president of the Veterinary Orthopedic Society, is president of the Gulf Coast Veterinary Education Foundation, serves on the credentials committee of the American College of Veterinary Surgeons, and is a member of AO-Vet.

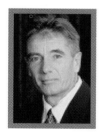

    Donald A. Hulse, DVM, Diplomate ACVS, Professor, Department of Small Animal Medicine and Surgery, College of Veterinary Medicine, Texas A&M University. Don is well recognized for his accomplishments in teaching and research in small animal orthopedics. He served as Section Chief of Small Animal Surgery from 1992 to 1996. He served on the examination committee of the ACVS from 1992 to 1996. He was a member of the board of directors of the Veterinary Orthopedic Society from 1984 to 1987. Don is an active member of AO-Vet and serves on the VEEG committee. He is a frequent national and international lecturer on orthopedic, arthroscopic, and physical rehabilitation topics.

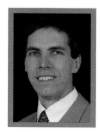

    Kurt S. Schulz, DVM, Diplomate ACVS, Assistant Professor, Department of Small Animal Medicine and Surgery, School of Veterinary Medicine, University of California, Davis. Kurt has an extensive research program and speaks internationally on arthroscopy, canine elbow dysplasia, and joint replacement. He served as Chief of Small Animal Surgery from 1999 to 2003. He is an active member of the Veterinary Orthopedic Society, AO-Vet, Orthopedic Research Society, and the ACVS.

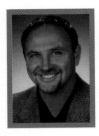

Wayne O. Whitney, DVM, Diplomate ACVS, Gulf Coast Veterinary Surgery, Houston, Texas. After completing his residency at the Animal Medical Center in New York, Wayne started with Gulf Coast Veterinary Specialists at its inception in 1989. There he developed a special interest in arthroscopy, the development of arthroscopic techniques, canine cruciate disease, and injuries of the athletic sporting breeds. He is a recognized speaker on these topics both nationally and internationally. Wayne chairs the arthroscopy seminar for the American College of Veterinary Surgeons, serves on the Gulf Coast Veterinary Education Foundation, and is a member of the Veterinary Orthopedic Society.

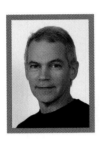

John Doval, Senior Artist, Department of Surgical and Radiological Sciences, School of Veterinary Medicine, University of California, Davis. John has been producing a variety of instructional and publication media since 1984. These include illustrations, photography and video, computer-based multimedia, and CD-ROM.

Contents

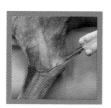

Small Animal Arthroscopy

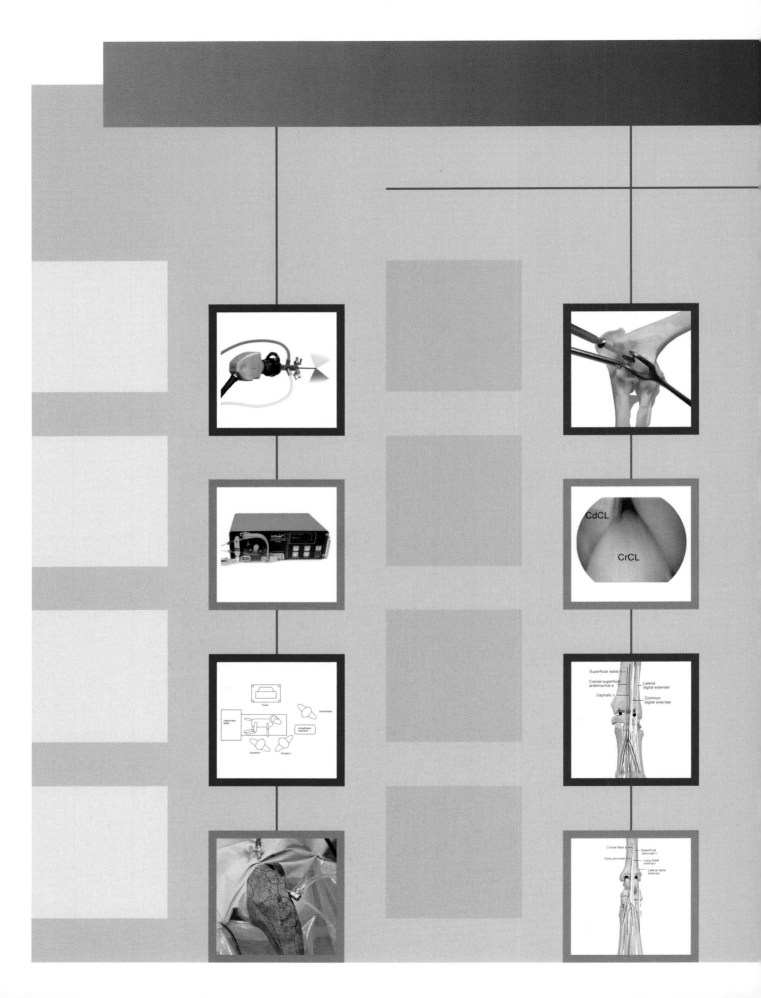

CHAPTER 1

History of Arthroscopy

Introduction

Curiosity about the inspection of body cavities can be traced to ancient Roman times, but it was not until the early 19th century that an instrument was developed to look into the human bladder. The instrument was called a *lichtleiter* and was presented by Bozzini to the Rome Academy of Science in 1806. The instrument generated much talk and curiosity, but was not accepted by the scientific community as a clinically useful item. During the early 19th century, few advances were made in the field of endoscopy, primarily because surgeons lacked an adequate source of illumination. Until the invention of the incandescent light bulb in 1879, the only sources of illumination were combustion of fuel and candlelight. Neither source provided adequate illumination, and combustion of fuel was often dangerous to the patient! Shortly after the invention of the light bulb, a cystocope was developed in Germany that used an incandescent light source. After that time, cystoscopy slowly developed and eventually was regarded as a reasonable diagnostic and therapeutic tool.

In the early 20th century, tuberculosis was a common cause of knee osteomyelitis and ankylosis in humans. A stiff knee was a serious disability for a population that relied on the ability to perform physical work. In Japan, Takagi attempted to diagnosis tuberculosis in its early stage in an effort to prevent late ankylosis. He was inspired to use a cystoscope to look inside the human knee and did so for the first time in 1918. Subsequently, Takagi began the development of the arthroscope. He continued to improve the design of the arthroscope and arthroscopic instrumentation until the outbreak of World War II. During the same period, Bircher from Switzerland and Kreuscher from the United States investigated the possibility of using arthroscopy to treat knee disorders in humans. Kreuscher is considered the first American pioneer in arthroscopy and was the first author to publish an article on arthroscopy in the English literature.

In the years just before World War II, several surgeons from the United States and Europe continued to investigate and publish reports on the use of rigid endoscopes to examine joints. The War brought a halt to advances in almost all biologic sciences, including arthroscopy. After the War, Wantanabe, of Tokyo, continued the work of Takagi and further advances in arthroscopy occurred. Wantanabe, who is considered the father of modern arthroscopy, developed arthroscopes using emerging technologies in Japanese optics and electronics. He developed a number of arthroscopes, and in 1959, he produced the first commercial arthroscope (the no. 21 arthroscope). The same year, Wantanabe also published the first atlas on arthroscopic surgery. In 1964, Jackson completed a surgical scholarship in Tokyo, and after observing Wantanabe, recognized the value of looking inside a joint. Jackson returned to Toronto with a no. 21 arthroscope and introduced arthroscopy to North America. Technology and expertise in human arthroscopy developed slowly through the late 1960s and 1970s. Surgeons responsible for pioneering arthroscopy in humans include such prominent orthopedists as O'Conner, who developed instrumentation for arthroscopic meniscectomy; Johnson, who introduced the needle arthroscope; and Jackson, who organized many instructional courses in diagnostic arthroscopy. Arthroscopic techniques and instrumentation continue to be refined, and today, arthroscopy is considered one of the most significant advances in human orthopedics.

Arthroscopy in veterinary surgery evolved similarly. In the early 1970s, the first reports of large animal arthroscopy appeared in the German and English European literature. In the United States, use of the arthroscope to diagnose equine carpal disorders was reported by Hall in 1974 and more extensively by McIlwraith in 1978. Early reports were met with skepticism, but by the mid-1980s, large animal arthroscopy was becoming more common. Although initially used as a diagnostic tool, as surgical expertise developed and equipment improved, therapeutic procedures became common. Prospective and retrospective studies have substantiated the value of therapeutic arthroscopy in large animal surgery. In general, the initial optimism and suggested advantages have been substantiated and criticisms refuted.

Small animal arthroscopy was slow to develop compared with the development of arthroscopy in humans and large animals. The belief that arthroscopy was not needed or was not practical in small animal orthopedics prevailed, and early reports in the literature were met with skepticism. The first report of arthroscopic surgery in small animal orthopedics was in 1978. Siemering used a 1.7-mm arthroscope to evaluate 180 stifle joints and concluded that arthroscopic examination of the stifle joint in dogs was both beneficial and useful. About the same time, Bennett and Kivumbi from the United Kingdom explored the usefulness of the arthroscope as a diagnostic aid in the stifle joints of dogs. They also concluded that arthroscopy was likely to become a useful tool in the assessment of joint disease. They wrote that arthroscopy in the canine required patience and a long, difficult learning curve. Small animal arthroscopy continued to be a topic of conversation, but few surgeons were interested in pursuing this new technology.

One of the few early pioneers in small animal arthroscopy was Person, who in the mid-1980s, began to publish a series of articles on the use of the arthroscope in small animal joint surgery. Person initially described the use of the arthroscope in the stifle joint of dogs. He described both normal and pathologic findings in 168 examinations and concluded that the arthroscope allowed a thorough, efficient, and atraumatic evaluation of the canine stifle joint. Person followed with a description of the normal arthroscopic anatomy of the canine shoulder joint and coxofemoral joint. In later reports, both Person and Goring described arthroscopic treatment of osteochondritis dissecans of the shoulder.

Even with these early reports of success, arthroscopy in small animal orthopedics did not gain widespread popularity. It was not until van Bree and van Ryssen reported the successful use of the arthroscope to treat joint pathology in dogs that arthroscopy began to receive attention from small animal orthopedists. These authors also offered the first courses on arthroscopic surgery.

Advantages and Disadvantages

Arthroscopy is a modality to perform joint surgery that offers the advantages of enhanced visualization, lower patient morbidity rates, and increased precision. Enhanced visualization and increased precision are possible because of the surgeon's view of the joint surfaces is magnified through the arthroscope. Additionally, the small size of the arthroscope and sheath allows the surgeon to place the arthroscope into various compartments of the joint for assessment. Decreased postoperative pain with arthroscopically assisted joint surgery is well documented in humans. Anecdotal information and early objective evidence suggest that the same is true for small animals. Small portal entrance sites through the inflamed joint capsule invade and transect fewer painful nerve endings than does conventional open arthrotomy. The use of smaller portals leads to much less postoperative pain, increased postoperative limb use, and improved recovery.

Although the advantages of arthroscopically assisted surgery outweigh the disadvantages, some important disadvantages deserve comment. The foremost disadvantage is the learning curve associated with arthroscopically assisted joint surgery. A number of factors contribute to this steep learning curve. First is the coordination needed to move the hand and instrumentation in the proper direction while viewing the instruments through a monitor. Second, canine joints offer little space in which to work. Skill and training are required to manipulate the arthroscope and instrumentation within the joint without causing iatrogenic injury to the cartilage surface. Skill can be increased through early participation in continuing education courses that offer cadaver laboratories. Perhaps early training should focus on the more accessible joints (shoulder and elbow). Once the surgeon is accomplished in procedures involving these joints, those requiring more skill and specialized instrumentation (knee and tarsus) can be studied. Practicing on cadaver specimens is recommended until the surgeon can easily establish egress, arthroscope, and instrument portals. The surgeon always should be prepared to convert the arthroscopic procedure to an open arthrotomy. The surgeon may choose to perform only diagnostic arthroscopy (egress and arthroscope portals) early in the period of training and to perform therapy with an open arthrotomy. As the surgeon gains experience in exploring the joint and identifying abnormal pathology without causing iatrogenic trauma, therapeutic arthroscopy can be used. The time needed to become skilled in diagnostic and therapeutic arthroscopy varies with the number of arthroscopic cases attempted. The surgeon must continue to practice, even though operative time initially will be longer than it would be for a similar procedure performed through an arthrotomy. With time and patience, arthroscopic procedures will require the same or less operative time compared with open arthrotomy.

A second disadvantage of arthroscopically assisted joint surgery is the cost associated with obtaining and maintaining the necessary equipment and instrumentation. For example, a pair of grasping forceps or a handheld curette may cost as much as 1000 US dollars. Motorized shavers and radiofrequency thermal probes are disposable items (although they can be reused if not damaged) and cost 100 to 500 US dollars each. Because the instruments and equipment needed for small animal arthroscopy are small, they can be damage easily. Breakage or damage can occur during setup, during surgery, or during cleaning and sterilization after surgery. Proper training of the technical staff in the handling, sterilization, and storage of instruments and equipment is essential.

Potential Complications

The most common complication of arthroscopic joint surgery is extravasation of fluid into the tissues surrounding the joint. Although unsightly, fluid accumulation outside the joint is a minor complication, and fluid usually is completely absorbed within 24 hours. Fluid extravasation causes the joint capsule to collapse into the joint. As a result, visualization is decreased, and the surgical procedure is prolonged. Extravasation of fluid outside the joint also causes collapse of the tissue walls of an instrument portal. If the surgeon is working through an open instrument portal or inadvertently dislodges a cannulated instrument portal, reentry into the joint may become increasingly difficult as the walls of the portal collapse. All of these factors increase both surgical time and the accumulation of fluid outside the joint.

Fluid extravasation usually is caused by lack of flow through the egress portal or excessive ingress fluid flow. Often, an egress portal becomes obstructed with debris or is dislodged from the joint early in the procedure, usually when a hypodermic needle is used for the egress cannula (shoulder or elbow). The surgeon must monitor fluid egress during the procedure and act quickly to correct a dislodged or obstructed needle. Often flushing the needle with sterile fluid corrects an obstruction, whereas redirecting a dislodged needle corrects a malpositioned egress needle. As the procedure progresses and an instrument portal is established, fluid egress occurs through this site. It is advisable to maintain an egress portal to help evacuate fluid. A large entry surrounding the arthroscope portal or instrument portal may allow fluid to leak around the arthroscope sheath or instrument cannula. This leakage can be prevented by using the scapel blade to incise the skin and subcutaneous tissues to a depth superficial to the joint capsule. The capsule is then penetrated with the arthroscope sheath and attached obturator. High ingress fluid pressure can cause fluid extravasation. This situation is more common with the use of a fluid pump and rarely occurs with gravity (pressure bag) flow. To prevent fluid extravasation associated with the use of an ingress pump, the surgeon must be familiar with the pump system being used. (See the discussion of fluid pumps in Chapter 2.)

The most common serious complication associated with arthroscopy is iatrogenic trauma of the articular surface. Most procedures cause minor abrasion of the surface (arthroscope tracks). These abrasions do not lead to degenerative arthritis. However, the potential for severe iatrogenic damage is real, and this damage is often caused by a combination of surgeon inexperience, inappropriate equipment, and small joint spaces (as seen in the canine). A common mistake is to force a large arthroscope into a small joint space (elbow or tarsus). In this situation, it may be possible to hear the arthroscope sheath grinding the surface as it enters the joint. The result is severe cartilage abrasion. This error is often caused by the use of an arthroscope or arthroscope sheath that is too large. Often, when initially purchasing equipment, the surgeon will purchase a single 2.7-mm arthroscope. However, smaller dogs and joints (elbow or tarsus) may not accommodate this size equipment. If the larger arthroscope is forced into the joint, significant damage is likely to occur. An accomplished arthroscopic surgeon must have arthroscopes and instruments for

joints and dogs of different sizes. Purchase of at least two arthroscopes is suggested: a 1.9- or 2.4-mm arthroscope (see Chapter 2) for smaller joints and animals and a 2.7- or 4.0-mm arthroscope for larger joints and animals. It is also important to know the outside diameter of the arthroscope sheath. Some manufacturers offer a small-diameter arthroscope (2.4 mm), but only a high-flow arthroscope sheath (3.2 mm). Although the arthroscope in the example is appropriate for small joints, the arthroscope sheath is not.

Another common error made by inexperienced surgeons is scarifying the articular cartilage by excessive movement of the arthroscope tip within the joint or by inappropriate movements with intra-articular instruments. This problem is particularly likely within the osteoarthritic cartilage because the surface is soft as a result of chondromalacia. This error can be avoided by adequate practice on cadavers before the surgeon performs clinical cases. Also, proper draping, patient positioning, and correct limb position during surgery are essential in preventing articular damage.

A third complication associated with inexperience is failure to recognize lesions or to treat them appropriately. All lesions may not be preventable. With the exception of 1- or 2-day arthroscopy courses for those beginning their training, most veterinary surgeons learn through experience. It is important to provide follow-up of all surgical cases. If the outcome is less than optimal or if a complication arises, a thorough workup is necessary to determine the reason for the failure. Perhaps the goal of the initial surgery was not accomplished.

Bipolar and monopolar radiofrequency units are becoming popular for use in canine arthroscopy. Bipolar units function by heating fluid between the electrodes in the tip of the ablation probe. Monopolar units function by heating interstitial fluid. These units are helpful, but must be used cautiously because both types can cause severe articular damage if they are not carefully controlled. Monopolar units must actually touch the cartilage to cause damage, whereas bipolar units cause cartilage damage even as far as 1 mm away from the surface.

Suggested Readings

Bircher E: Die arthroendoskopie. Zentralbl Chir 48:1460–1461, 1921.

Burman MS: Arthroscopy or direct visualization of joints. An experimental cadaver study. J Bone and Joint Surg 13:669–695, 1931.

Jackson RW: The introduction of arthroscopy to North America. Clin Orthop 374:183–186, 2000.

Kreuscher P: Semilunar cartilage disease: a plea for early recognition by means of the arthroscope and early treatment of this condition. Ill Med J 47:290–292, 1925.

McIlwraith CW: Diagnostic and Surgical Arthroscopy in the Horse, 2nd ed. Philadelphia, Lea and Febiger, 1989.

Smith M: Arthroscopy in large animals. Proceedings of the 11th Conference for the European Society of Veterinary Surgery, 1975.

Takagi K: Practical experience using Takagi's arthroscope. J Jpn Orthop Assoc 14:359–441, 1933.

Wantanabe M: The development and present status of arthroscopy. J Jpn Med Instr 25:11, 1954.

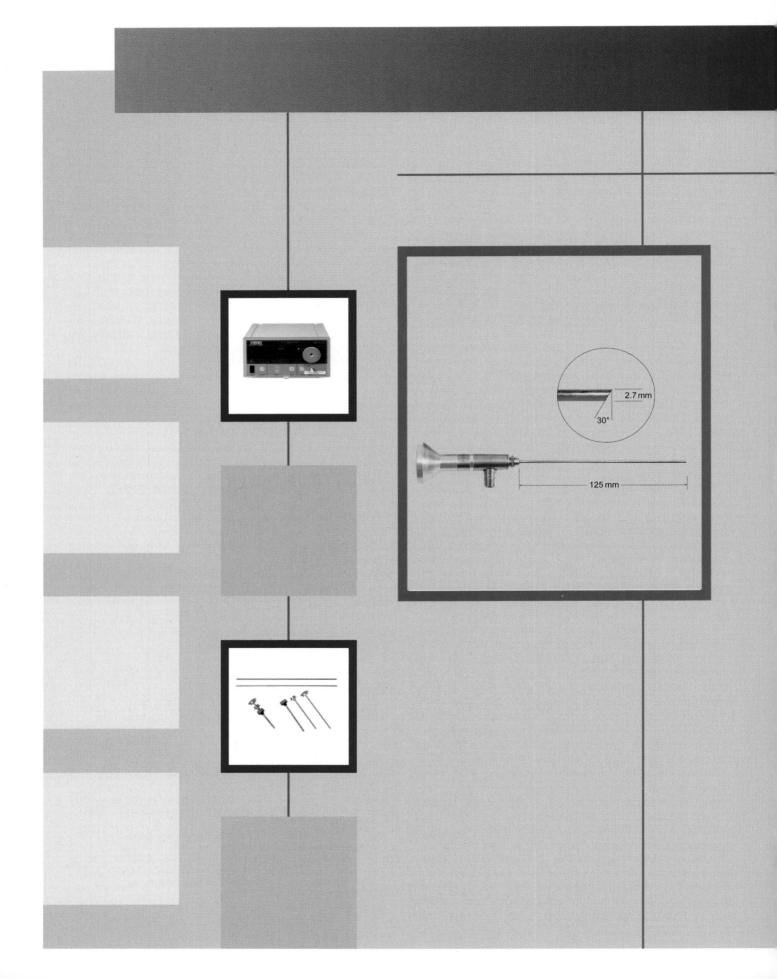

2.7 mm

30°

125 mm

CHAPTER 2

Arthroscopic Instrumentation

Introduction

The technique of arthroscopy was pioneered in the early 1920s by Kenji Takagi, a Japanese physician at the University of Tokyo who adapted a cystoscope for examination of the knee. Starting with a 7.3-mm–diameter scope, his design progressed to a 3.5-mm system that included lenses for magnification. Independently, Eugene Bircher of Switzerland used a laparoscope to examine the knee joint in 1921. The first full arthroscopic surgery was performed by Masaki Watanabe, a student of Takagi. In 1955, Watanabe successfully removed a necrotizing xanthomatous giant cell tumor from a patient's knee. Watanabe's development of the "needlescope," a fiberoptic instrument with tip diameters of 2.2 mm and 1.7 mm, marked the beginning of the modern age of arthroscopy and the evolution of instrumentation that permits evaluation of small joints, including those of the dog.

Understanding arthroscopic equipment and selection of appropriate equipment are vital to the success of an arthroscopy program. Of primary importance is the quality of the optical system. The equipment must provide an excellent image to enable precise visualization, diagnosis, and therapy. The quality of the visualization is supported by appropriate fluid management. To maintain visualization during the procedure, adequate fluid flow must be established and maintained. Fluid flow is dependent on the ingress and egress (inflow and outflow) system and the gravity or fluid pump system. Finally, success in biopsy or therapy requires small, high-quality hand instruments. Appropriate selection and care of the appropriate equipment will permit years of accurate arthroscopic diagnosis and therapy with minimal iatrogenic joint trauma.

Arthroscopes

The modern arthroscope is a fine-diameter telescope that includes an outer fiberoptic portion that transmits light into the joint and a series of inner lenses that transmit an image to the eye or camera (Fig. 2–1).

Arthroscopes are commonly described by three measurements: telescope diameter, distal lens angle (viewing angle), and working length (Fig. 2–2). The telescope diameter is the outer diameter of the tubular portion of the arthroscope without the accompanying cannula. Arthroscope diameters commonly used in canine arthroscopy include 1.9 mm, 2.3 mm, and 2.7 mm. These instruments are commonly considered to be forms

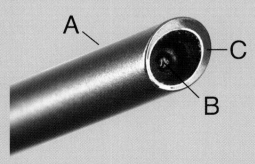

FIGURE 2–1 A 2.7-mm long 30-degree oblique arthroscope. *A*, Telescope; *B*, lens; *C*, fiberoptic light fibers.

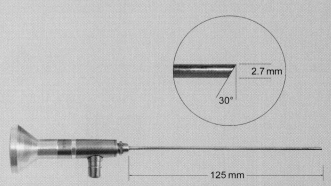

FIGURE 2–2 A 2.7-mm long 30-degree oblique arthroscope, demonstrating bevel angle, length, and diameter.

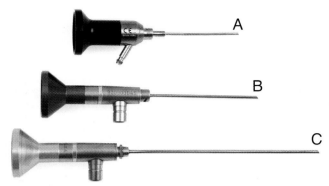

FIGURE 2–3 *A*, 1.9-mm short 30-degree oblique (Dyonics) arthroscope; *B*, 2.3-mm short 30-degree oblique (Stryker Endoscopy) arthroscope; *C*, 2.7-mm long 30-degree oblique (Stryker Endoscopy) arthroscope.

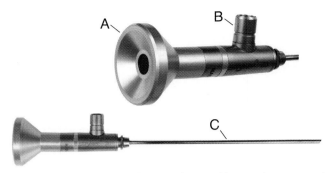

FIGURE 2–5 A 2.7-mm long 30-degree oblique arthroscope with a close-up view of the external end. *A*, Eyepiece; *B*, light post; *C*, telescope (Stryker Endoscopy).

of needle scopes or small-joint arthroscopes (Fig 2–3). Smaller arthroscopes minimize joint trauma and allow greater mobility in small joints, such as the elbow or hock. Larger arthroscopes permit a larger field of view and offer greater resistance to bending and, therefore, greater durability.

The selection of appropriate arthroscopes is discussed in the following chapters. Generally, arthroscopy of the shoulder is performed with a 2.7-mm long arthroscope in most dogs; however, in some smaller dogs, the use of a 2.3-mm scope may be more appropriate. Arthroscopy of the elbow is usually performed with a 1.9-mm short arthroscope. Larger scopes, including 2.7 mm, are also used for this procedure, but the smaller scope provides excellent visualization, improved manipulation, and significantly less iatrogenic trauma than larger arthroscopes. Arthroscopy of the knee is most often performed with a 2.7-mm long arthroscope, although the use of a 2.3-mm or smaller arthroscope may be appropriate in miniature and small breed dogs.

Lens angle is the angle between the center of the viewing range and the axis of the telescope (see Fig. 2–2). The most common angles available in arthroscopes are 0 degrees, 30 degrees, and 70 degrees. The 30-degree arthroscope is the most common type used in canine arthroscopy. Working length is the overall length of the shaft of the telescope and is usually designated as "short" or "long." Short arthroscopes have a working length of approximately 8.5 cm; long arthroscopes have a working length of approximately 13 cm (Fig. 2–4).

Both short and long arthroscopes are used in small animal orthopedics. Short arthroscopes allow greater ease of handling in smaller joints, such as the elbow, and these scopes may be less susceptible to damage from bending. Longer arthroscopes are necessary for larger and deeper joints, such as the shoulder and knee.

The external end of the scope includes an eyepiece, a light source post, and a cannula interlock (Fig. 2–5). The arthroscopic image can be viewed directly through the eyepiece, but because of concerns about sterility and ease of visualization, this method is impractical for modern arthroscopy. Instead, the eyepiece is connected directly to a camera and the image projected onto a monitor.

The connection between the arthroscope and the camera is available in two styles. The most common type is a standard or clip-on adapter (Fig 2–6). The other type is a direct-coupling, or "glass-on-glass," system (Fig 2–7). The standard system has a spring-loaded clip that attaches to the eyepiece of a traditional arthroscope. The direct-coupling system is connected by screwing the arthroscope onto the camera. The arthroscope and the camera used for this type of system are unique in that the arthroscope does not have an eyepiece for direct viewing (without video) and the direct-coupling camera cannot be connected to a traditional arthroscope. It is

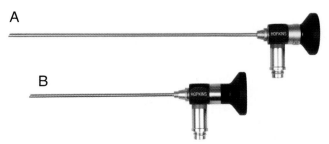

FIGURE 2–4 *A*, 2.7-mm long 30-degree oblique (Karl Storz GmbH & Co) arthroscope; *B*, 2.7-mm short 30-degree oblique (Karl Storz GmbH & Co) arthroscope.

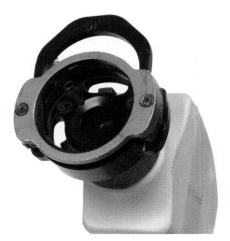

FIGURE 2–6 Clip-on arthroscopy system.

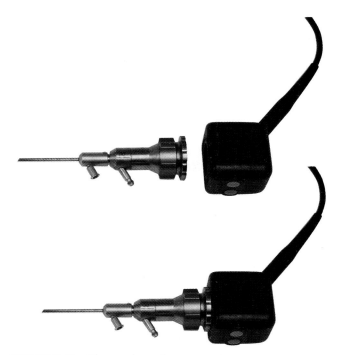

FIGURE 2–7 Glass-on-glass arthroscopy system.

separating the light post from the remainder of the arthroscope.

Cannula interlock designs vary between manufacturers, with designs ranging from simple J-locks to more complex spring-lock mechanisms. Familiarity and dexterity in handling the interlock is an important basic skill in assembly of the arthroscopy system. J-locks are simple to operate; however, they require a flexible washer that can be lost or dropped if it becomes loose. More complex spring-loaded designs do not require a washer but can be slightly more difficult to assemble.

Arthroscopes are available from numerous manufacturers, with moderate variations in design and cost. (See the Appendix.) The choice of which arthroscope to purchase is affected by numerous factors. The first consideration is the diameter and length of arthroscope that is desired. If arthroscopy of all three of the most common joints (shoulder, elbow, stifle) will be performed, then it is advisable to purchase both 1.9-mm short and 2.7-mm long scopes (see Fig. 2–3). If a large volume of arthroscopic cases is anticipated, then it is advantageous to have a 2.3-mm short scope available, although this size is not commonly used. Generally, all small animal arthroscopy is performed with 30-degree scopes, and although other angles are available, they are not frequently used.

Both 1.9-mm–diameter and 2.7-mm–diameter arthroscopes are available from most manufacturers. The choice of manufacturer should depend on the quality and reputation of the product; the warranty and repair record; the price of the individual arthroscopes, either individually or combined with an arthroscopy package; and surgeon preference. The optical quality of the arthroscopes of the companies listed in the Appendix is excellent, and it may be difficult for beginning arthroscopists to recognize a significant difference. Most arthroscopes come with full, long-term warranties against scope failure except for that caused by misuse or inadvertent damage. Typically, most damage to arthroscopes is caused by the surgeon and not as a result of manufacturing problems. Regardless of the cause of damage, however, the manufacturer or a qualified repair company should be able to provide a loaner unit for use while the primary arthroscope is being repaired. Excellent and responsive service is a high priority in the use of arthroscopy equipment. Used and restored arthroscopes are often available for less cost; however, it is imperative to ensure that the units still have outstanding optics and are backed by an adequate warranty.

The only differences in handling of arthroscopes from different manufacturers are slight variations in telescope length and the manner of interlock of the cannula and light post. Familiarity with a particular model or preference for one system over another may affect the purchase. Some manufacturers provide demonstration equipment that can be used clinically for several days or weeks to aid in the selection of equipment. Although most surgeons purchase their original equipment primarily from one manufacturer, it is possible to select different components of the arthroscopy system from multiple manufacturers. Most arthroscopes are adaptable to any

estimated that 50% to 90% of human arthroscopists use standard clip-on arthroscopes because of the ease of switching arthroscopes during a procedure and the lower cost of the system. In general, direct-coupling arthroscopes are more expensive. The potential advantages of glass-on-glass arthroscopes are more reliable coupling and decreased incidence of fogging as a result of water penetration. Fogging of arthroscopes occurs infrequently, but can be frustrating because it significantly obscures the operator's view. Fogging is caused by two mechanisms. The most common is differences in temperature (δT) between the tip of the scope, inside the joint, and the opposite end of the arthroscope. This type of fogging is not entirely eliminated with the glass-on-glass system. Cameras designed for standard mounting may have a suction port on the side to help control fogging. Fogging may also occur if water from the surgical procedure infiltrates the scope-to-camera linkage. This type of fogging is substantially limited by the glass-on-glass system. Some brands offer improved image clarity with the glass-on-glass system. Selection of the glass-on-glass system versus the standard system should be based on cost and consultation with a reputable arthroscopy equipment representative.

The light post is the site of attachment of the fiberoptic cable that provides lighting within the joint (see Fig. 2–5). Light post connections are available in threaded and snap-on varieties, and adaptors are available to accommodate various cable designs. Familiarity with the function of the light post can be important in the selection of compatible light cables and in avoidance of problems with assembly and disassembly of the arthroscopy system. Specifically, it is important that the light cable be separated from the light post versus

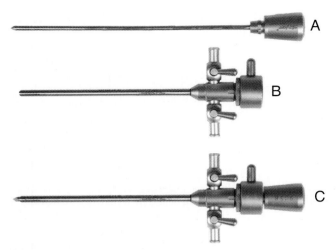

FIGURE 2–8 Large arthroscope cannula system. A, Trocar; B, cannula; C, assembled cannula and trocar (Stryker Endoscopy).

video camera system; however, light cable attachments may vary from manufacturer to manufacturer, and it is important to ensure that an adaptor is available or to purchase a separate light cable.

Arthroscopic Cannulas

The arthroscope is inserted into the joint through a cannula that serves multiple functions (Figs. 2–8 and 2–9). The cannula is a steel tube that is slightly larger than the arthroscope. It permits fluid to run into the joint in the space between the telescope and the cannula. The far end of the cannula is beveled to the angle of the arthroscope. The near end of the cannula has an interlock mechanism that allows connection to the arthroscope and attachment of a fluid line. Cannulas are designed to match a specific arthroscope and usually are not interchangeable. The cannula and arthroscope interlocks must be compatible, and the length and diameter of the

cannula must be appropriate for the arthroscope as well. Because cannulas are specifically designed for their accompanying arthroscope, there are few options in their selection; however, manufacturers offer cannulas of different diameters to allow different levels of fluid ingress. For example, Storz manufactures a high-flow cannula for its 1.9-mm and 2.4-mm arthroscopes.

The functions of the cannula include maintenance of the arthroscope portal, protection of the arthroscope, and ingress of fluid. An arthroscope should never be inserted into a joint without a cannula because the lens may be damaged and the telescope bent during insertion. The cannula is inserted first to establish a portal into the joint. The portal is initiated by incision with a scalpel blade, followed by insertion of the cannula combined with an obturator or trocar (Fig. 2–10). The trocar reinforces the cannula during insertion and provides a tip for ease of insertion. Sharp and blunt trocars are available for most cannulas (Fig. 2–11). Blunt trocars are used most frequently in small animal arthroscopy; sharp trocars tend to cause greater cartilage damage. Sharp trocars are rarely necessary, but it is helpful to have them available in case they are needed. Like the arthroscope and the cannula, the trocar and cannula are specifically designed for each other and must have appropriate interlocks, lengths, and diameters.

Care and Handling of the Arthroscope and Cannula

The arthroscope is likely the most fragile and expensive component of the arthroscopic equipment. It may be damaged during surgery or at any other time by bending the telescope shaft or by cracking or scratching the lens. Specific protocols should be established to avoid damage to the arthroscope. It is advisable to have small cases for each arthroscope that can secure the

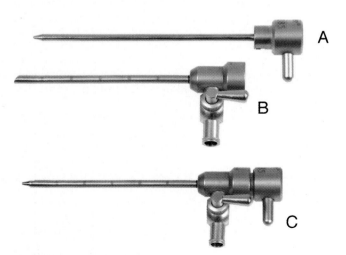

FIGURE 2–9 Small arthroscope cannula system. A, Trocar; B, cannula; C, assembled cannula and trocar.

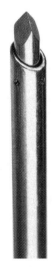

FIGURE 2–10 Close-up view of the tip of an arthroscopic cannula and a sharp trocar (Stryker Endoscopy).

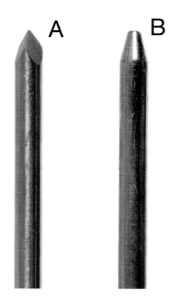

FIGURE 2-11 Close-up view of trocar tips. *A,* Sharp; *B,* blunt (Stryker Endoscopy).

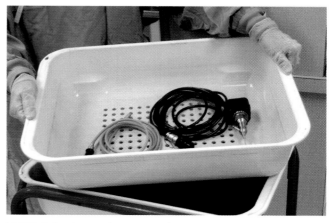

FIGURE 2-13 Soaking process for enzymatic cleaner.

arthroscope, cannula, and trocars for sterilization and storage (Fig. 2–12). The cases should be sturdy and have a means to secure the instruments within the case. The arthroscope should be returned to the case immediately after use to avoid damage while the remainder of the surgical table is cleared. All junctions on the arthroscope, including those between the light post and the scope or between the eyepiece and the telescope, should be checked regularly for tightness. Loose junctions may permit fluid to leak in and impede light or image transmission. Bending of an arthroscope may be evident by the appearance of a black crescent at the periphery of the field of view. A bend will also result in the arthroscopic image migrating across the monitor screen as the arthroscope is rotated. Severe bending will cause complete obliteration of the view. A bent instrument should be sent to a qualified repair facility. Unqualified personnel who attempt to straighten the instrument may cause permanent damage.

Arthroscopes should be cleaned by hand with an enzymatic cleaner and distilled water. Cleaning should be performed as soon as possible after the procedure to remove blood or other body fluids or tissues. The lens

and eyepiece may be gently cleaned with a cotton ball and distilled water. The cannulas and trocars are cleaned in a similar fashion. Sterilization may be performed by several methods. Cold sterilization is performed by placing the arthroscope, cannula, and trocars in a 14-day glutaraldehyde solution (e.g., Cidex, Johnson & Johnson) for no more than 30 minutes (Figs. 2–13 and 2–14). The arthroscope also may be sterilized by ETO gas, Steris, or Sterad, depending on the recommendations of the manufacturer. Most arthroscopes are not autoclavable; even those that are may be damaged by repeated autoclaving because it causes gradual destruction of the glue.

Arthroscopic Cameras

The image from the arthroscope is projected onto a television screen with an endoscopic video camera system. The camera system includes a control unit and a camera head (Figs. 2–15 and 2–16). The camera head includes an electronic chip and a lens adaptor that clip onto the ocular end of the arthroscope and a cable that connects this assembly to the control box. The electronic chip is a semiconductor that converts the image to an

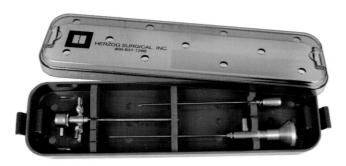

FIGURE 2-12 Arthroscope case (Herzog Surgical).

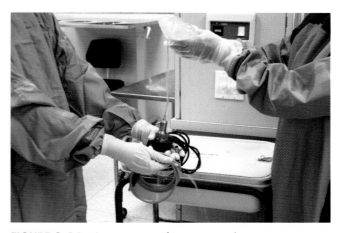

FIGURE 2-14 Rinsing process for enzymatic cleaner.

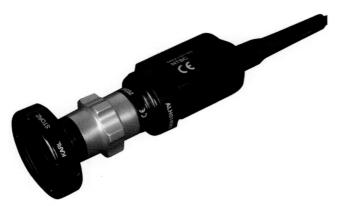

FIGURE 2-15   Camera head for veterinary video camera system (Karl Storz GmbH & Co).

electronic signal. Most cameras contain either one or three semiconducting chips. Three-chip cameras give greater resolution than one-chip cameras; however, three-chip cameras can be significantly more expensive. Single-chip cameras provide an excellent image and are appropriate for most applications. Most camera heads fit most arthroscopic eyepieces, regardless of manufacturer, although it is advisable to ensure compatibility before purchasing components from different manufacturers. Some camera heads have controls that permit white balance, image printing, or zoom. These camera heads may be significantly more expensive, however, and these features are not necessary for basic arthroscopy. The end of the cable that plugs into the control box has a cap that protects the connecting pins or card edge connector from damage during sterilization and handling. During an arthroscopic procedure, the cap should not be removed by the surgeon because the inside is not sterilized. Instead, a technician removes the cap after this end of the cable is passed off the table.

The control box converts the electronic image information into a standard video signal and relays the image to the monitor. The control box is usually specific to the camera head; therefore, the camera head and control box must be from the same manufacturer. The box may have controls that specify the type of endoscopy, color balance, and white balance. In most cases, only the white balance function is used once the

unit is set up for arthroscopy. When purchasing an initial camera system, a single-chip camera with a simple control box is adequate.

The cost of camera systems (head and control box) varies primarily based on the number of digital chips and functions. Secondhand or rebuilt equipment may be adequate if it has been restored to excellent operating condition.

The camera head and cable may be damaged by dropping or mishandling. The camera head contains a lens and a prism that may be damaged if dropped or handled roughly. The camera cord contains delicate wires, and the connection may have fine pins. The camera cord should never be bent or wound too tightly, and the cap should be replaced on the connector when it is not in use. Camera heads may be sterilized by autoclave, ETO gas, or cold sterilization, according to manufacturer's recommendations.

Monitors

The final arthroscopic image is visualized on a standard analog color monitor. Most monitors sold in the medical field are manufactured by the Sony Corporation and are of very high quality. These monitors may be purchased independently or in combination with an entire arthroscopy package. Monitors for arthroscopy should have a high horizontal resolution of at least 450 lines and a tube size of 33 cm or larger. Most monitors have S-VHS or composite inputs that allow higher-quality video imaging. No other design factors need to be considered in the selection of a monitor. Used or reconditioned monitors are adequate if the picture quality is not compromised.

Light Sources

Light sources provide illumination within the joint for visualization. The light source box contains the lamp and intensity regulators (Fig. 2–17). Lamps may be tungsten-halogen or xenon. Most new light sources

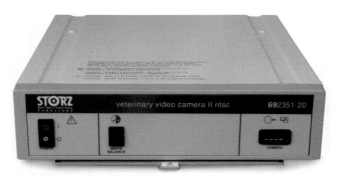

FIGURE 2-16   Control box for veterinary video camera system (Karl Storz GmbH & Co).

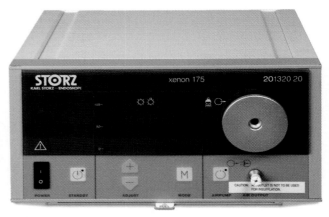

FIGURE 2-17   Xenon 175 light source (Karl Storz GmbH & Co).

use xenon rather than tungsten-halogen lamps. Xenon lamps provide increased light intensity and higher color temperature and, therefore, higher visual clarity and color rendition. Xenon light sources are more expensive but are recommended for superior image quality. Most light sources include automatic intensity control through feedback from the camera video output system. This feature is important for maintaining appropriate image intensity throughout an arthroscopic procedure. Lamp wattage may vary from 175 to 250 W, depending on the manufacturer. Lamps may last a year or longer, depending on usage. Newer units may provide lamp-hour displays, and it is important to have a supply of spare lamps in case of burnout during a procedure. Used units are often available and often are adequate. Recommendations for the selection of a light source include a xenon lamp with limited controls and a lamp-hour display.

The light from the light source is conveyed to the arthroscope through a fiberoptic cable that attaches to the light post on the arthroscope (Fig. 2–18). The connection on the light source may be specific to the manufacturer; however, many light sources have a spring-release connection that permits use with almost any fiberoptic light cable. The type of connection between the light cable and the arthroscope varies with the manufacturer and the size of the arthroscope. For example, the Dyonics 1.9-mm arthroscope uses a small-diameter light cable that screws onto the arthroscope, whereas the Stryker arthroscope uses a larger-diameter cable that snaps onto the arthroscope. In some situations, more than one type of light cable may be needed. Alternatively, appropriate adaptors can be used. Light cables may cost as much as several hundred dollars when purchased new. They may be obtained more inexpensively either used or as part of packages that include a light source. Used fiberoptic light cables are not recommended because degradation or fiber breakage may occur. Light cables may be sterilized by ETO gas, soaking, or autoclave, depending on manufacturer recommendations. A light cable is composed of numerous glass fibers that may be broken if the cable is bent

or wound too tightly. Fiberoptic cables also heat up significantly and should not be placed directly against the patient because it may cause burning.

Documentation

Documentation of arthroscopic procedures provides a permanent visual record that allows historical archiving of arthroscopic findings and therapy and facilitates client and professional communication. Applicable media for arthroscopic imaging include videotape recording, digital capture of still images, and color printing. Each system has advantages and disadvantages, and although one system is adequate for most arthroscopy programs, some surgeons may elect to use more than one method.

Video Recording

Videotape or digital video recording of arthroscopic procedures allows the entire surgical procedure to be recorded with minimal interruption. Unlike with other modes of imaging, the surgeon does not need to remember to capture specific images. Video recording is particularly valuable for demonstration, review, or teaching of arthroscopic techniques and therapies. However, it is less practical for documentation of specific lesions and client communication. Disadvantages of analog video recording include the complexity of creating print images from videotape recording and the necessity to review the tape to find specific images of interest. Advanced digital video systems simplify the process of reviewing and printing images.

Video recording of arthroscopic procedures should be performed with a high-quality system to optimize image resolution. S-VHS and digital systems are recommended and are compatible with most arthroscopic camera systems. The most practical method is to use a separate videotape or disc for each patient, noting in bilateral cases the order of joint operation. The recorder should be placed high on the arthroscopic tower to avoid potential water damage. Medical-grade recording equipment is not necessary, and no advanced features are required, unless video editing is anticipated.

Video Printers

For many years, video printers were the standard method for capturing arthroscopic images (Fig. 2–19). These units produce a 5 × 7-inch glossy color print from the video signal that exits the camera. Most of these units are manufactured by Sony and vary in price. Used units are available for substantially lower prices. A video printer can quickly provide a full-color print without the need for other hardware. In addition, when purchased in combination with a camera system, the camera may have an integrated remote control button for making prints. Disadvantages of video printers include the relative high cost per print and the potential for image

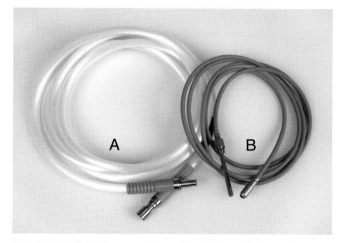

FIGURE 2–18 Fiberoptic light cables. A, Large (Stryker Endoscopy); B, small (Dyonics).

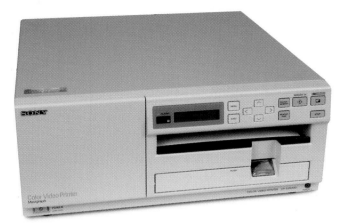

FIGURE 2–19 Arthroscopy printer (Sony Corp.).

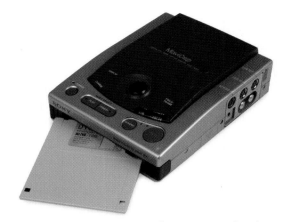

FIGURE 2–20 Device to capture still images (Sony Corp.).

fading with time. If multiple copies of an image are needed, they must be made at the time of the procedure or reproduced with digital scanning or color copying.

Because most printers are manufactured by the same company (Sony), few options are available. There are minor differences in resolution, with most units producing more than 700 lines. Similarly, there are minor differences in printer speed, with most units printing the image in less than 30 seconds. If video printing is the only means of documentation, then an adequate supply of printer ink and paper cartridges should be available.

Digital Capture of Still Images

Digital capture of still images is rapidly becoming a preference in arthroscopic imaging. This method may be used independently or in combination with video recording (Figs. 2–20 and 2–21). In these systems, small or medium file–size images are captured and stored on digital media. These systems offer numerous advantages over other methods of documentation. Digital images may be enhanced with either Macintosh or PC-based computers. Most systems store images as JPEG or TIFF files. These files can easily be imported into software, such as Adobe Photoshop, which can improve image quality through cropping or alteration of contrast or color. Digital images may be incorporated into slide presentations, linked to e-mail, or incorporated into Web pages. These images can often be used in conjunction with computer-based medical records systems. If a color printer is available, digital images also permit greater flexibility in reproducing the image. The two broad categories of digital image capture systems are professional medical systems and consumer items. Medical systems, such as the Stryker system, store images on Iomega Zip disks or CDs in standard file formats (see Fig. 2–21).

Storage of digital images is more convenient than storage of prints, and the images are more durable. Each patient may be assigned a single floppy disk or CD that can be accessed with a personal computer. Disks are readily copied and sent to clients or colleagues. Large volumes of images can be cataloged for numerous uses with software programs, such as Extensis Portfolio, that provide a thumbnail of each image, methods for assigning key words, and search functions that permit the user to find all of the images of one type, for example, images of a torn meniscus.

Arthroscopic Irrigation

Constant, reliable flow of fluid across the tip of the arthroscope and through the joint is vital to adequate visualization. Fluid expands the joint, provides clear fluid for visualization, and clears the joint of debris and contamination. Irrigation also provides a tamponade effect to minimize bleeding during the procedure. Irrigation systems must provide enough pressure to distend the joint and maintain flow without increasing the extravasation of fluid into the soft tissue. The recommended pressure in most human arthroscopic procedures is between 40 mm Hg and 100 mm Hg. Fluid is directed into a Luer-Lok connector on the arthroscopic cannula. It enters the joint through the space between the telescope and the cannula. In some cases, a separate inflow cannula may be used to introduce larger volumes of fluid. Indications for the use of a separate inflow cannula include lavage of a blood-filled or septic joint. Fluid usually must be pushed into the joint under pressure to achieve adequate flow. Fluid may be pressurized by gravity flow or with an electric fluid pump. Both systems have advantages, and selection often depends on the joint being operated on as well as surgeon preference.

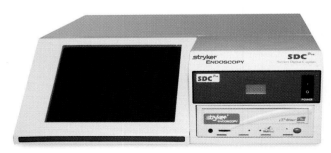

FIGURE 2–21 Digital video camera and device to capture still images (Stryker Endoscopy).

Gravity is an effective method of fluid delivery for procedures that do not involve fluid suction or long-term use of shaving devices. Gravity flow is appropriate for diagnostic procedures and procedures with lower fluid outflow rates. Hospitals that anticipate a high volume of arthroscopic procedures will likely require a fluid pump system.

Gravity and Gravity Assist

Gravity flow is administration of fluid directly from the fluid bag to the cannula with a simple administration set. The diameter of the administration set determines the fluid flow rate. Large-diameter tubing for arthroscopy is available. The rate of fluid flow also may be increased by placing the fluid bag in a pressure bag (Fig. 2–22). Gravity flow also may be increased with commercially available gravity assist devices. These sterile bulbs are placed in line with the fluid administration set and permit intermittent increases in fluid flow. Advantages of gravity flow include the relative simplicity of the system, low cost, and safety against overpressurization. Gravity systems are easy for the surgeon and technician to learn and to use. In addition, they are easy to maintain and do not require additional space in the operating room or on the arthroscopy tower.

Disadvantages include poor control of pressure, relatively low maximum pressures, and the inability to maintain high fluid pressures and flow during the

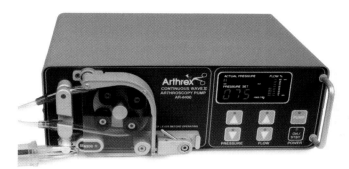

FIGURE 2–23 Control box for an arthroscopic pump (Arthrex).

course of long surgical procedures. Gravity and gravity assist systems require much greater user attention than do pump systems once the system is started. Use of a 3- or 5-L bag may improve pressure and decrease the need for a technician to replace fluid bags or reinflate pressure bags. Also, Y-adaptors permit multiple bags to be hooked up at the initiation of the surgical procedure. Elevation of fluid bags to as high as 8 or 9 feet is recommended to achieve adequate pressures. However, gravity systems may not be able to keep up with fluid outflow if suction devices are applied to the joint.

Fluid Pumps

Fluid pumps permit precise control over inflow rate, inflow pressure, and in some cases, outflow rate (Fig. 2–23). Fluid pumps permit selection of both fluid flow rate and fluid pressure. Most are pressure priority, which means that the selected pressure in the joint will be maintained, and when the pressure drops below this level, the fluid will be pumped in at the selected flow rate. Fluid pumps are superior to gravity at maintaining pressure when suction or shaver systems are in use. When the pump improves visualization and clarity, significantly less time may be needed for the surgical procedure.

Disadvantages of fluid pumps include their initial cost and the cost of the administration sets, the moderate complexity of tube setup, and the space requirements. Many manufacturers supply the pump free of charge with the purchase of a minimum number of tubing sets. Some tubing systems include additional extensions that permit the same basic tubing set and fluids to be used for other patients within 24 hours.

The most basic pump designs, pressure control pumps, maintain articular pressure at a preset flow rate. Newer pumps, known as inflow control pumps, allow selection of both inflow pressure and flow rate. More sophisticated pumps (inflow/outflow control) also allow selection of outflow rate, although this expensive, complicated feature is not necessary for most small animal arthroscopy. Additional features include pressure-relief mechanisms and air-infusion protection systems. Most pumps operate by either a centrifugal impeller or a peristaltic roller. Peristaltic systems provide better pressure maintenance and therefore are preferable to impeller-driven devices. A peristaltic inflow control pump is usually preferred

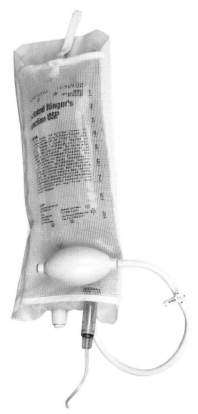

FIGURE 2–22 Fluid compression bag.

for small animal arthroscopy. The selection of a pump is determined by the features desired, the frequency of use, and the tube or pump contract rate.

Egress Systems

Adequate outflow, or egress, must be established to maintain appropriate fluid flow through the joint during arthroscopy. Maintenance of fluid outflow can be particularly challenging in small animal arthroscopy because of the small size of the joints. The use of standard outflow cannulas in smaller joints, particularly the elbow, may cause significant iatrogenic cartilage trauma. The use of needles or catheter stylets may minimize trauma due to size, although the sharp tips may damage the cartilage and the thin diameter may become clogged frequently. Selection of the appropriate outflow instrument is based primarily on the size of the joint.

Commercially available outflow cannulas are steel tubes with outer diameters that range from approximately 2.5 mm to more than 6.0 mm (Fig. 2–24). The far tip of the cannula usually is not beveled, and the tip may have multiple side fenestrations to increase fluid flow. The close end of the cannula may have a Luer-Lok for attaching tubing. The close end also may have a stopcock mechanism to control flow. Cannulas are sold with an appropriately sized sharp or blunt trocar. Other commercially available fluid cannulas are made of clear or opaque plastic, and some have threads or a flange to prevent them from falling out. More complex cannulas have side ports at the close end to permit fluid inflow or outflow while the cannula is used for instrumentation.

For arthroscopy of small joints, such as the human wrist or canine elbow, standard outflow cannulas may be too large for the joint space. In these cases, needles or catheter stylets may be used. Relatively large gauges (14–18) are used to minimize clogging with synovium or shavings. Plastic catheters also may be used if they are large enough and stiff enough to avoid clogging and bending. General recommendations for outflow cannulas in small animal arthroscopy include the following:

Shoulder: large-gauge catheter stylet, small outflow catheter, or teat cannula

Elbow: large-gauge needle

Hip: large-gauge catheter stylet or spinal needle

Stifle: multifenestrated outflow cannula

Fluid may be scavenged from the outflow in several ways. In some situations, the table and drapes can be positioned so that fluid from the cannula drips into a wastebasket on the floor. Alternatively, the fluid may be allowed to flow onto the floor and then be scavenged by a suction device. Numerous reusable floor suction devices are available, and selection often depends on which one performs best given the specific flooring material (Fig. 2–25). A tube may be attached to the outflow cannula or needle and then connected to a suction device or drained into a wastebasket. This technique

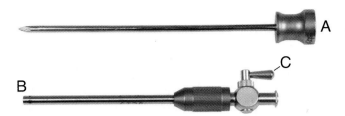

FIGURE 2–24 Multifenestrated outflow cannula. *A,* Trochar; *B,* fenestrations; *C,* stopcock (Stryker Endoscopy).

can be effective, although there are two precautions. First, in small joints, the weight and presence of the tube may cause needle tips to contact the articular cartilage and result in more iatrogenic damage. Second, when gravity flow is used, the outflow rate increases as a result of siphoning. As a result, air may be drawn into the joint if the flow rate from the gravity system cannot keep up with the outflow rate. When an outflow tube is used, it is helpful also to use a clamping device to slow the outflow rate. The clamp reduces the amount of air that is drawn into the joint, decreases the turbulence of fluid in the joint, and permits greater pressurization when desired.

Hand Instruments

Hand instruments for small-joint arthroscopy must combine small diameter with excellent mechanics to provide high accuracy and reliability while minimizing the likelihood of iatrogenic trauma and instrument failure. The basic recommended arthroscopic hand tools include probes, grasping forceps, and biting forceps. Most probes are of a right-angle design with a tip that is approximately 3 mm long (Fig. 2–26). Probes are used to palpate surfaces and manipulate tissues within the joint. In small animal arthroscopy, right-angle probes are used to palpate articular cartilage to detect pathology and to manipulate osteochondritis dissecans flaps, meniscal injuries, and bone fragments. Probes are manufactured in variable thicknesses, and it is recommended to purchase one of moderate stiffness to avoid bending and breaking of the instrument. It is also

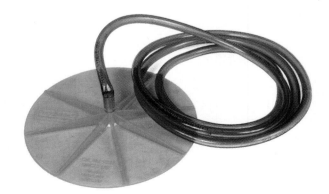

FIGURE 2–25 Floor suction unit (Linvatec).

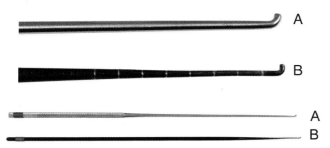

FIGURE 2-26 Right-angle probes with close-up views of the tips. *A,* Plain (Dr. Fritz GmbH); *B,* measured (Arthrex).

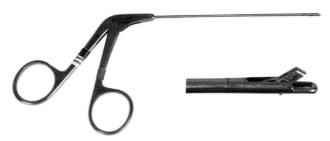

FIGURE 2-28 Arthroscopic punch forceps with a close-up view of the tip (Stryker Endoscopy).

recommended to purchase a probe with measurement markers on the shaft. These markings aid determining the size of lesions within the joint. Probes and other instruments are available in silver, black, or gold. Some manufacturers claim that black or gold instruments create less glare than silver during the arthroscopic procedure. Grit blasting and other surface-roughening techniques are used on some instruments to reduce glare. Manufacturers often provide a handle that may be attached to the probe and other instruments, such as hooks and knives.

Grasping forceps are available as locking and nonlocking types (Fig. 2–27). Nonlocking types include standard alligator forceps and those designed specifically for arthroscopic use. Most grasping forceps designed for arthroscopic use have an enclosed operating mechanism that avoids interference between the mechanism and surrounding tissues. However, standard surgical alligator forceps are adequate for some small animal arthroscopic techniques. Graspers vary in size and length, and selection depends on the joint, the specific procedure being performed, and the preference of the surgeon. Arthroscopic graspers tend to be larger than surgical alligator forceps because of the enclosed mechanism and also because most arthroscopic instruments are designed for human use. However, newer designs for veterinary surgery and human wrist surgery have outer diameters as narrow as 2 mm. The smaller-diameter forceps have distinct advantages in procedures on small animal joints. However, these instruments may bend or break within the joint, and the smaller mechanism provides less grasping power. It is therefore recommended

that a basic arthroscopic surgery pack include a very narrow alligator forceps and a slightly larger and sturdier arthroscopic grasping forceps. The grasping surface may be with or without teeth and blunted or pointed. For most small animal applications, pointed forceps without teeth are recommended.

Locking forceps are advantageous in many arthroscopic procedures involving the removal of bone or cartilage flaps. Locking mechanisms vary significantly, and the choice may be based on cost and surgeon preference. Many forceps designs are available in long and short lengths. Again, selection is based primarily on surgeon preference, although a shorter working length is recommended for smaller joints.

Biting, or punch, forceps are used to débride soft tissues and also may be referred to as basket forceps (Fig. 2–28). Punch forceps have a sharp, hollow lower anvil and an upper punch that is used to remove small pieces of soft tissue, including synovium and meniscus. Variations in design include straight and side-biting and differences in diameter and length. A small- or medium-diameter straight punch forceps is useful in small animal arthroscopy for débriding synovium that is obscuring the view, obtaining a synovial biopsy specimen, and débriding a meniscal injury. Suction punch forceps provide suction at the tip to immediately remove the débrided material (Fig. 2–29). These instruments are larger and much more expensive than standard punch forceps, and they currently have limited application in small animal arthroscopy.

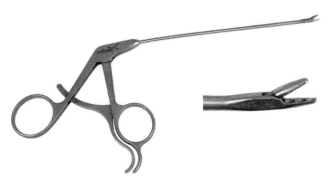

FIGURE 2-27 Arthroscopic grasping forceps with a close-up view of the tip (Arthrex).

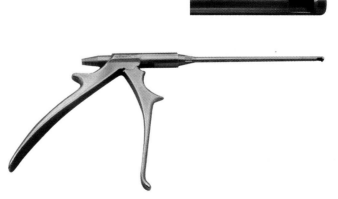

FIGURE 2-29 Arthroscopic suction punch.

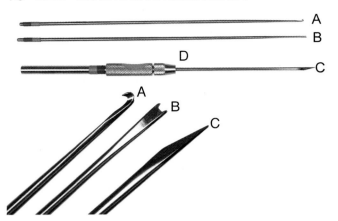

FIGURE 2–30 *Arthroscopic knives. A, Hook knife; B, meniscal knife; C, bayonet knife; D, handle (Dr. Fritz GmbH).*

Arthroscopic knives are useful in small animal arthroscopy for treating meniscal injuries, performing tenodesis, and cutting soft tissue attachments to bony fragments (Fig. 2–30). Knives may be straight, curved, or hooked, and the choice depends on the procedure being performed. Manufacturers often also provide a handle for the knife, but the handle is not necessary for most procedures. A knife set is not mandatory for basic small animal arthroscopy, although purchase of straight and hook knives is recommended for advanced techniques.

Small-diameter curettes are useful in small-joint arthroscopy. These instruments are used to elevate bone fragments and débride cartilage and bone (Fig. 2–31). In most cases, a small (5–0) surgical curette works, although the large diameter of the shaft limits its use to portals without a cannula. Smaller-diameter (2.5-mm) arthroscopic curettes are available that may fit through larger cannulas. A straight curette is easier to insert into the joint and is adequate for most applications. An angled curette is more difficult to insert through the portal, but may be useful for working at difficult angles. Loop or ring curettes are also available specifically for arthroscopic use. These instruments are recommended for advanced arthroscopic techniques, including cartilage débridement.

Curettage and abrasion of bone or cartilage can be performed with a hand burr available from Dr. Fritz

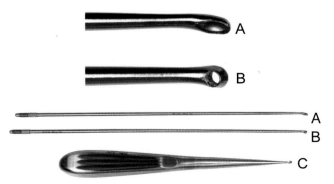

FIGURE 2–31 *Arthroscopic ring (A) and closed (B) curettes with close-up view of the tips (Dr. Fritz GmbH); C, 5–0 surgical curette.*

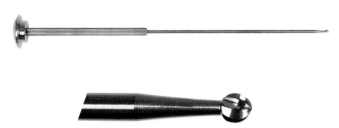

FIGURE 2–32 *Arthroscopic hand burr with a close-up view of the tip (Dr. Fritz GmbH).*

(Fig. 2–32). The instrument is a round burr on the end of an arthroscopic handle. Alternatively, a burr from a power shaver may be used.

In human arthroscopy, microfracture of the subchondral bone bed is routinely performed with angled awls and a mallet. Awls for small animal use are available from Storz (Fig. 2–33). Alternatively, a small (0.035- to 0.045-inch) K-wire may be bent at the tip and secured in a Jacobs chuck for small-joint microfracture.

Instrument Cannulas

Arthroscopic instruments may be inserted into the joint through a portal with or without a cannula. The major advantage of working through a cannula is the ease of instrument insertion. Without a cannula, it may be difficult to switch instruments and identify the portal, particularly if the portal was poorly made. Repeated attempts to insert an instrument through a poorly defined portal can lead to soft tissue trauma and fluid extravasation. The major disadvantage of using a cannula is that some instruments may be too large to permit insertion.

Instrument cannulas are available in numerous diameters and lengths (Fig. 2–34). For small-joint

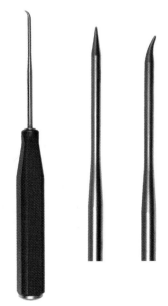

FIGURE 2–33 *Arthroscopic micropick and a close-up view of the tip angles (Karl Storz GmbH & Co).*

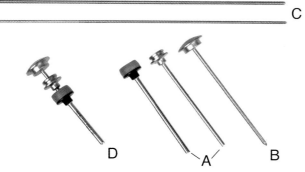

FIGURE 2-34 Veterinary small-joint cannula system. *A,* Cannulas; *B,* trocar; *C,* switching sticks; *D,* assembled system (Dr. Fritz GmbH).

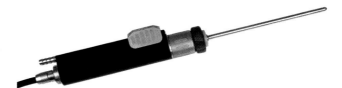

FIGURE 2-36 Small-joint handpiece for an arthroscopic shaver (Karl Storz GmbH & Co).

arthroscopy, cannulas with an inner diameter of 2.3 to 3.5 mm are most appropriate. Lengths of 4 to 5 cm are appropriate. Most cannulas come with both sharp and blunt obturators, although the blunt obturator should be used whenever possible. Some larger cannulas also may have a removable diaphragm that permits insertion of the instrument while limiting loss of fluid from the joint.

Small-joint cannula systems should include a set of switching sticks or tubes (see Fig. 2–34). This system permits progressive dilation of the portal and subsequent insertion of larger cannulas. To use this system, a relatively small cannula, with an obturator, is inserted into the joint. A switching stick is placed through the cannula, and the cannula is withdrawn. A larger cannula or dilation tube is placed over the stick, and the process is repeated until the desired cannula is in place. The use of cannulas depends on the joint, the instruments being used, and the surgeon's preference. Although a cannula system is not necessary for small-joint arthroscopy, it is useful to have a system available for special situations, and it may be easier for beginning arthroscopists to work through cannulas.

Power Shavers

Power shavers are designed to rapidly débride soft and hard tissues. Power shavers are separated into small- and large-joint instruments. Small-joint shavers are appropriate for procedures on the small animal elbow, shoulder, and knee. Large-joint shavers are used in the canine knee for débridement of the fat pad.

Power shavers include a control box, a handpiece, and a shaver tip. The control box includes the power supply and basic operational controls (Fig. 2–35). Most shavers permit the operator to vary both the speed and the direction of the instrument, and options include forward, reverse, and oscillation. Speed control is important because different tissues require different approaches. Variation in direction may not be necessary in small-joint procedures, but this feature is standard on most units. Controls may be located on a foot pedal or the handpiece.

The handpiece secures the shaver to the unit (Fig. 2–36) and should have an insertion point for tubing that directs suction to the tip of the shaver. A suction regulator may be found on the handpiece as well. The handpiece is supplied by an electrical cord that has a capped connector that inserts into the control box. As with all arthroscopic electrical connections, the cap should be removed by a nonsterile assistant rather than by the surgeon because the inside of the cap is not sterile.

Shaver tips are available in numerous styles that are designed for either soft tissue or hard tissue débridement (Fig. 2–37). Soft tissue shavers include guarded sharp cutters and aggressive cutters. Sharp cutters have a simple sharp-edged cup, whereas aggressive cutters

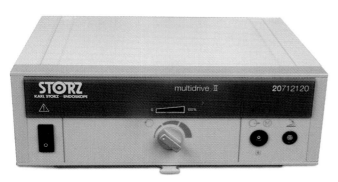

FIGURE 2-35 Control box for an arthroscopic shaver (Karl Storz GmbH & Co).

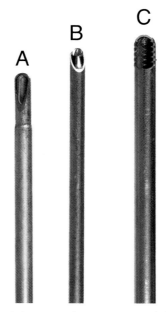

FIGURE 2-37 Arthroscopic shaver tips. *A,* Radial shaver; *B,* burr; *C,* aggressive shaver (Linvatec).

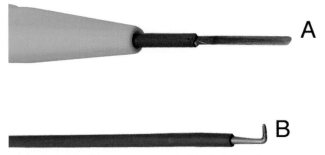

FIGURE 2–38 Electrocautery tips. *A*, Standard; *B*, arthroscopic.

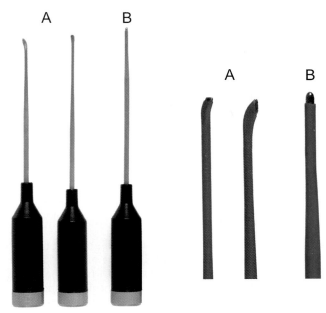

FIGURE 2–40 Unipolar radiofrequency instruments with a close-up view of the tips. *A*, Ablation; *B*, shrinkage (Oratec).

have a toothed cup. The toothed cup is more useful for débridement of fat or synovium in small joints. When an aggressive cutter is used to débride the fat pad of the stifle, limited suction is used and the shaver is operated at a relatively slow speed. Operation of the shaver at higher speeds limits the amount of tissue that can be drawn into the blade. Shaver tips used for débridement of bone are round or oval guarded burrs.

Shaver systems are available either new or used. Many manufacturers supply the handpiece and control box free of charge with a minimum contract for purchase of the shaver tips. The shaver tips are intended for single use, but may be reused if they are resterilized by Sterad or gas. Shaver tips are two-piece units that are separated for cleaning.

Electrocautery and Radiofrequency Devices

Electrocautery and radiofrequency are used to generate heat for cauterization of vessels, débridement of tissues, or shrinking of collagen. Electrosurgical tips specifically designed for underwater arthroscopic application are available for use with standard eletrocautery generators (Fig 2–38). These instruments may be used for cautery of small vessels, and special tips are designed to cut soft tissues.

Radiofrequency devices transfer energy by using electromagnetics to produce molecular friction in the intracellular and extracellular environment. Monopolar units generate an alternating current that runs from the tip of the probe to the joint capsule or other surface,

through the body, to a grounding plate (Figs. 2–39 and 2–40). Heat is generated in the tissues because their resistance is higher. Bipolar units create an arc of energy through the arthroscopic fluid that can be directed through tissues (Figs. 2–41 and 2–42).

Joint capsule collagen is primarily type I. When radiofrequency probes are used on a joint capsule, collagen undergoes denaturation in response to the heating in association with breaking of some crosslinks within the triple-helix structure. Crosslinks between collagen molecules are maintained and cause contraction, or shrinking, of the tissue.

The effect of radiofrequency on shrinkage and tissue strength depends in part on the temperature of the probe. Optimum temperatures are from 65°C to 75°C. Higher temperatures cause greater weakening of tissues. Collagen and the tissues undergoing shrinkage are weaker than normal for 6 to 12 weeks after the procedure. In addition, it is not know how long shrinkage of treated

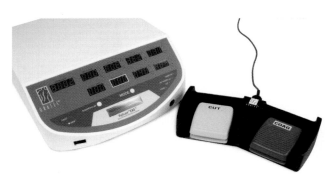

FIGURE 2–39 Unipolar radiofrequency unit (Oratec).

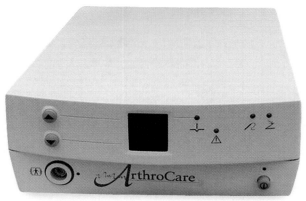

FIGURE 2–41 Bipolar radiofrequency unit (ArthroCare).

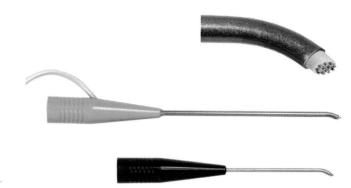

FIGURE 2-42 Bipolar radiofrequency tips (Arthrocare).

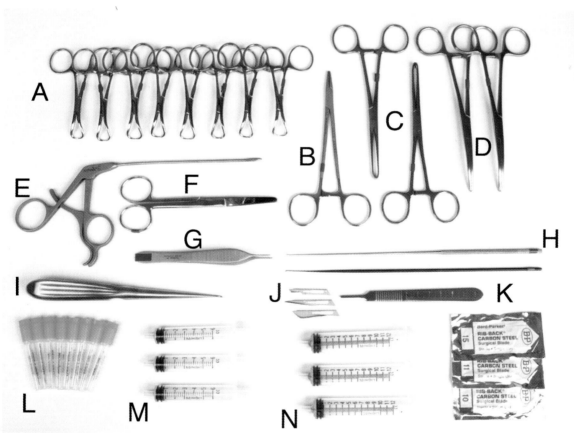

FIGURE 2–43 Basic arthroscopy tray. *A*, Towel clamps (8); *B*, needle driver (1); *C*, Allis tissue forceps (2); *D*, Carmalt tissue forceps (2); *E*, small-joint grasping forceps (1); *F*, suture scissors (1); *G*, Brown Adson tissue forceps (1); *H*, right-angle probes (1 or 2); *I*, 5–0 curette; *J*, surgical blades (blade nos. 11 and 15); *K*, blade handle (1); *L*, 18-gauge needles (8); *M*, 6-mL syringes (3); *N*, 12-mL syringes (3).

tissues persists. In human orthopedics, the most common use of radiofrequency is in the management of shoulder instability in association with rotator cuff injuries. In these cases, the joint capsule of the shoulder is treated, causing immediate shrinkage of tissue accompanied by increased stability. Although shrinkage of as much as 50% can be achieved experimentally, clinical shrinkage is normally 15% to 25%.

In addition to shrinkage, a radiofrequency unit may be used to ablate tissues, including proliferative synovium, torn or damaged meniscus, or partial-thickness cartilage lesions. Routine applications in human orthopedics include imbrication of the shoulder joint by capsular shrinkage, thermal chondroplasty to remove partial-thickness cartilage, partial meniscectomy, débridement of damaged ligaments, synovectomy, and débridement of labral injuries in the shoulder and hip joints.

Radiofrequency probes were only recently introduced into veterinary arthroscopy and orthopedics; however, several useful applications have been identified and numerous experimental applications are being considered. In the stifle joint, radiofrequency is used in combination with power shavers to rapidly remove the fat pad and permit evaluation of the joint. Radiofrequency probes also are used to perform partial meniscectomy of torn meniscus and to débride damaged cranial cruciate ligaments. Potential uses include imbrication of joint capsules in combination with other stabilizing techniques or tibial plateau leveling osteotomy.

Radiofrequency units include a control box, a connecting cable, and a tip. Most manufacturers supply the control box with a contract to purchase a minimum number of tips. Variations in tip design include shrink tips versus ablation tips, and tips are available in different shapes, sizes, and angles. Tips can be resterilized, although they cannot be reused if the insulating cover is damaged.

Instrumentation Sets

Numerous methods are used to organize arthroscopic equipment for surgery, but it is important to limit equipment to what is needed for the procedure so that instruments may be found quickly and easily. The surgeon may elect to have specific packs for each type of joint (i.e., elbow pack, shoulder pack, knee pack) or may choose to have a standard arthroscopy pack, with other equipment packaged separately. The contents of these packs must be cleaned and sterilized routinely.

A standard arthroscopy pack (Fig. 2–43) includes the following:

Alligator forceps (1)
Allis tissue forceps for securing cords (2)
Blade handle (1)
5-0 curette (1)
Grasping forceps (1)
No. 11 and no. 15 blades (2 each)
Needle holder

Right angle probes (1)
Suture scissors (1)
Tissue forceps (1)
Towel clamps for surgical drapes (8)
6-mL and 12-mL syringes (4 each)
18-gauge needles (4)

Additional equipment needed for a shoulder or elbow pack may include an instrument cannula set. Additional equipment for a knee pack may include an egress cannula set.

Towers

An arthroscopic tower is the cart and associated control boxes and monitor. Used carts are often available. Purchase of a heavy-duty cart is important because the control boxes and monitor are heavy (Fig. 2–44).

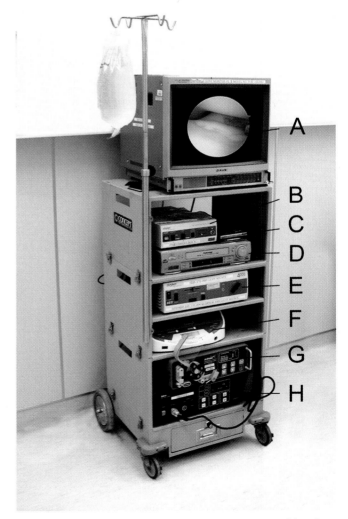

FIGURE 2–44 Arthroscopic tower. *A,* Monitor; *B,* control box for a camera; *C,* device to capture still images; *D,* videocassette recorder; *E,* light source; *F,* radiofrequency unit; *G,* fluid pump; *H,* control box for a shaver.

Suggested Readings

Chamness CJ: Endoscopic instrumentation. In Tams TR (ed): Small animal endoscopy, 2nd ed. St. Louis, Mosby, 2001, pp. 1–16.

Editors: Arthroscopic irrigation/distention systems. Health Devices 28:242, 1999.

Ogilvie-Harris DJ, Weislander L: Fluid pump systems for arthroscopy: a comparison of pressure control versus pressure and flow control. Arthroscopy 11:591, 2001.

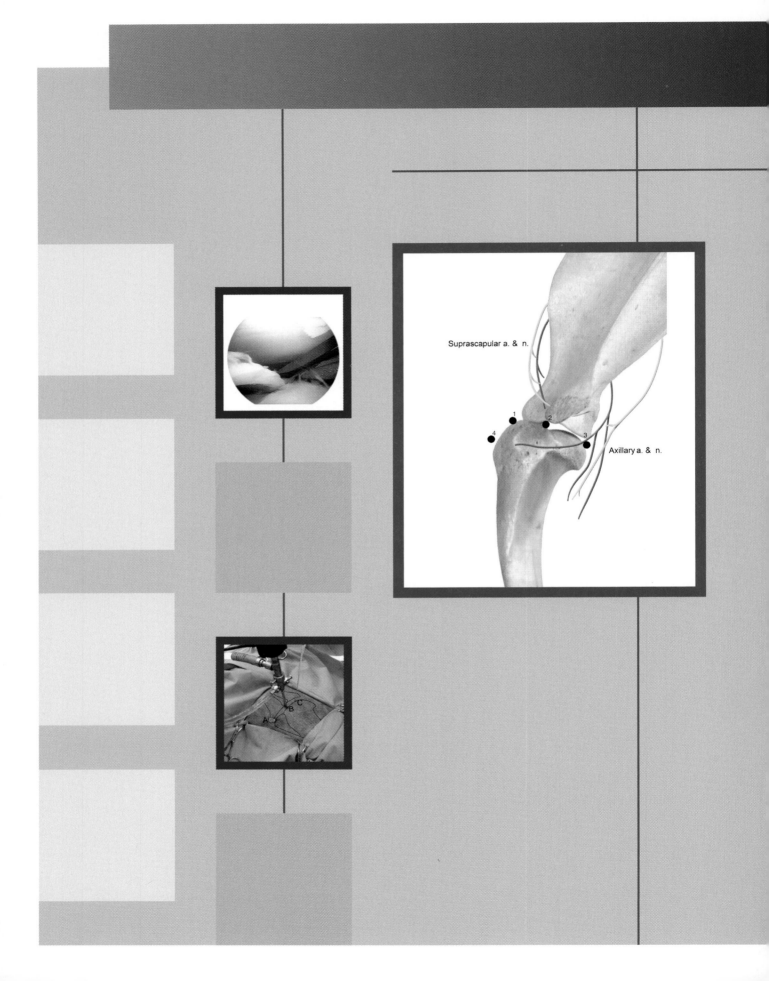

Suprascapular a. & n.

Axillary a. & n.

Arthroscopically Assisted Surgery of the Shoulder Joint

Introduction

Arthroscopy of the shoulder joint is one of the most common indications for rigid endoscopy in the dog. Juvenile orthopedic condition (OCD) and diagnostic arthroscopy (ligament or muscle injury) are two conditions for which rigid endoscopy is useful. As veterinary surgeons become more adept with the arthroscope and instrumentation, new treatment modalities will emerge. The advantage of arthroscopy for the shoulder joint is the same as for the other joints: decreased morbidity, visualization, and the ability to thoroughly inspect the joint. The latter is particularly evident when one considers the occurrence of ligament and soft tissue injuries about the joint.

The specific aims of this chapter are to introduce the reader to the proper placement of portals and manipulation of the camera and light post used to explore all structures in the joint and to discuss common conditions affecting the shoulder joint.

Arthroscopic Surgery of the Shoulder Joint

Equipment and Instrumentation. The surgical table should be capable of being lowered, raised, and tilted in at least one direction. During shoulder arthroscopy, the table should be adjusted to a position that allows the surgeon and assistants to hold the arms as close to the body as is possible. The shoulders should be in neutral position, with the elbows close to 90 degrees. This position prevents fatigue and improves efficiency. The imaging tower is positioned opposite the surgeon for unilateral procedures and at the head or end of the surgical table for bilateral shoulder procedures (Fig. 3–1). A well-

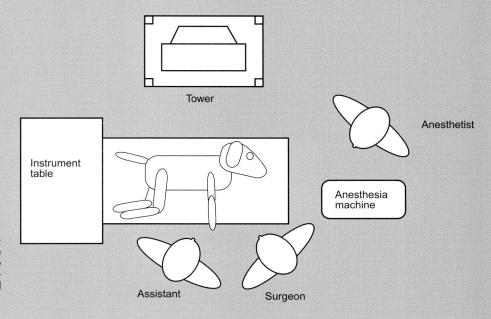

Tower

Anesthetist

Instrument table

Anesthesia machine

Assistant

Surgeon

FIGURE 3–1 Arrangement of the operating room for a unilateral procedure. Note the positions of the operating team and the monitor. Figure 4–1 shows the arrangement of the operating room for a bilateral shoulder procedure.

organized instrument stand should be within easy reach of the surgeon to prevent accidental dropping of delicate arthroscopy instruments. Fluid ingress is achieved with a pressurized gravity bag or an infusion fluid pump that is introduced through the arthroscope cannula (see Chapter 2). Fluid can be evacuated by allowing it to flow freely through the egress needle (or working cannula); evacuation of fluid can be assisted with suction attached to the egress needle (or cannula). Suction must be set at a low level, or bubbles will be produced that obscure the surgeon's view.

A 30-degree fore-oblique arthroscope is commonly used in the shoulder joint. In most dogs, a 2.7-mm arthroscope is easily inserted into the joint space (Fig. 3–2A). In small breeds, the use of a 2.4-mm or a 1.9-mm arthroscope is suggested to prevent iatrogenic damage to the cartilage during insertion or manipulation of the cartilage during surgery. In giant breeds, shoulder arthroscopy can be performed with a 4.0-mm arthroscope. The larger scope offers superior viewing area and depth of focus. Whichever size arthroscope is chosen, it is important to consider the outside diameter of the arthroscopic cannula because it too must enter the joint. Each arthroscopic cannula is fitted with a blunt obturator and a sharp trocar. If a sharp trocar is used, caution must be exercised when entering the joint to prevent iatrogenic damage to the cartilage. In most cases, it is not necessary to use the sharp trocar to enter the joint, and a conical, blunt obturator is recommended.

An assortment of hand instruments is necessary for shoulder arthroscopy. Recommended are instruments to assist in the inspection of intra-articular structures (probes), grasping forceps for removal of free bodies, biopsy forceps, and instruments for surface abrasion (see Fig. 3–2D to F). Instruments commonly used for abrasion arthroplasty are handheld burrs, curettes, and

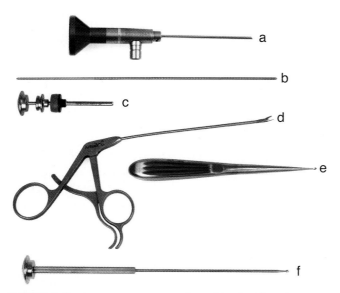

FIGURE 3–2 Instrumentation commonly used for shoulder arthroscopy. Arthroscope (a), switching stick (b), instrument cannula system (c), graspers (d), small curette (e), and small handheld burr (f).

motorized shavers. Instruments can be inserted into the joint through an open instrument port, instrument cannulas, or a combination of the two. The use of an instrument cannula requires the availability of cannulas of different sizes and switching sticks (see Fig. 3–2B and C). An assortment of operating cannulas of different diameters and lengths is ideal because the cannula must be long enough to enter the joint (e.g., shoulder, hip).

Anesthetic Considerations and Perioperative Pain Management. Preoperative laboratory workup is based on the patient's physical status and surgical risk. Most dogs undergoing shoulder arthroscopy are young, healthy patients with no underlying systemic problems. These patients require minimal laboratory workup. Older dogs should undergo a complete blood screen, urinalysis, chest radiographs, and electrocardiogram. Table 3–1 shows a standard anesthetic protocol, including preemptive pain medication. Postoperative pain is controlled with cold therapy, opioids, and nonsteroidal anti-inflammatory drugs (NSAIDs). If arthroscopy is completed early in the day, the patient may be dismissed from the hospital that same afternoon; if arthroscopy is completed later in the afternoon, the patient is discharged the next day. In all cases, during recovery, cold therapy is applied to the operative site by alternating 15 minutes on and 10 minutes off for two applications. A commercial cold pack or a package of frozen vegetables (e.g., peas) can be used. To increase comfort, a thin layer (e.g., towel, tissue) is placed between the cold pack and the skin surface. The cold pack is applied, followed by layers of towels to insulate the area from surrounding room temperature. Cold therapy is continued by the client at home for the first 2 days after surgery, using the same protocol.

All patients receive preemptive analgesic drugs as part of their premedication protocol. Buprenorphine is preferred by this author because of its relatively long mode of action (6 to 8 hours) and its effectiveness in patients that experience mild to moderate postoperative pain. When the dog is dismissed from the hospital, NSAIDs and oral butorphanol (Table 3–2) are dispensed for administration at home. NSAIDs are continued for 5 days, and butorphanol is discontinued after 48 hours. If the dog remains in the hospital overnight, a second dose of buprenorphine is administered in the evening. NSAIDs and butorphanol are prescribed for home administration. Alternate methods of pain management, such as transdermal fentanyl patches, are available. The fentanyl patch can be applied the day before surgery.

Patient Preparation and Positioning. The patient is clipped and prepared for open shoulder arthrotomy in case the arthroscopic procedure must be aborted for technical reasons and an open arthrotomy performed. This situation is most likely when the surgeon is beginning to learn arthroscopy. Two methods for limb preparation are used, with the choice of method depending on the desired level of limb maneuverability. For maximum maneuverability of the limb during surgery, a hanging limb preparation is recommended.

TABLE 3–1
Suggested Protocols for General Anesthesia and Preemptive Pain Management

PURPOSE		MEDICATION AND DOSAGE
Premedication		Glycopyrrolate 0.005–0.011 mg/kg SC or IM or atropine 0.02–0.04 mg/kg SC or IM
Preemptive pain management		Hydromorphone 0.1–0.2 mg/kg SC or IM or oxymorphone 0.05–0.1 mg/kg SC or IM plus acepromazine 0.05 mg/kg, not to exceed a total dose of 1 mg SC or IM Buprenorphine 0.005–0.02 mg/kg IM, SC or IV q 4–8 hr
Alternative preemptive pain medication		Epidural morphine (preservative free) 0.1 mg/kg Intra-articular bupivacaine 1 mg/kg or morphine (preservative free) 0.1 mg/kg, with the dose for each drug adjusted to accommodate the total joint volume Brachial plexus block (bupivacaine, maximum 2 mg/kg)
Induction		Thiopental 10–12 mg/kg IV to effect or propofol 4–6 mg/kg IV to effect
Maintenance		Isoflurane, sevoflurane, or halothane

Postoperative pain management	First 24 hr	If a morphine epidural was used, monitor for pain breakthrough; otherwise,
		   administer one of the following during recovery: single-dose IV NSAIDs
		or carprofen 4 mg/kg
		or meloxicam 0.2 mg/kg) *Note: None of these are approved for use in the dog
		   or cat in the US.*
		Morphine 0.4 mg/kg SC or IM q 4–6 hr
		Oxymorphone 0.1 mg/kg SC or IM q 4–6 hr

	After 24 hr	Carprofen 1 mg/lb bid or 2 mg/lb PO qd for 5–7 days Deracoxib 3–4 mg/kg PO qd for 5–7 days Etodolac 5–7 mg/kg PO qd for 5–7 days Butorphanol 0.5 mg/kg PO q 4–6 hr PRN plus NSAID if needed for additional comfort

IM, intramuscularly; IV, intravenously; NSAID, nonsteroidal anti-inflammatory drug; q, every; SC, subcutaneously.

As the surgeon becomes more experienced and adept at shoulder arthroscopy, less maneuverability is needed and a lateral limb preparation can be done for each limb (Fig. 3–3). The lateral limb preparation is still done in a way that allows the surgeon to perform an open

procedure if necessary. The dog is positioned in lateral recumbency, with the limb to be operated on uppermost (Fig. 3–4). The limb is supported in a neutral position (humerus parallel to the ground) or slightly adducted. If both limbs need arthroscopic intervention, the dog is

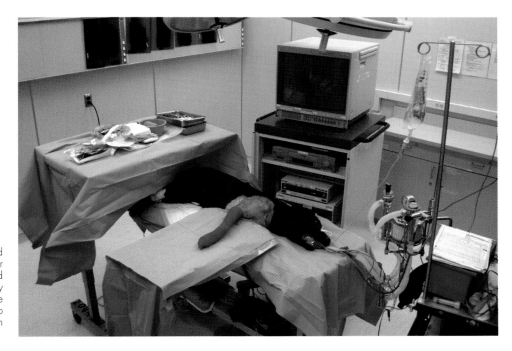

FIGURE 3–3 Lateral position and lateral limb preparation for shoulder arthroscopy. The limb is clipped and prepared so that a lateral arthrotomy may be performed if needed. The lower limb is supported on a Mayo stand to keep the shoulder joint in neutral position.

TABLE 3-2

Suggested Protocol for Postsurgical Rehabilitation

PHASE	DURATION AND GOALS	THERAPY
1	The duration varies with procedures and cases. The goal is to have the dog bearing weight with each step while walking at a normal pace (20 minutes 2–3 times daily).	*Always assess limb function at the beginning of each session!* Warm up for 2–4 minutes with gentle massage and small flexion and extension movements of the involved joint. On day 5, heat therapy is added to the warmup session. For the first week, exercise therapy is limited to slow leash walking on a flat surface for 10 minutes. Teach the dog to walk beside the owner on a loose lead; do not let the dog "drag" the owner around for 10 minutes! The walking pace must be slow enough that the dog bears weight with each step. (It is more difficult for the dog to "skip" off the leg at a slow pace.) If the dog does not bear weight with each step, slow the pace. If the dog is not using the leg properly, the owner can "bait" the dog with a low-calorie treat to allow them to walk one step at a time and keep the dog's mind focused on something other than the leg! Increase the walking time and pace as the days pass; if, at any time, the dog skips off the leg, return to a slower pace. If the dog will not bear weight on the leg and no problem is noted with the surgical site, a syringe cap can be taped between the footpads on the normal limb. The cap will not hurt the dog but will cause an unusual sensation that makes the dog take weight off the normal limb and place it on the operated limb. After walking, use cold therapy to provide comfort and prevent rebound swelling. The exercise session is repeated 2–3 times daily, depending on the client's availability. Between sessions, the dog is confined to a small area and allowed no free activity.
2	The duration varies with procedures and cases. At the end of phase 2, the dog should be able to bear weight with each step while walking at a brisk pace or trotting for 10 minutes. The exercise surface is high grass or brush. The height of the grass can vary, but should be at least above the carpus or tarsus.	*Always assess limb function at the beginning of each session!* As in phase 1, warm up with heat therapy, massage, and small joint movements. Exercise therapy begins with a walk at a brisk pace on an even surface for 2–3 minutes. Then move onto a grass surface and walk briskly for 2–3 minutes. Finally, move to a surface of higher grass or brush and walk for 1–2 minutes. The high surface is used to increase the range of joint motion and the endurance of muscles. Alternative exercises are swimming, walking in shallow water, and using an underwater treadmill. After the walking exercises are completed, static strength and balance exercises are initiated. The forelimb muscles are strengthened with a "wheelbarrow" stance (simply raise the dog's hindquarters and push forward). The rear limb muscles are strengthened by dancing (simply raise the dog's forelimbs and push backward). A good strength exercise is a "down-to-sit" motion. When moving from a down position to a sitting position, the dog will push weight from the hindquarters to the forelimbs. The number of repetitions will vary between dogs; begin with 1–3 and increase to 10. Balance and proprioception are achieved with a physio ball; place the rear limbs (or forelimbs) on the ball and allow the dog to maintain this position as best as possible. After the exercises are completed, passive stretch is applied. Place the joint through a comfortable range of motion. At the limit of extension, hold the position for 5 seconds; at the limit of flexion, hold the position for 5 seconds. Repeat the passive stretch 4–5 times. This exercise session is repeated 2–3 times daily, depending on the client's availability. Between sessions, the dog is confined to a small area.
3	The duration varies between procedures and cases. At the end of phase 3, the dog should be able to undergo controlled exercise for 20 minutes and free activity for 10 minutes. No lameness should be noticeable at the end of the therapy session.	*Always assess limb function at the beginning of each session!* Warm up with heat therapy, massage, and walking. Exercise therapy begins with the same exercises as in phase 2; the difference between phase 1 and phase 2 is the pace and amount of time spent in each activity. The exercises may vary, but each exercise session should include activities to increase range of motion, strength, endurance, and balance.

rolled over to the opposite side and the second side prepared for sterile surgery.

Portal Sites. Two or three portal sites are used for shoulder arthroscopy, depending on the purpose of arthroscopic intervention. If visual exploration of the shoulder joint is all that is required, an egress portal and an arthroscope portal are necessary. However, if tissue biopsy or treatment of joint pathology is needed, then an additional instrument portal is required.

The egress portal is established first. Either a hypodermic needle (16- or 18-gauge, 1.5-inch) or an egress cannula (2.4 to 2.7 mm) is used. Most surgeons prefer a hypodermic needle. The shoulder is palpated to locate the superior ridge of the greater tubercle, and the needle is inserted at the craniocaudal midpoint of the ridge.

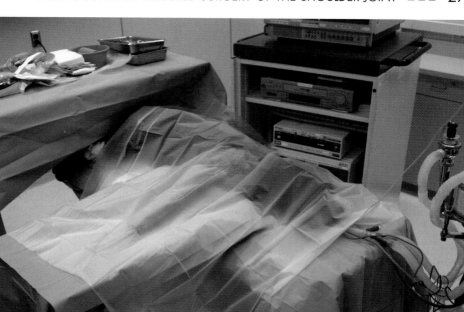

FIGURE 3–4 Proper sterile draping procedure. A clear adhesive drape is used to cover the shoulder and the dog.

The needle is directed caudally and medially at a 70-degree angle from the perpendicular (Figs. 3–5, *1*; 3–6, *a*; and 3–7*A*). To ensure placement within the joint, a syringe is attached to the needle and the synovial fluid aspirated. In most cases, when the egress portal is properly placed, synovial fluid is easily aspirated. If synovial fluid is not aspirated and the surgeon believes that the joint has been entered, lactated Ringer's

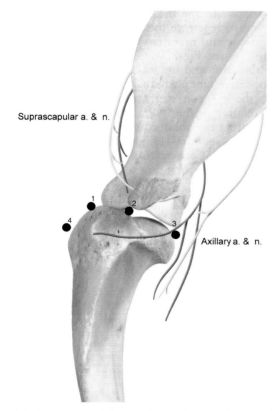

FIGURE 3–5 Position of the portal sites relative to bony landmarks and neurovascular structures. *1*, egress portal; *2*, arthroscope portal; *3*, instrument portal; *4*, portal site for access to the biceps tendon.

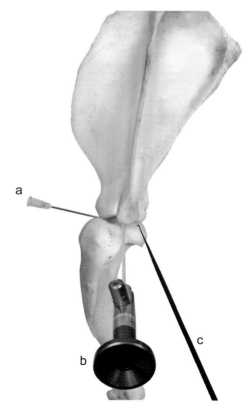

FIGURE 3–6 Placement of the egress needle (*a*), arthroscope (*b*), and instrument probe (*c*) within the proper portal sites.

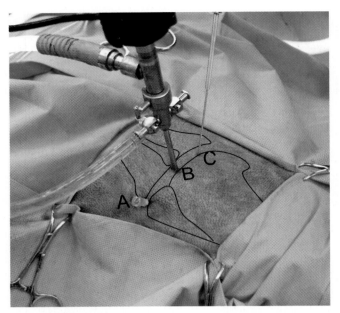

FIGURE 3–7 Surgical preparation showing the egress needle (A), arthroscope (B), and instrument (C) in the portal sites relative to bony landmarks.

solution can be instilled into the joint.
located in the joint, fluid is easily instill
joint cavity begins to fill with fluid, rev
felt on the syringe plunger from the inst
pressure also ensures proper placement
into the joint. The joint cavity is distenc
12 mL lactated Ringer's solution, and the
maintained by leaving the syringe attachec
needle (the assistant must maintain pre
plunger). Distension simplifies correct posi
arthroscope portal. Once the arthroscop
ingress are established, the syringe is remo
needle to allow evacuation of fluid. This e
fluid maintains fluid flow through the join
visualization. Intravenous (IV) or suction tu
attached to the needle to capture fluid as i
joint. Alternatively, fluid is allowed to spi
floor to be captured by a floor suction unit c

The arthroscope portal is established se ... The
arthroscope cannula, with the attached trocar, conical
obturator, or blunt obturator, is inserted first. In most
cases, the conical blunt obturator is used. The proper
position for the arthroscope portal is directly distal or
1 to 2 mm cranial to the acromial process of the scapula
(see Figs. 3–5,2 and 3–6,b). The acromium is located,
and the space just craniodistal to its border is palpated.
A 20-gauge (1.5-inch) needle is used to confirm the
position. The needle is inserted perpendicular to the
skin surface, and this orientation is maintained through
the soft tissues as the needle enters the joint. Lactated
Ringer's solution (previously used to distend the joint)
flows through the needle once the joint is entered,
marking the point of entry for the arthroscope. A no. 11
Bard-Parker blade is used to make a small entry wound
through the skin and the superficial soft tissues adjacent

to the needle. It is not advisable to enter the joint with
the scalpel blade because extravasation of fluid outside
the joint cavity is more likely. The needle is removed,
and the arthroscope is inserted with the attached conical
blunt obturator. When the arthroscope cannula is
inserted, the limb should be in neutral position
(humerus parallel to the table) and the assistant should
place slight traction on the limb. These maneuvers make
insertion easier and decrease the likelihood of iatrogenic
damage to the cartilage. When a conical blunt obturator
is used, pressure must be applied to penetrate the joint
capsule. Holding the cannula with the thumb and index
finger approximately 1 inch from the tip prevents
overpenetration into the joint. With experience, the
surgeon will learn to feel when the joint is entered. After
the joint is entered, the obturator is removed from the
cannula. Fluid will flow freely from the cannula,
confirming correct placement. The fluid ingress line is
attached to the cannula, and the arthroscope is inserted
(see Fig. 3–7B).

The instrument portal is established, if necessary. The
craniocaudal and proximodistal positions of the instrument portal relative to the acromium can be estimated
from the lateral radi̶o̶ This site is often approxi-
y distal to the caudal edge
bers are only estimates,
dog and the size of the
ɔ learn to triangulate the
to the position of the
t. A 20-gauge, 2- or 3-
uide needle to locate the
nent portal. The guide
surface at a 75- to 90-
ɔrientation through the
3–6C). As the needle
ie monitor (as long as
ɔd toward the point of
he placement of the
needle appears to be
his illusion is created
ɔscope and does not
. The most common
.ppropriate instrument
.ʊ ᴄ̶ɪitering the skin and soft tissue at too
oblique an angle. When the angle of entry is too oblique,
the triangulation needle (to locate the instrument port)
"crosses" the arthroscope and cannot be visualized on
the monitor. If the triangulation needle cannot be seen,
the needle should be inserted at a different location and
at a 75- to 90-degree angle to the skin surface.

After the appropriate site for the instrument portal is
confirmed by observation of the needle on the monitor,
the portal site is prepared as appropriate for the surgery
being performed. For example, to remove loose cartilage associated with an osteochondritis dissecans
(OCD) lesion, a no. 11 Bard-Parker scalpel blade can
be inserted adjacent to the needle. The opening can then
be enlarged with Metzenbaum scissors or a series of
cannulas of increasing diameter (see Fig. 3–7C).
Alternatively, the surgeon may reduce the size of the
cartilage flap with curettes or an arthroscopic knife

T = 100.7°

P = 95

R = sniffing

Storm

inserted through a cannula. If different-sized cannulas are needed, a switching stick is used to change the cannulas.

Surgical Anatomy. Because it is a ball-and-socket joint, the shoulder joint is well suited for movement in all directions. Although it is capable of movement in all directions, however, the shoulder primarily moves in flexion and extension. Joint stability is provided through a combination of passive and active mechanisms. Passive mechanisms include the medial and lateral glenohumeral ligaments, surrounding joint capsule, joint conformation, and synovial fluid cohesion. The medial collateral ligament (MCL) commonly appears as a Y-shaped figure, with the cranial arm coursing caudally from its origin at the medial surface of the supraglenoid tubercle (Fig. 3–8). The caudal arm of the MCL originates from the medial surface of the scapular neck and joins the cranial arm to insert onto the humeral neck. The lateral collateral ligament (LCL) originates from the lateral rim of the glenoid and extends ventrally to insert onto the humerus at the caudal region of the greater tubercle (see Fig. 3–8). The joint capsule originates from the periphery of the glenoid cavity. Medially, the joint capsule forms a synovial recess because it is attached several millimeters proximal to the glenoid rim. The concavity of the glenoid and the fit of the humeral head into the glenoid provide joint stability, particularly when compression across the joint is enhanced by active muscle contraction. Dynamic active glenohumeral stability is provided by contraction of the surrounding cuff muscles. These include the biceps brachii muscle, subscapularis muscle, teres minor muscle, supraspinatus muscle, and infraspinatus muscle. Active contraction of all or selective cuff muscles induces compression across the shoulder joint and increases tension in the joint capsule.

When the arthroscope enters the joint, the camera is positioned in a way that provides proper spatial orientation on the monitor. Orientation is correct when the monitor shows right to the right, left to the left, ventral down, and dorsal up. The fore-oblique direction is dependent on the surgeon's preference, but most prefer to initially view 30 degrees down (with the light post in the dorsal position). Proper spatial orientation and the fore-oblique view are obtained when the buttons on the camera head are upright and the light post is in the upright position. With the camera and light post in this position, the initial view will be just cranial to the apex of the humeral head dome. Often, the tip of the arthroscope initially lies close to the medial joint capsule, giving a view of soft tissue only. The arthroscope is slowly retrieved to visualize the articular cartilage of the humeral head. Once the articular surface of the humeral head is identified, spatial orientation is easier to achieve. As the surgeon views straight ahead (medially), the cranial arm of the MCL, subscapularis tendon of insertion, and medial joint capsule are visible (Fig. 3–9A). The position of the camera head is maintained, and the light post is rotated to the ventral position to view the articular surface of the medial glenoid (Fig. 3–10A and B). Next, the light post is rotated caudally and the camera head is moved slightly caudal to visualize the cranial compartment of the shoulder. As the light post is turned ventrally, the origin of the biceps tendon is seen (Fig. 3–11A and B). As the light post is turned dorsally, the tendon is seen as it courses down the bicipital groove (Fig. 3–12A and B). As the arthroscope tip is moved cranial and lateral to the biceps tendon and the light post is turned, the joint compartment cranial to the biceps tendon is seen (see Fig. 3–12C).

The arthroscope and light post are returned to the original entry position to begin exploration of the caudal compartment of the joint. The camera head is moved cranially and the light post adjusted to view the articular surface of the caudal glenoid (light post is moved ventrally) or the articular surface of the humeral head (light post is moved dorsally; Fig. 3–13A and B). The tip of the arthroscope is moved medially to view the medial compartment between the humeral head and joint capsule.

The limb is abducted and then adducted to allow inspection of the medial joint capsule. The operator gently advances the tip of the arthroscope caudally and rotates the light post to view the caudal, medial, and lateral surfaces of the humeral head. Often, the assistant must adjust the limb position to make inspection easier. The tip of the arthroscope is advanced along the caudal slope of the humeral head until the caudal and medial gutters are visualized. The capsular recess is adjacent to the insertion of the joint capsule onto the humeral head (Fig. 3–14A and B). The camera head and light post are returned to the original entry position. The arthroscope is slowly withdrawn to visualize the lateral joint compartment (Fig. 3–15A). The light post is adjusted to view the lateral articular surface of the glenoid and humeral head, craniolateral joint capsule, and caudolateral joint capsule. Caution must be used when viewing the lateral joint compartments because the tip of the arthroscope is easily displaced from the joint, and extravasation of

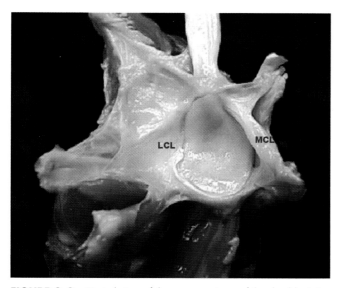

FIGURE 3–8 Ventral view of the gross anatomy of the shoulder joint. Note the position of the medial collateral ligament (MCL) and lateral collateral ligament (LCL).

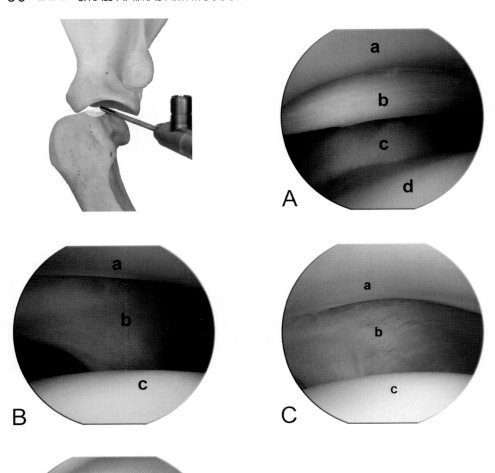

FIGURE 3–9 *A,* Arthroscopic view of the craniomedial compartment of the shoulder joint. Glenoid (*a*), cranial arm of the medial collateral ligament (MCL) (*b*), subscapularis tendon (*c*), and humeral head (*d*). *B,* Arthroscopic view of the centromedial compartment of the shoulder joint. Glenoid (*a*), centromedial area of the MCL (*b*), and humeral head (*c*). *C,* Arthroscopic view of the caudomedial compartment of the shoulder joint. Glenoid (*a*), caudomedial area of the MCL (*b*), and humeral head (*c*). *D,* Arthroscopic view of the cranial compartment of the shoulder joint. Cranial arm of the MCL (*a*), insertion of the subscapularis tendon (*b*), and humeral head (*c*).

fluid is more likely when the tip of the arthroscope is in the lateral compartment. For this reason, the lateral compartment is usually inspected last.

Indications for Arthroscopic Surgery of the Shoulder Joint

Arthroscopy is a relatively new treatment modality in small animal surgery, and numerous indications for shoulder arthroscopy are described in the literature. As small animal surgeons become more adept at arthroscopy, it will be used to treat more conditions, either alone or as an assistive modality. Indications for

shoulder arthroscopy include OCD, bicipital tenosynovitis, shoulder instability (e.g., joint capsule or ligament tears), and diagnostic examination (e.g., biopsy of bone, cartilage, or the soft tissue envelope).

Osteochondritis Dissecans

OCD is a manifestation of osteochondrosis in which a fragment of cartilage is lifted from the articular surface. Osteochondrosis is thought to result from a disturbance in endochondral ossification. Aberrant endochondral ossification leads to multiple areas of cartilage islands on the surface and within the humeral epiphysis that have not undergone normal maturation to bone

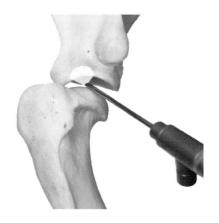
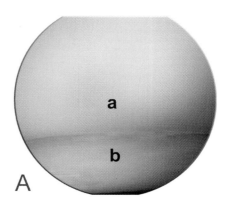
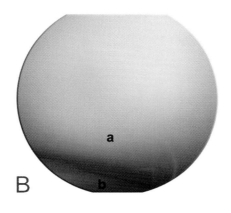

FIGURE 3-10 *A,* Arthroscopic view of the mediocentral glenoid. Mediocentral glenoid (*a*) and cranial arm of the medial collateral ligament (*b*). *B,* Arthroscopic view of the central glenoid. Mediocentral glenoid (*a*) and cranial arm of the medial collateral ligament (*b*).

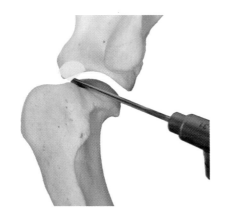
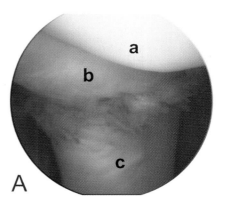

FIGURE 3-11 *A,* Arthroscopic view of the biceps origin. Supraglenoid tuberosity (*a*), labral origin of the biceps (*b*), and biceps tendon (*c*). *B,* Arthroscopic view of the biceps origin. Supraglenoid tuberosity (*a*) and lateral labral origin of the biceps (*b*).

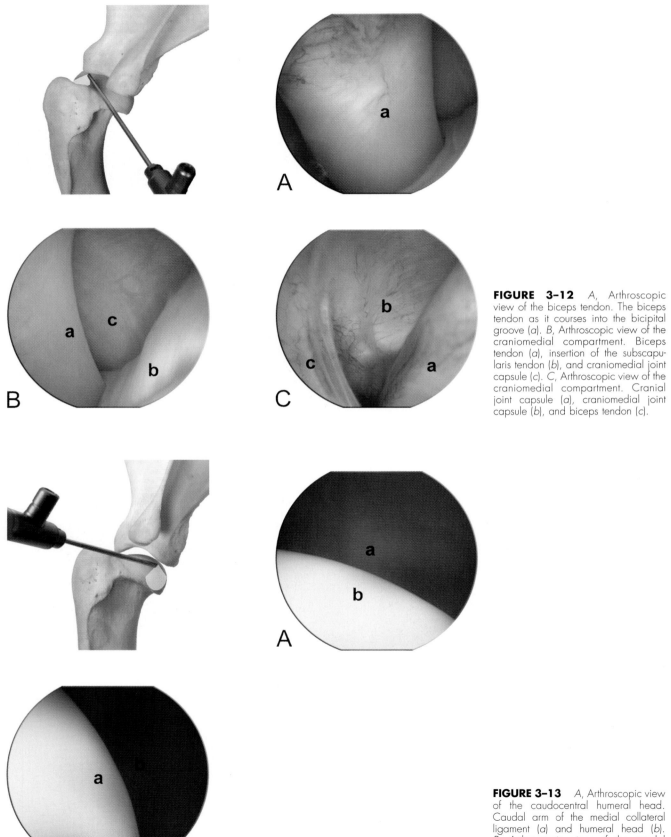

FIGURE 3-12 *A,* Arthroscopic view of the biceps tendon. The biceps tendon as it courses into the bicipital groove (*a*). *B,* Arthroscopic view of the craniomedial compartment. Biceps tendon (*a*), insertion of the subscapularis tendon (*b*), and craniomedial joint capsule (*c*). *C,* Arthroscopic view of the craniomedial compartment. Cranial joint capsule (*a*), craniomedial joint capsule (*b*), and biceps tendon (*c*).

FIGURE 3-13 *A,* Arthroscopic view of the caudocentral humeral head. Caudal arm of the medial collateral ligament (*a*) and humeral head (*b*). *B,* Arthroscopic view of the caudal humeral head. Humeral head (*a*) and medial joint capsule (*b*).

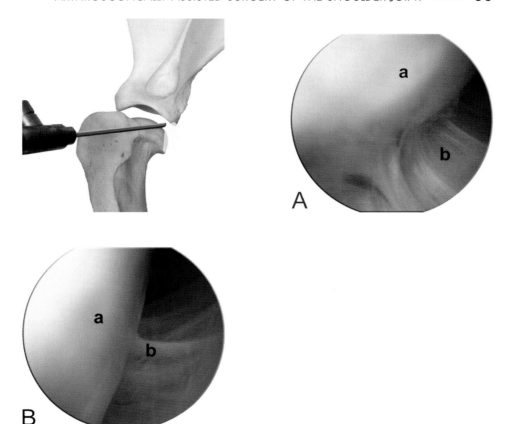

FIGURE 3-14 *A*, Arthroscopic view of the caudal humeral head. Humeral head (*a*) and caudomedial joint capsule (*b*). *B*, Arthroscopic view of the medial gutter. Humeral head (*a*) and medial gutter (*b*).

(Fig. 3–16). Zones of abnormal ossification lead to increased thickness of the articular cartilage and are susceptible to fissure and loosening. The abnormal cartilage may fissure as the deeper chondrocytes undergo necrosis as a result of an inadequate nutrient supply. The peripheral area of thickened cartilage separates because of increased local shear stress. As a result, a loose fragment of cartilage elevates into the joint or completely detaches from the underlying bone. Free cartilage becomes lodged in the caudomedial joint pouch or, less commonly, adjacent to the biceps tendon. Despite unilateral lameness, this condition is often bilateral.

History and Signalment. Large and giant breed dogs are commonly affected, and males are more often affected than females. Clinical signs often develop between 4 and 8 months of age; however, some dogs may not present for evaluation until they are mature or middle-aged. Affected animals are presented for examination because of unilateral forelimb lameness. Owners usually report a gradual onset of lameness that improves after rest and worsens after exercise.

Physical Examination Findings. On physical examination, the shoulder is palpated and moved through a complete range of motion. Crepitation or palpable

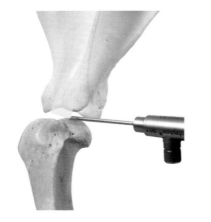

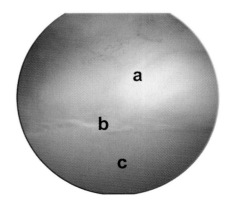

FIGURE 3-15 *A*, Arthroscopic view of the lateral collateral ligament. Lateral collateral ligament (*a*), insertion of the lateral collateral ligament onto the glenoid rim (*b*), and glenoid (*c*).

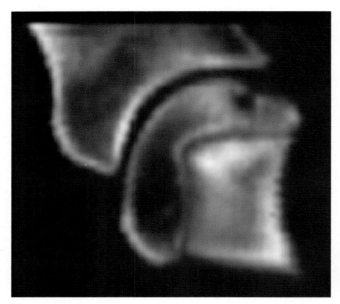

FIGURE 3–16 Computed tomography of a shoulder diagnosed with osteochondritis dissecans. Note the radiolucent zone extending from the surface deep into the humeral epiphysis.

swelling of the joint is seldom evident, but affected animals may exhibit pain when the shoulder is moved into hyperextension or extreme flexion. Often the examiner detects muscle atrophy of the forelimb when muscle mass is lost adjacent to the spine of the scapula.

Differential Diagnosis. The differential diagnosis includes osteochondrosis, bicipital tenosynovitis, shoulder instability, osteoarthritis, panosteitis, and elbow dysplasia.

Radiographic Findings. Despite apparent lameness in one limb, both shoulders are radiographed. Sedation may be required to obtain quality radiographs, particularly in large, hyperactive dogs. The earliest radiographic sign of OCD is flattening of the caudal humeral head (Fig. 3–17). This flattening is caused by thickening of the articular cartilage and deviation of the subchondral bone line. As the disease progresses, a saucer-shaped radiolucent area in the caudal humeral head may be visualized. Calcification of the flap may allow visualization of the flap, either in situ or within the joint, if it has detached from the underlying bone. In chronic cases, large, calcified joint mice are often observed in the caudoventral joint pouch or cranially within the bicipital groove. Osteophytes are occasionally noted adjacent to the bicipital groove or the caudal region of the glenoid. Computed tomography of the shoulder shows multiple areas of abnormal ossification throughout the epiphysis.

Diagnosis. A complete orthopedic examination is essential because other juvenile orthopedic conditions, such as elbow dysplasia [fragmented medial coronoid process (FCP) or ununited anconeal process (UAP)],

panosteitis, hypertrophic osteodystrophy, bicipital tenosynovitis, and shoulder instability, can occur concurrently with shoulder OCD. The diagnosis of OCD is based on signalment and history and physical findings, and confirmed radiographically.

Treatment. Medical treatment of OCD consists of anti-inflammatory medication and moderate exercise. An early hypothesis of treatment was that exercise would dislodge the cartilage flap that would then undergo enzymatic resorption. One difficulty with this hypothesis is that the inflammatory process cannot distinguish between normal cartilage and the dislodged cartilage flap. Additionally, ongoing inflammation could lead to osteoarthritis. Surgical intervention is the treatment of choice. Nevertheless, conservative management may be necessary if financial constraints preclude surgical intervention. Removal of loose or dislodged cartilage coupled with curettage or microfracture of the lesion bed leads to an excellent prognosis for return of clinical function.

Anesthetic Considerations and Perioperative Pain Management. Most dogs with shoulder OCD are young, healthy patients, and require minimal preoperative laboratory screening. Table 3–1 shows a standard anesthetic protocol, including preemptive pain medication.

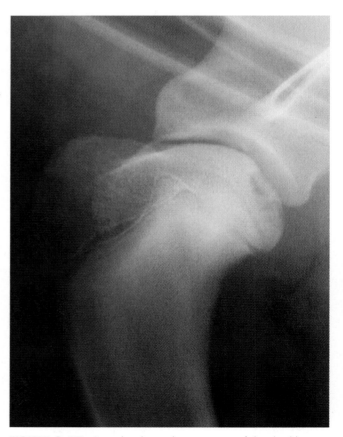

FIGURE 3–17 Lateral radiographic projection of the shoulder joint in a case with osteochondritis dissecans. Note the flattening and the radiolucent zone of the caudal humeral head.

Surgical Intervention. Surgery is the treatment of choice. Portal sites and surgical anatomy were discussed earlier. With the advent of arthroscopy, both shoulders are treated at the same time if the condition is bilateral. The operative site is clipped and prepared according to the amount of limb maneuverability desired during surgery. A hanging limb preparation provides the greatest degree of freedom for manipulating limb position. A lateral limb preparation allows less maneuverability, but requires less time and provides a more cosmetic appearance (see Fig. 3–4). Even with a lateral limb preparation, liberal clipping and thorough sterile preparation are needed because an open arthrotomy may be required. In most cases, a 2.7-mm, 30-degree fore-oblique arthroscope is used. Basic instrumentation includes probes to inspect the cartilage surface or help raise a cartilage flap, graspers to remove the cartilage flap, and a hand curette or hand burr to prepare the lesion bed (see Fig. 3–2A to F). If the surgeon chooses to work through an instrument cannula, different-sized cannulas and switching sticks facilitate surgery. A motorized shaver can be helpful, but is not essential for arthroscopic débridement of the lesion bed. The dog is positioned in lateral recumbency, with the leg to be operated on uppermost. The limb is supported in neutral position to prevent excessive adduction or abduction, which will close the joint line between the glenoid and humeral head.

Egress is established with a needle or cannula, lactated Ringer's solution is instilled to distend the joint, and the arthroscope site is established (see Fig. 3–7B). The arthroscope is inserted, and ingress flow is established through the arthroscope cannula. The medial compartment is inspected for evidence of inflammation, followed by inspection of the cranial compartment. The region of the biceps tendon is thoroughly inspected for inflammation and the presence of free cartilage pieces (Fig. 3-18B). The camera head and light post are positioned to identify and determine the extent of the OCD lesion (see Fig. 3–18C to E). The arthroscope is placed such that the lesion is clearly visible, and a guide needle is used to triangulate the position for the instrument port (see Fig. 3–18G). The most common reason for failing to visualize the guide needle inside the joint is "crossing" the arthroscope. Once the position for the instrument portal is established, the surgeon must decide whether to work through an open instrument portal, an instrument cannula, or a combination of the two. If the surgeon chooses to work through an open portal site, a no. 11 Bard-Parker scalpel blade is used to make a 0.5- to 1-cm soft tissue tunnel adjacent to the guide needle (Fig. 3–19). Small Metzenbaum scissors can be used to enlarge the opening through the joint capsule. If the cartilage fragment is still attached (usually cranial or medial), a probe or elevator is inserted to begin freeing the edge of the fragment. The fragment is not freed completely but is left attached at one site. Grasping forceps are inserted and used to hold the cartilage fragment. To facilitate removal of the fragment, the forceps are twisted to fold the fragment along its long axis. Pushing the cartilage fragment forward helps to break any remaining peripheral attachment. When it is twisted

and pushed, the fragment may break off as a single large piece. In many cases, it breaks off and is removed in two or three sections (Fig. 3–20). Whether the fragment is removed as one large section or two or three smaller sections, the surgeon must be careful when extracting it through the capsule opening. If the opening is not large enough or if the surgeon does not have a firm hold on the fragment, it may slip from the forceps and become a free joint mouse. Removing a free fragment often increases operative time and iatrogenic trauma.

As an alternative to the open portal, the surgeon may choose to work through an instrument cannula. If so, the small instrument cannula with a sharp trocar is inserted into the joint adjacent to the guide needle. Larger cannulas are placed with the use of switching sticks, but the smallest instrument cannula through which the surgeon can treat the lesion is used. A hand curette, hand burr, or motorized shaver is passed through the cannula and used to break the cartilage flap into small pieces. In most cases, the pieces are small enough to flow out the instrument cannula. If a piece is too large to pass freely through the cannula, small grasping forceps are inserted and used to capture the fragment. The fragment is pulled next to the instrument cannula, and the cannula and forceps are removed at the same time. The instrument port is reestablished by placing a switching stick and then the cannula into the joint. The surgeon continues to break the cartilage flap into small pieces until the cartilage that lines the periphery of the lesion bed is firmly attached to the underlying subchondral bone.

Occasionally, the cartilage fragment is no longer attached at the lesion periphery. When this occurs, the fragment is most commonly located in the medial joint recess (Fig. 3–21B to D). The free fragment is retrieved before the lesion bed is addressed. As surgery time passes, the joint villa becomes increasingly inflamed and may obscure vision adjacent to the joint capsule. To capture the free fragment, fluid ingress is increased and the instrument cannula is positioned to serve as a vacuum. The free fragment moves in the direction of fluid outflow. Once the fragment is seen, the ingress flow is slowed, and graspers are inserted through the instrument cannula. Care must be taken to ensure that the opening in the joint capsule will accommodate extraction of the free fragment. If possible, the fragment is grasped and twisted on its long axis; most times, the fragment has lost flexibility and does not roll. If the fragment is located too far cranially to allow access through a caudal instrument port, the surgeon must switch the arthroscope and instrument portals. The cranial instrument port will allow access to fragments that are displaced in the craniomedial recess or those adjacent to the biceps tendon.

Whether an open portal or an instrument cannula is used to facilitate removal of the cartilage flap, treatment of the lesion bed is best accomplished through an instrument cannula. If the surgeon has worked through an open portal to remove the cartilage flap, an instrument cannula must be inserted over a switching stick. The surface of the lesion must be treated with abrasion or

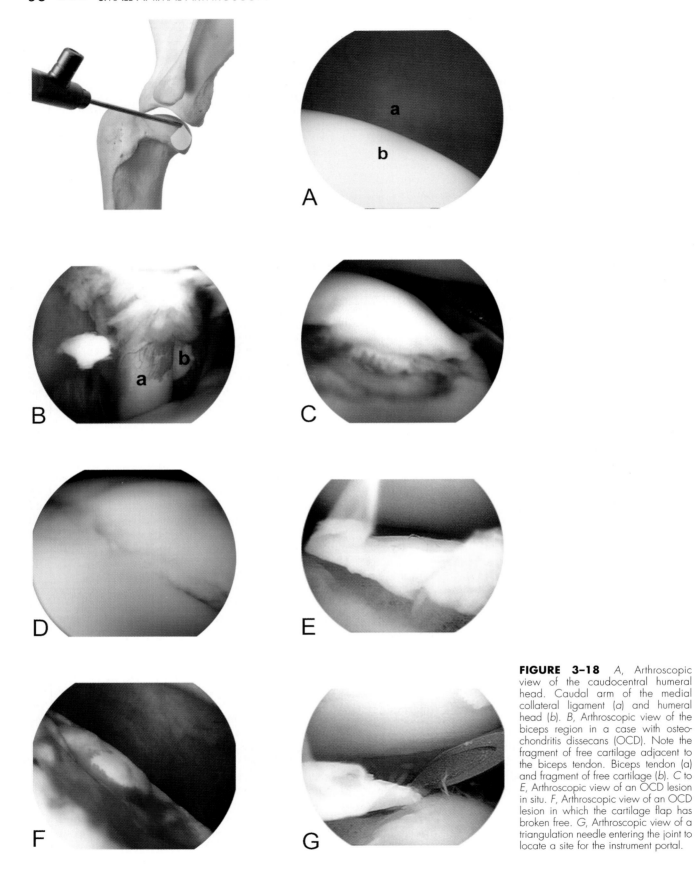

FIGURE 3-18 *A,* Arthroscopic view of the caudocentral humeral head. Caudal arm of the medial collateral ligament (*a*) and humeral head (*b*). *B,* Arthroscopic view of the biceps region in a case with osteochondritis dissecans (OCD). Note the fragment of free cartilage adjacent to the biceps tendon. Biceps tendon (*a*) and fragment of free cartilage (*b*). *C* to *E,* Arthroscopic view of an OCD lesion in situ. *F,* Arthroscopic view of an OCD lesion in which the cartilage flap has broken free. *G,* Arthroscopic view of a triangulation needle entering the joint to locate a site for the instrument portal.

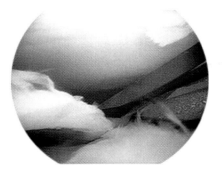

FIGURE 3-19   Arthroscopic view of a no. 11 scalpel blade entering the joint to establish an open instrument portal.

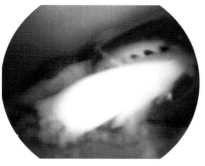

FIGURE 3-20   Arthroscopic view of a grasping forceps holding free cartilage associated with an osteochondritis dissecans lesion.

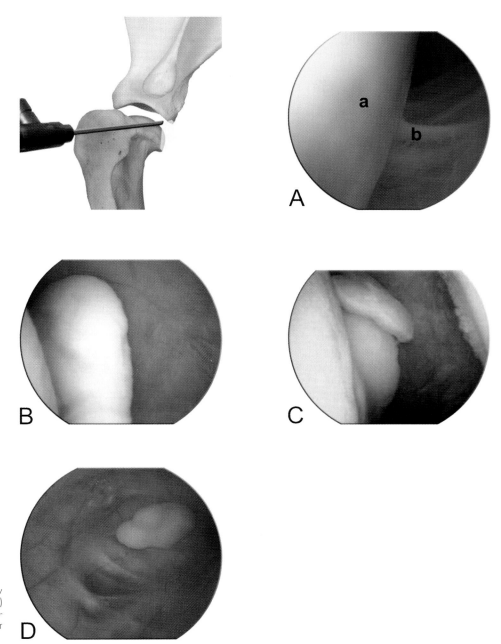

FIGURE 3-21   *A*, Arthroscopic view of the medial gutter. Humeral head (*a*) and medial gutter (*b*). *B to D*, Arthroscopic view of the caudomedial gutter showing fragments of free cartilage.

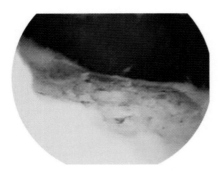

FIGURE 3–22 Arthroscopic view after curettage of the lesion. Note the small bleeding vessels in the lesion bed.

microfracture techniques (Fig. 3–22). Surface abrasion is performed with a hand curette, hand burr, or motorized shaver. The surgeon continues to abrade the surface until the underlying bone bleeds freely. It may be necessary to stop the ingress fluid to observe the extent of bleeding bone. Although it is important to avoid abrading the surface too aggressively, abrasion should continue until bleeding is observed throughout the lesion surface. A microfracture pick and mallet are used to treat the lesion bed with this technique. The point of the microfracture pick is positioned, and the handle is tapped with the mallet until the point impales the surface to a depth of 1 to 2 mm. After surface abrasion or microfracture is completed, small bone or cartilage fragments are flushed from the joint by increasing the ingress flow and allowing egress through a large instrument cannula. The joint is inspected for remaining bone or cartilage fragments and the arthroscope and instrument cannula are removed. Finally, the portals are sutured with nonreactive, non-absorbable suture material.

Postoperative Care. Cold therapy is applied to the shoulder during recovery to provide pain relief and reduce swelling. Cold therapy is applied by alternating 15 minutes on and 10 minutes off for two applications. Commercial cold packs or a commercial circulating cold water pack can be used. Alternatively, ice wrapped in a towel or packs of frozen vegetables can be used. To increase comfort, a thin towel is placed next to the skin surface before the ice pack is positioned. Next, a thick layer of towels is placed to prevent loss of cold to the environment. If the dog is dismissed from the hospital the day of surgery, NSAIDs and oral butorphanol (see Table 3–2) are dispensed for administration at home. If the dog remains in the hospital overnight, buprenorphine is administered in the evening and NSAIDs and butorphanol are dispensed for administration at home. NSAIDs are continued for 5 days, whereas butorphanol is discontinued after 48 hours. Cold therapy is continued by the client at home for the initial 2 days after surgery using the protocol described earlier. After the surgical swelling is gone (48 to 72 hours), the owner should begin heat therapy and passive motion and stretch exercises. The owner should apply moist heat to the shoulder region with a commercial heat pack or moistened warm towel. The owner should be instructed to hold the warm pack

against the inside of his own elbow for 30 seconds to ensure that it is not too hot. Then the warm pack is placed over the animal's shoulder area for 10 minutes. Afterward, the warm pack is removed and gentle flexion and extension movements of the shoulder joint are begun. The owner is instructed to begin with small movements and gradually increase movements to the limit of comfort over a 1- to 2-minute period. At the limit of comfort, the joint is held in position for 10 seconds. The motion and stretch exercise is repeated five times two or three times daily. In addition, the owner should examine the portal sites daily for signs of irritation or drainage.

Exercise is limited to controlled walking on a leash for the first 4 weeks after surgery. Dogs undergoing arthroscopy will use the affected leg immediately after surgery. To increase the weightbearing load on the limbs, walking at a slow pace is recommended. As postoperative time increases, the pace can be hastened. To increase the range of motion in the shoulder when walking, ask the client to walk the dog in high grass (e.g., weeds), thereby forcing the dog to pick up the feet and step high with the legs. After 4 weeks, the owner should begin limited amounts of free activity with controlled walking, starting with 5 minutes of free activity and increasing to 30 minutes over the next 2 weeks. After 6 to 8 weeks, free activity is gradually increased to normal levels. If during any exercise period (controlled or free activity), the dog becomes sore at the end of the exercise period or is sore the next day, the owner should decrease the pace and return to controlled activity for 2 to 3 days.

Complications. Complications are unusual after shoulder arthroscopy. Occasionally, in the immediate postoperative period, excessive fluid extravasation occurs and results in swollen soft tissues around the shoulder. This fluid resorbs within the first 24 hours. Residual mild swelling adjacent to the portal sites may be noticeable for the first 48 hours.

Prognosis. The prognosis for normal limb function with OCD of the shoulder is good. After surgery, most dogs become sound within 4 to 8 weeks. In one study of 44 shoulders treated with open arthrotomy to remove cartilaginous flaps, 75% had excellent function and 22.5% had good function on long-term evaluation (Rudd, Whitehair, Margolis, 1990).

Bicipital Tenosynovitis

Bicipital tenosynovitis is an inflammation of the biceps brachii tendon and its surrounding synovial sheath. It is caused by either direct or indirect trauma to the bicipital tendon or tendon sheath. Direct trauma from repetitive injury may be an inciting factor and may cause partial or complete tearing of the tendon. Indirect trauma as a result of proliferative fibrous connective tissue, osteophytes, or adhesions between the tendon and sheath limit motion and cause pain. Mineralization of the supraspinatus tendon also may cause secondary mechanical bicipital tenosynovitis.

History and Signalment. Affected dogs are usually medium to large and middle-aged or older. Working and active dogs are more commonly affected, and there is no predisposition for either sex. Intermittent or progressive forelimb lameness that worsens after exercise is common. The owner may relate the lameness to trauma, but usually there is slow onset of clinical signs.

Physical Examination Findings. Forelimb lameness is usually evident. The animal is weightbearing, but is visually lame during ambulation. Pain may be elicited during direct palpation over the bicipital tendon, especially with flexion and rotation of the shoulder joint. Atrophy of the supraspinatus and infraspinatus muscles may be palpable.

Differential Diagnosis. The differential diagnosis includes acute or chronic strain of the supraspinatus tendon, shoulder instability, OCD, calcifying tendinopathy of the biceps tendon, and elbow dysplasia.

Radiographic Findings. Radiographic views should include standard lateral projections of both shoulders. A craniocaudal projection of the humerus with the shoulder flexed (skyline view) can be used to identify the bicipital groove. Bone proliferation or resorption of the supraglenoid tuberosity at the origin of the biceps tendon indicates inflammation at the origin of the biceps tendon. This inflammation is usually caused by complete or partial rupture of the biceps tendon. Calcification of the biceps tendon sheath or osteophytes in the intertubercular groove may be evident. Arthrography can be used to outline the tendon and show irregularities and filling defects that suggest synovial hyperplasia, tendon rupture, and joint mice. Caution must be exercised when interpreting the finding of mineralization adjacent to the bicipital groove as being within the biceps tendon sheath. More often, mineralization in this area involves the tendon of insertion of the supraspinatus muscle.

Diagnosis. A complete orthopedic examination is essential because other orthopedic conditions may be found concurrently with bicipital tendon injury. OCD, elbow dysplasia (FCP, UAP), panosteitis, hypertrophic osteodystrophy, and acute or chronic strain of the supraspinatus tendon are some of these conditions. The diagnosis of bicipital tendon injury is based on signalment and history, physical findings, and radiographic appearance consistent with acute or chronic bicipital tendon injury. Ultrasonographic changes also may be evident in contrast to the opposite normal limb. The diagnosis is confirmed through direct visualization during arthroscopy.

Treatment. Both medical and surgical approaches are successful in the treatment of bicipital tenosynovitis. Medical treatment consists of injecting methylprednisolone acetate into the tendon sheath and restricting activity for 3 weeks. In one report, Stobie (1995) reported that the outcome was good to excellent in 50% of dogs treated medically and in all dogs treated surgically. Given

these results, initiating treatment with one or two steroid injections is a reasonable approach. If the outcome is not favorable, surgical intervention is advised; if steroids had been used previously, white intra-articular deposits may be present.

Anesthetic Considerations and Perioperative Pain Management. Preoperative laboratory workup is based on the patient's physical status and surgical risk. Young, healthy patients with no underlying systemic problems require minimal laboratory workup. Older dogs should undergo a complete blood screen, urinalysis, chest radiographs, and electrocardiogram. Table 3–1 shows a standard anesthetic protocol, including preemptive pain medication.

Surgical Intervention. Portal sites and surgical anatomy were discussed earlier. The operative site is clipped and prepared as necessary to provide the desired amount of limb maneuverability during surgery. A hanging limb preparation provides the greatest degree of freedom for manipulating limb position. Liberal clipping and thorough sterile preparation are necessary because an open arthrotomy may be required. In most cases, a 2.7-mm, 30-degree fore-oblique arthroscope is used. Basic instrumentation includes probes to inspect the biceps tendon and a handheld cutting instrument to release the tendon. If the surgeon chooses to work through an instrument cannula, different-sized cannulas and switching sticks facilitate the surgery. A motorized shaver can be helpful to débride synovial proliferation, but it is not essential. The dog is positioned in lateral recumbency, with the leg to be operated on uppermost. The limb is supported in neutral position to prevent excessive adduction, which will close the joint line between the glenoid and humeral head.

Egress is established with a needle or cannula, and lactated Ringer's solution is instilled to distend the joint. A guide needle is used to locate the joint line and correct the position for the arthroscope portal. The surgeon may find it beneficial to establish the arthroscope portal more caudal than the standard position when operating on the cranial shoulder joint. To place the arthroscope portal more caudal, a site 0.5 to 1 cm caudal to the acromium is used. The arthroscope is inserted, and ingress flow is established through the arthroscope cannula. The arthroscope and light post are positioned to visualize the cranial compartment. The origin of the biceps tendon is inspected for partial or complete tears, and the bicipital groove is inspected for fibrous proliferation and osteophyte formation (Fig. 3–23A to C). The arthroscope is positioned such that the biceps tendon is clearly visible, and the guide needle is used to triangulate the position for the instrument port. The instrument port is located either just cranial to the acromium (cranial to the arthroscope portal) or medial to the lateral humeral tuberosity over the proximal bicipital groove. The latter is shown as portal position 4 in Figure 3–5. The guide needle is visualized as it enters the joint. Once the position for the instrument portal is established, the surgeon must decide whether to work

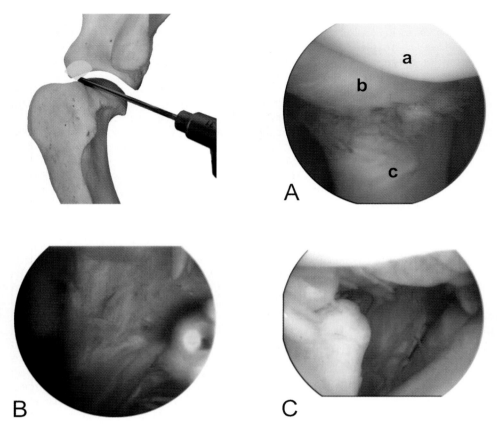

FIGURE 3-23 *A,* Arthroscopic view of the biceps origin. Supraglenoid tuberosity (*a*), labral origin of the biceps (*b*), and biceps tendon (*c*). *B,* Arthroscopic view of an injured biceps tendon. Note the frayed appearance of the ligament. *C,* Arthroscopic view of an injured biceps tendon. Note the stumps of complete ligament tear.

through an open instrument portal, an instrument cannula, or a combination of the two. If the surgeon chooses to work through an open portal site, a no. 11 Bard-Parker scalpel blade is used to make a 0.5- to 1-cm soft tissue tunnel adjacent to the guide needle. Blunt dissection with a pair of small Metzenbaum scissors may be used to establish or enlarge the instrument portal. A probe is inserted through the instrument portal to allow inspection of the biceps tendon and surrounding soft tissue. A motorized shaver may be inserted through the instrument portal to débride synovial and tendon hyperplasia. The bicipital tendon may show partial tearing of either the tendon fibers or the fibrocartilaginous origin of the biceps tendon at the supraglenoid tuberosity. If the biceps tendon shows evidence of partial or complete tearing, the tendon is released from its origin at the supraglenoid tuberosity. Likewise, if there is evidence of synovial proliferation, mineralization, and osteophyte formation within the bicipital groove, the tendon is released from its origin. Tendon release may be performed with a blade instrument (e.g., banana knife, no. 11 scalpel blade), motorized shaver, or radiofrequency unit. After the tendon is released, the joint is flushed by increasing the ingress flow and allowing fluid egress through a large instrument cannula. The joint is inspected for remaining pathology, and the arthroscope and instrument cannula are removed. The portals are sutured with nonreactive, nonabsorbable suture material. Some surgeons make a small craniomedial incision for bicipital tendon tenodesis; others do not. Tenodesis is

the standard technique, but recent clinical experience indicates that it is not necessary.

Postoperative Care. Cold therapy is applied to the shoulder during recovery to relieve pain and reduce swelling. Cold therapy is applied by alternating 15 minutes on and 10 minutes off for two applications. Commercial cold packs or a commercial circulating cold water pack can be used. Alternatively, ice wrapped in a towel or frozen packs of vegetables can be used. If the dog is dismissed from the hospital the day of surgery, NSAIDs and oral butorphanol are dispensed for administration at home. If the dog remains in the hospital overnight, buprenorphine is administered in the evening and NSAIDs and butorphanol are dispensed for administration at home. NSAIDs are continued for 5 days, but butorphanol is discontinued after 48 hours. Cold therapy is continued by the client at home for the first 2 days after surgery using the protocol described earlier. After the surgical swelling is gone (48 to 72 hours), the owner should begin heat therapy and passive motion and stretch exercises. For post-op rehabilitation, see Table 3–2. The owner applies moist heat to the shoulder region with a commercial heat pack or moistened warm towel. The owner should hold the warm pack against the inside of her own elbow for 30 seconds to ensure that it is not too hot. Then the owner places the warm pack over the dog's shoulder area for 10 minutes. Afterward, the owner removes the warm pack and begins gentle flexion and extension movements of the shoulder joint. These exercises begin with small movements, gradually increasing movements to the limit of comfort over a 1- to 2-minute period. At the limit of comfort, the joint is held in position for 10 seconds. The motion and stretch exercise is repeated five times. Additionally, the client should examine the portal sites daily for signs of irritation or drainage.

Exercise is limited to controlled walking on a leash for the first 4 weeks after surgery. Dogs undergoing arthroscopy use the affected leg immediately after surgery. To increase the weightbearing load on the limb, walking at a slow pace is recommended. As postoperative time increases, the pace can be hastened. To increase the range of motion in the shoulder when walking, the client should walk the dog in high grass (e.g., weeds), shallow water, or sand, thus forcing the dog to pick up the feet and step high with the legs. After 4 weeks, the owner should begin limited amounts of free activity with controlled walking, starting with 5 minutes free activity and increasing to 30 minutes free activity over the next 2 weeks. After 6 to 8 weeks, free activity is gradually increased to normal levels. If the dog becomes sore during any exercise period (controlled or free activity) or is sore the next day, the owner should decrease the pace and return to controlled activity for 2 to 3 days.

Complications. Complications are unusual after shoulder arthroscopy. Occasionally, in the immediate postoperative period, excessive fluid extravasation occurs and leads to swollen soft tissues around the shoulder. This fluid resorbs within the first 24 hours. Residual mild swelling adjacent to portal sites may be noticeable for the first 48 hours.

Prognosis. The prognosis for normal limb function with bicipital tenosynovitis of the shoulder is dependent on the degree of pathology. In most cases, with bicipital tendon release, the source of discomfort is eliminated and good to excellent function is restored. After surgery, most dogs become sound within 4 to 8 weeks.

INJURY OF THE SOFT TISSUES OF THE SHOULDER JOINT

The fibrous joint capsule, collateral ligaments, and surrounding cuff muscles of the shoulder joint are sometimes injured. If the joint capsule or collateral ligaments are torn, shoulder instability occurs. If one of the surrounding cuff muscles is strained, fibrosis and mineralization of the muscle tendon unit can occur.

Shoulder Instability

History and Signalment. Dogs present with chronic foreleg lameness, some as long as 2 years before diagnosis and treatment. Often, the patient has no history of a single traumatic event. Lameness does not respond to anti-inflammatory medication. Any age or breed of dog can be affected, and either medial or lateral instability may be present. In one series (Bardet, 2000), the ages of the dogs ranged from 18 months to 13 years, with a mean of 5 years.

Physical Examination Findings. Gait analysis may show obvious lameness; more often, however, lameness is difficult to detect during walking or trotting and is apparent only after exercise. Pain on manipulation of the shoulder and muscle atrophy are evident in most cases. In toy breeds, circumduction of the shoulder may elicit subluxation. Circumduction rarely elicits instability of the shoulder in large breeds. Examination with anesthesia shows a side-to-side difference in abduction/adduction stability and craniocaudal stability. To perform an abduction/adduction test, the animal is placed in lateral recumbency. The elbow and shoulder joints are positioned in extension, and the scapula is stabilized with one hand. With the limb in extension, an abduction force (upward) is exerted on the limb, followed by an adduction force (downward). If the joint is unstable, excessive abduction or adduction is present relative to the normal contralateral side. To perform a craniocaudal stability test, one hand is positioned to stabilize the scapula and the other hand is placed to exert a craniocaudal force on the shoulder joint. The normal shoulder is compared with the affected shoulder to detect abnormal craniocaudal translation.

Differential Diagnosis. The differential diagnosis includes OCD, bicipital tenosynovitis, and acute or chronic strain of the supraspinatus tendon.

Radiographic Findings. Radiographic views should include standard lateral projections of both shoulders. The findings may be unremarkable except for the finding of degenerative osteoarthritis in long-standing cases (Fig. 3–24). Arthrography can be used to outline the joint and show irregularities and filling defects that suggest synovial hyperplasia, tendon rupture, and joint mice.

Diagnosis. A complete orthopedic examination is essential to exclude other shoulder problems. Abduction/adduction and craniocaudal stability of the shoulder should be assessed with the dog anesthetized. Often, the diagnosis is made by exclusion of other, more common shoulder lesions and verification of a torn ligament or capsule through arthroscopy.

Treatment. Medical management usually is not successful in cases with shoulder instability as a result of capsule or ligament injury. Arthroscopic diagnosis followed by open medial or lateral reconstruction is the most common surgical intervention. Arthroscopic reconstruction of capsular tears is often carried out in humans and is in the future for larger dogs. Capsular thermal contracture is also carried out to treat mild to moderate joint laxity in humans. Thermal contracture is feasible in the dog with laxity as a result of capsular or ligament stretching.

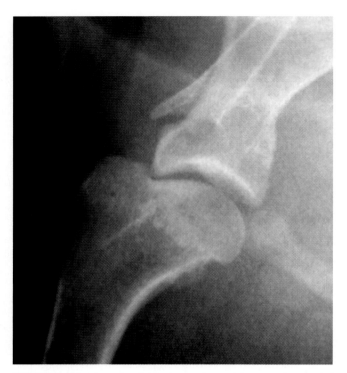

FIGURE 3–24 Lateral radiograph of a dog with long-standing medial instability. Note the mild radiographic changes characteristic of degenerative joint disease.

Anesthetic Considerations and Perioperative Pain Management. The preoperative laboratory workup is based on the patient's physical status and surgical risk. Young, healthy patients with no underlying systemic problems require minimal laboratory workup. Older dogs should undergo a complete blood screen, chest radiographs, and an electrocardiogram. Table 3–1 shows a standard anesthetic protocol, including preemptive pain medication.

Surgical Intervention. Portal sites and surgical anatomy were discussed earlier. The operative site is clipped and prepared according to the amount of limb maneuverability desired during surgery. A hanging limb preparation provides the greatest degree of freedom for manipulating the limb position. Liberal clipping and thorough sterile preparation are necessary because an open arthrotomy may be required. In most cases, a 2.7-mm, 30-degree fore-oblique arthroscope is used. Basic instrumentation includes probes to inspect the joint capsule. If the surgeon chooses to work through an instrument cannula, different-sized cannulas and switching sticks facilitate the surgery. A motorized shaver is helpful to débride synovial proliferation, but this instrument is not essential. If tissue ablation or thermal contracture is indicated, a radiofrequency unit is necessary. The dog is positioned in lateral recumbency, with the leg to be operated on uppermost. The limb is supported in neutral position to prevent excessive adduction, which closes the joint line between the glenoid and humeral head.

Egress is established with a needle or cannula, and Ringer's lactated solution is instilled to distend the joint (see Fig. 3–7). A guide needle is used to locate the joint line and the correct position for the arthroscope portal. The arthroscope is inserted, and ingress flow is established through the arthroscope cannula. The arthroscope and light post are positioned to visualize the medial compartment. With a guide needle, the surgeon triangulates the position for the instrument port. The most common reason for failure to visualize the guide needle in the joint is crossing the arthroscope. To prevent crossing the arthroscope with the guide needle, the needle is inserted perpendicular to the skin surface and this position is maintained through the soft tissues. Once the position for the instrument portal is established, a probe is inserted through a cannula or open portal. The MCL and adjacent medial joint capsule are visualized and inspected with the probe (see Fig. 3–9B). Next, the arthroscope tip is positioned cranially and the light post is turned caudally to view the craniomedial joint capsule and subscapularis tendon (see Fig. 3–9A). The instrument probe is then used to inspect the latter structures. Next, the arthroscope is positioned caudal to the dome of the humeral head and the light post is turned caudally to visualize the insertion of the medial joint capsule at the humeral neck (see Fig. 3–14B). Finally, the LCL and lateral joint capsule are visualized (see Fig. 3–15A).

Tears in the ligament or capsule may be partial or complete (Fig. 3–25A to E). If a partial tear is identified, a thermal probe is used to ablate the torn ligament or capsule remnants. Ablation is followed by thermal contracture of the remaining ligament or capsule (see Fig. 3–25F). If a complete tear is identified, it is best to stop the arthroscopic procedure immediately to prevent excessive extravasation of fluid through the torn joint capsule into the surrounding soft tissue. A medial arthrotomy is performed to reconstruct the medial joint restraints. An approach to the craniomedial shoulder joint is used to expose the luxated joint. If the labrum is worn, the prognosis for successful stabilization of the shoulder is poor. The tendon of the coracobrachialis muscle may be torn and retracted with traumatic luxations. The joint is reduced, and the capsule and subscapularis tendon are imbricated with nonabsorbable mattress sutures. In addition, the MCL is reconstructed with suture anchors and nonabsorbable suture material (see Fig. 3–25G). Additional support may be achieved through transposition of the biceps brachii tendon. The transverse humeral ligament is incised over the biceps tendon. A small incision is made in the joint capsule under the biceps tendon to free this tendon and move it medially. A small groove is created in the humerus at the site at which the tendon will be transposed. The tendon is secured to the humerus with a bone screw and a spiked washer. The same techniques can be used to treat LCL or capsular injuries. An approach to the cranial region of the shoulder joint is used to expose the luxated or subluxated joint. This approach is also used to approach cranial luxations of the shoulder. It may be helpful to reduce the joint before the approach is made to reestablish normal anatomic relationships. The skin

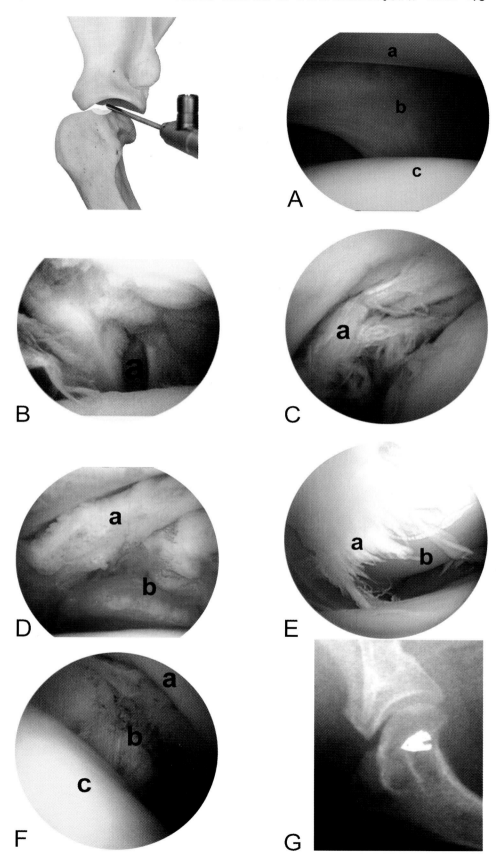

FIGURE 3–25 *A,* Arthroscopic view of the centromedial compartment of the shoulder joint. Glenoid (*a*), centromedial area of the medial collateral ligament (MCL) (*b*), and humeral head (*c*). *B,* Arthroscopic view of a complete tear (*a*) in the central body of the MCL. *C,* Arthroscopic view showing a partial tear and fraying of the MCL. Cranial arm of the MCL (*a*). *D,* Arthroscopic view showing a partial tear of the cranial arm of the MCL (*a*) and tearing of the subscapularis tendon (*b*). *E,* Arthroscopic view showing a partial tear of the lateral collateral ligament (*a*). Lateral rim of the glenoid (*b*). *F,* Arthroscopic view of the MCL after radiofrequency capsulorraphy. Glenoid (*a*), MCL (*b*), and humeral head (*c*). *G,* Postoperative radiograph after reconstruction of the MCL with a suture anchor.

and subcutaneous tissues are incised, and the incision is deepened through the pectoral muscles. An osteotomy of the greater tubercle is performed and includes the supraspinatus muscular insertion. The joint is reduced, and the capsule is imbricated with nonabsorbable mattress sutures. The LCL is reconstructed with suture anchors and nonabsorbable suture material. Additional support can be achieved by transposition of the biceps brachii tendon. A small incision is made in the joint capsule under the biceps tendon to free this tendon and move it laterally across the osteotomy site. While the tendon is held in place, the osteotomy is reduced and stabilized with Kirschner wires and a tension-band wire or lag screw.

Postoperative Care. Cold therapy is applied to the shoulder during recovery for pain relief and to reduce swelling. Cold therapy is applied by alternating 15 minutes on and 10 minutes off for two applications. Commercial cold packs or a commercial circulating cold water pack may be used. Alternatively, ice wrapped in a towel or frozen packs of vegetables can be used. If the dog is dismissed from the hospital on the day of surgery, NSAIDs and oral butorphanol (see Table 3–2) are dispensed for administration at home. If the dog remains in the hospital overnight, buprenorphine is administered in the evening. NSAIDs and butorphanol are dispensed for administration at home. NSAIDs are continued for 5 days, and butorphanol is discontinued after 48 hours. Cold therapy is continued by the client at home for the first 2 days after surgery. After the surgical swelling is gone (48 to 72 hours), the owner should begin heat therapy and passive motion and stretch exercises. The owner should apply moist heat to the shoulder region with a commercial heat pack or a moistened warm towel. The owner should hold the warm pack against the inside of his own elbow for 30 seconds to ensure that it is not too hot. Then the warm pack is placed over the shoulder area for 10 minutes. Afterward, the warm pack is removed and gentle flexion and extension movements of the shoulder joint are begun. The owner should begin with small movements that gradually increase to the limit of comfort over a period of 1 to 2 minutes. At the limit of comfort, the joint is held in position for 10 seconds. The motion and stretch exercise is repeated five times. In addition, the owner should examine the portal sites daily for signs of irritation or drainage.

Exercise is limited to controlled walking on a leash for the first 4 weeks after surgery. Dogs undergoing arthroscopy use the leg immediately after surgery. If an open arthrotomy was performed, the dog may be unable to bear weight for as long as 1 week. To increase the weightbearing load on the limb, walking at a slow pace is recommended. As postoperative time increases, the pace can be hastened. To increase the range of motion in the shoulder when walking, the client should walk the dog in high grass (e.g., weeds), which forces the dog to pick up the feet and step high with the legs. After 4 weeks, the owner should begin limited amounts of free activity with controlled walking. Free activity

should begin with 5 minutes and increase to 30 minutes over the next 2 weeks. After 6 to 8 weeks, free activity is gradually increased to normal levels. If during any exercise period (controlled or free activity), the dog becomes sore or is sore the next day, the owner should decrease the pace and return to controlled activity for 2 to 3 days.

Complications. Complications are unusual after shoulder arthroscopy. Occasionally, excessive fluid extravasation occurs and causes swollen soft tissues around the shoulder in the immediate postoperative period. This fluid resorbs within the first 24 hours. Residual mild swelling adjacent to the portal sites may be noticeable for the first 48 hours. Complications with shoulder arthrotomy are also uncommon. Occasionally, a screw used for tenodesis of the biceps tendon becomes loose. This situation is resolved by removal of the screw.

Prognosis. The prognosis for normal limb function with shoulder instability varies depending on the degree of injury of the medial or lateral restraints. If stretching of the soft tissues is the only pathology, treatment with imbrication or thermal contracture is usually successful. In the case of more extensive soft tissue injury or wearing of the labrum, the prognosis is fair to good.

Strain of the Supraspinatus Insertion

History and Signalment. Dogs present with chronic foreleg lameness. Some dogs exhibit periods of lameness and inability to bear weight. Any age or breed of dog can be affected, but the condition is more common in large breeds.

Physical Examination Findings. Gait analysis usually shows visible lameness. Some dogs are lame only after exercise. Manipulation of the shoulder (e.g., flexion, extension, rotation) may elicit discomfort in most dogs.

Differential Diagnosis. The differential diagnosis includes OCD, bicipital tenosynovitis, and shoulder instability.

Radiographic Findings. Radiographic views should include standard lateral projections of both shoulders. Mineralization is seen adjacent to the greater tubercle of the humerus. Patterns of mineralization are either irregular and nonhomogeneous or well circumscribed with dense foci (Fig. 3–26). A skyline view of the bicipital groove is helpful to delineate the location of dystrophic mineralization (Fig. 3–27). Arthrography can be used to outline the bicipital groove to determine whether irregularities or filling defects that suggest bicipital tenosynovitis are present. Computerized tomography of the shoulder is an excellent method to delineate the position of dystrophic mineralization.

Diagnosis. The diagnosis is based on radiographic findings and direct observation of mineralized foci in the tendon of insertion of the supraspinatus muscle.

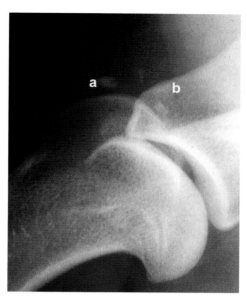

FIGURE 3-26 Lateral radiograph showing mineralization (a and b) near the insertion of the supraspinatus tendon.

History and signalment and physical findings typically are compatible with chronic strain of the supraspinatus tendon of insertion.

Treatment. Medical management is not successful in many cases. Arthroscopic intervention to visualize the biceps tendon and bicipital groove is recommended to determine whether local pathology is present. If the bicipital groove is irregular and has caused a bicipital tenosynovitis, tendon release is recommended. If the bicipital groove and tendon are normal, the arthroscopic procedure is discontinued. After arthroscopic intervention, a medial approach is made to the insertion of the supraspinatus tendon insertion site. The tendon is isolated and a tenectomy of the supraspinatus insertion performed.

Anesthetic Considerations and Perioperative Pain Management. Preoperative laboratory workup is

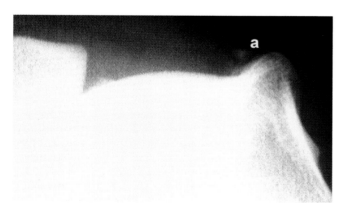

FIGURE 3-27 Skyline view of the case shown in Figure 3-26 showing mineralization near the insertion of the supraspinatus tendon (a).

based on the patient's physical status and surgical risk. Young, healthy patients with no underlying systemic problems require minimal laboratory workup. Older dogs should undergo a complete blood screen, chest radiographs, and electrocardiogram. Table 3–1 shows a standard anesthetic protocol, including preemptive pain medication.

Surgical Intervention. Surgical intervention entails inspection of the joint to confirm the absence of significant pathology. The surgeon must carefully inspect the cranial compartment in the region of the biceps tendon. Portal sites and surgical anatomy were discussed earlier. The operative sites are clipped and prepared according to the amount of limb maneuverability desired during surgery. A hanging limb preparation provides the greatest degree of freedom to manipulate limb position. Liberal clipping and thorough sterile preparation are necessary because an open arthrotomy may be required. A 2.7-mm, 30-degree fore-oblique arthroscope is used in most cases. Basic instrumentation includes probes to inspect the joint capsule. If the surgeon chooses to work through an instrument cannula, different-sized cannulas and switching sticks facilitate the surgery. A motorized shaver is helpful to débride synovial proliferation but is not essential. The dog is positioned in lateral recumbency with the leg to be operated on uppermost. The limb is supported in neutral position to prevent excessive adduction, which closes the joint line between the glenoid and humeral head.

Egress is established with a needle or cannula, and lactated Ringer's solution is instilled to distend the joint (see Fig. 3–7). A guide needle is used to locate the joint line and the correct position for the arthroscope portal. The arthroscope is inserted, and ingress flow is established through the arthroscope cannula. The arthroscope tip is positioned cranially, and the light post is turned caudally to view the biceps tendon and bicipital groove. It is important to inspect the area cranial to the tendon and deep within the bicipital groove (see Figs. 3–11 and 3–12). If pathology is found, bicipital tendon release is performed through an instrument portal. After arthroscopic intervention, a craniomedial incision is made to expose the insertion of the supraspinatus tendon at its insertion onto the greater tubercle of the humerus. After the tendon is isolated, it is released by removing a 1- to 2-cm section of tendon at its insertion (Fig. 3–28). The surgical wound is closed with standard methods.

Postoperative Care. Cold therapy is applied to the shoulder during the recovery period to provide pain relief and reduce swelling. Cold therapy is applied by alternating 15 minutes on and 10 minutes off for two applications. Commercial cold packs or a commercial circulating cold water pack may be used. Alternatively, ice wrapped in a towel or frozen packs of vegetables can be used. If the dog is dismissed from the hospital the day of surgery, NSAIDs and oral butorphanol (see Table 3–2) are dispensed for administration at home. If the dog remains in the hospital overnight, buprenorphine is administered in the evening and NSAIDs and butorphanol

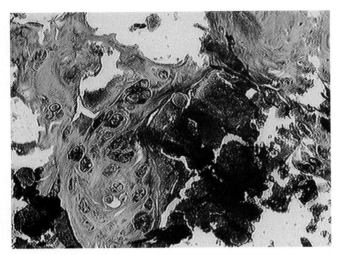

FIGURE 3–28 Histologic specimen showing chronic mineralization of the insertion of the supraspinatus tendon characteristic of chronic insertional strain.

are dispensed for administration at home. NSAIDs are continued for 5 days, and butorphanol is discontinued after 48 hours. Cold therapy is continued by the client at home for the first 2 days after surgery. After the surgical swelling is gone (48 to 72 hours), the owner should begin heat therapy and passive motion and stretch exercises. Moist heat is applied to the shoulder region with a commercial heat pack or a moistened warm towel. The owner should hold the warm pack against the inside of her own elbow for 30 seconds to ensure that it is not too hot. The warm pack is then placed over the dog's shoulder area for 10 minutes. Afterward, the warm pack is removed and gentle flexion and extension movements of the shoulder joint are begun, starting with small movements and gradually increasing movement to the limit of comfort over a period of 1 to 2 minutes. At the limit of comfort, the joint is held in position for 10 seconds. Five repetitions of this exercise are performed two or three times daily. The client also should examine the portal sites daily for signs of irritation or drainage.

Exercise is limited to controlled walking on a leash for the first 4 weeks. Dogs undergoing arthroscopy use the leg immediately after surgery. To increase the weightbearing load on the limb, walking at a slow pace is recommended. As postoperative time increases, the pace can be hastened. To increase the range of motion in the shoulder when walking, the owner should walk the dog in high grass (e.g., weeds), thus forcing the dog to pick up the feet and step high with the legs. After 4 weeks, the owner can introduce limited amounts of free activity with controlled walking. Free activity should begin with 5 minutes and increase to 30 minutes over the next 2 weeks. After 6 to 8 weeks, free activity is gradually increased to normal levels. If during any exercise period (controlled or free activity), the dog becomes sore or is sore the next day, the owner should decrease the pace and return to controlled activity for 2 to 3 days.

Complications. Complications are unusual after shoulder arthroscopy. Occasionally, excessive fluid extravasation occurs and causes swollen soft tissues around the shoulder immediately after surgery. This fluid resorbs within the first 24 hours. Residual mild swelling adjacent to portal sites may be noticeable for the first 48 hours. Complications with shoulder arthrotomy are also uncommon.

Prognosis. The prognosis for normal limb function with chronic supraspinatus sprain is good to excellent.

Incomplete Fusion of the Caudal Glenoid Ossification Center

The presence of a secondary caudal glenoid ossification center is described in the dog. Incomplete fusion appears radiographically as a small radiodense projection located just caudal to the glenoid. In most cases, incomplete fusion of the caudal ossification center may be an incidental finding on radiographic examination of the shoulder. Lameness occurs when an osteochondral fragment is loosely embedded in the joint capsule. An unstable osteochondral fragment acts as a free body in the joint and causes synovitis and pain.

History and Signalment. Most cases occur in large breeds (e.g., rottweiler, German shepherd), but the condition is seen in small breeds as well (terrier, corgi). The age at the time of clinical onset varies, but the condition is usually diagnosed in young dogs. Low-grade and periodic lameness may be present from a few weeks to more than a year before diagnosis.

Physical Examination Findings. Weightbearing lameness is associated with pain on flexion and extension of the shoulder. Mild to moderate muscle atrophy is evident as well, depending on the duration of clinical signs.

Differential Diagnosis. The differential diagnosis includes acute or chronic strain of the supraspinatus tendon, shoulder instability, OCD, calcifying tendinopathy of the biceps tendon, and elbow dysplasia.

Radiographic Findings. Radiographic views should include standard anteroposterior and lateral projections of both shoulders and both elbows. The lateral projection of the shoulder will show a radiodense projection adjacent to the caudal edge of the glenoid (Fig. 3–29). Care is taken to exclude other causes of shoulder and elbow pathology as a cause for the lameness because incomplete ossification can be an incidental radiographic finding. Lameness can be attributed to incomplete fusion only after other causes of forelimb lameness are excluded and a loose osteochondral fragment is found arthroscopically. A nuclear scan is useful to exclude other sources of inflammation, as is computed tomography of the elbows to exclude in situ osteomalacic medial coronoid.

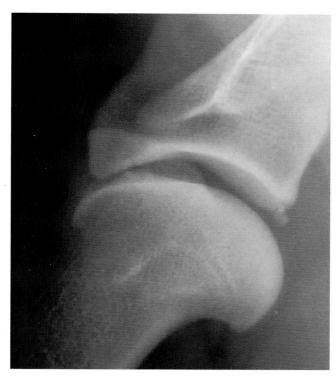

FIGURE 3-29 Lateral radiographic projection showing a radiodense fragment adjacent to the caudal edge of the glenoid.

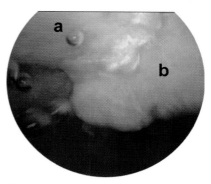

FIGURE 3-30 Arthroscopic view showing the caudal edge of the glenoid (a) and a large, unstable osteochondral fragment (b) adjacent to the glenoid.

Diagnosis. A complete orthopedic examination is essential because other orthopedic conditions may be seen concurrently with incomplete fusion of the caudal ossification center. OCD, elbow dysplasia (FCP, UAP), panosteitis, hypertrophic osteodystrophy, and acute or chronic strain of the supraspinatus tendon are some of these conditions. The diagnosis is based on history and signalment, physical findings, radiographic appearance, and the arthroscopic confirmation of a loose osteochondral fragment. As noted before, this condition may be an incidental finding, so other, more common causes of forelimb lameness must be excluded before the diagnosis can be made.

Surgical Intervention. Portal sites and surgical anatomy were discussed earlier. The operative site is clipped and prepared according to the amount of limb maneuverability desired during surgery. A hanging limb preparation provides the greatest degree of freedom for manipulating limb position. Liberal clipping and thorough sterile preparation are necessary because an open arthrotomy may be required. A 2.7-mm, 30-degree fore-oblique arthroscope is used in most cases. Basic instrumentation includes probes to inspect the osteochondral fragment and a handheld cutting instrument (e.g., banana knife) to remove the fragment. If the surgeon chooses to work through an instrument cannula, different-sized cannulas and switching sticks facilitate the surgery. A motorized shaver is helpful to débride synovial proliferation and remove the loose osteo-

chondral fragment. The dog is positioned in lateral recumbency, with the leg to be operated on uppermost. The limb is supported in neutral position to prevent excessive adduction, which closes the joint line between the glenoid and the humeral head.

Egress is established with a needle or cannula, and lactated Ringer's solution is instilled to distend the joint. A guide needle is used to locate the joint line and the correct position for the arthroscope portal. The arthroscope is inserted, and ingress flow is established through the arthroscope cannula. All compartments of the joint are thoroughly examined. The arthroscope and light post are positioned to visualize the caudal glenoid. The osteochondral fragment is probed to determine its stability and then removed by severing any capsule attachments (Fig. 3-30).

Postoperative Care. Cold therapy is applied to the shoulder during recovery to relieve pain and reduce swelling. Cold therapy is applied by alternating 15 minutes on and 10 minutes off for two applications. Commercial cold packs or a commercial circulating cold water pack can be used. Alternatively, ice wrapped in a towel or frozen packs of vegetables can be used. If the dog is dismissed from the hospital the day of surgery, NSAIDs and oral butorphanol (see Table 3-2) are dispensed for administration at home. If the dog remains in the hospital overnight, buprenorphine is administered in the evening and NSAIDs and butorphanol are dispensed for administration at home. NSAIDs are continued for 5 days, and butorphanol is discontinued after 48 hours. Cold therapy is continued by the client at home for the first 2 days after surgery. After the surgical swelling is gone (48 to 72 hours), the owner should begin heat therapy and passive motion and stretch exercises. The owner should apply moist heat to the shoulder region with a commercial heat pack or a moistened warm towel. The owner should hold the warm pack against the inside of her own elbow for 30 seconds to ensure that it is not too hot, then place the warm pack over the dog's shoulder area for 10 minutes. Afterward, the warm pack is removed and gentle flexion and extension movements of the shoulder joint are started, beginning with small movements and gradually increasing movements to the limit of comfort over a period of 1 to 2 minutes. At the limit of comfort, the joint is held in position for 10 seconds. The motion and stretch exercises are performed for five repetitions. The owner should examine the portal sites daily for signs of irritation or drainage.

For the first 4 weeks after surgery, exercise is limited to controlled walking on a leash. Dogs undergoing arthroscopy use the affected leg immediately after surgery. To increase the weightbearing load on the limb, walking at a slow pace is recommended. As postoperative time increases, the pace can be hastened. To increase the range of motion in the shoulder when walking, the client should walk the dog in high grass (e.g., weeds), shallow water, or sand, thereby forcing the dog to pick up the feet and step high with the legs. After 4 weeks, the owner should resume limited amounts of free activity with controlled walking, beginning with 5 minutes free activity and increasing to 30 minutes free activity over the next 2 weeks. After 6 to 8 weeks, free activity is gradually increased to normal levels. If the dog becomes sore during any exercise period (controlled or free activity) or is sore the next day, the owner should decrease the pace and return to controlled activity for 2 to 3 days.

Suggested Readings

Barber FA, Byrd JW, Wolf EM, et al: How would you treat the partially torn biceps tendon. Arthroscopy 17: 636–639, 2001.

Bardet J: Arthroscopy of the shoulder in dogs and cats: A six year retrospective study of 221 cases. Proceedings of the Veterinary Orthopedic Society, Val d'Isere, France 2000, p 19.

Cook JT: Arthroscopic treatment of shoulder instability using radiofrequency induced thermal modification. Proceedings of the Veterinary Orthopedic Society, Lake Louise, Canada 2001, p 37.

Goring RL, Pierce C: Arthroscopic examination of the canine scapulohumeral joint. J Am Anim Hosp 3:551–555, 1986.

Innes JF: Advanced arthroscopy in the dog. Proceedings of European Society of Veterinary Orthopedics and Traumatology, Munich, Germany 2000, p 51.

Kriegleder H: Mineralization of the supraspinatous tendon: Clinical observations in 7 dogs. VCOT 8:91, 1995.

Olivieri M, Vezzoni A, Marcellin-Little D: Incomplete fusion of the caudal glenoid ossification center in 5 dogs. Proceedings of the Veterinary Orthopedic Society, Val d'Isere, France 2000, p 20.

Person MW: Arthroscopy of the canine shoulder. Comp Cont Ed 8:537–546, 1986.

Person MW: Arthroscopic treatment of OCD in the canine shoulder. Vet Surg 18:3, 175–189, 1989.

Rudd RG, Whitehair JG, Margolis JH: Results of management of osteochondritis dissecans of the humeral head in dogs: 44 cases (1982–1987). J Am Anim Hosp Assoc 26(2):173–178, 1990.

Stobie D, Wallace L, Lipowitz A, et al: Chronic bicipital tenosynovitis in dogs: 29 cases. JAVMA 207:201–207, 1995.

van Bree H, van Ryssen B: OCD lesions of the canine shoulder: Correlation of arthrography and arthroscopy. Vet Radiol Ultrasound 33:342–347, 1992.

van Ryssen B, van Bree H: Successful arthroscopic treatment of shoulder OCD in the dog. J Small Anim Pract 34:521–528, 1993.

Viguier E: Arthroscopic study of shoulder diseases in the dog. Proceedings of the European College of Veterinary Surgeons, Velbert, Germany 2001, p 49.

Whitney WO, Beale B, Hulse DA: Arthroscopic release of the biceps tendon for treatment of bicipital injury in the dog. Proceedings of the Veterinary Orthopedic Society, Lake Louise, Canada 2001, p 3.

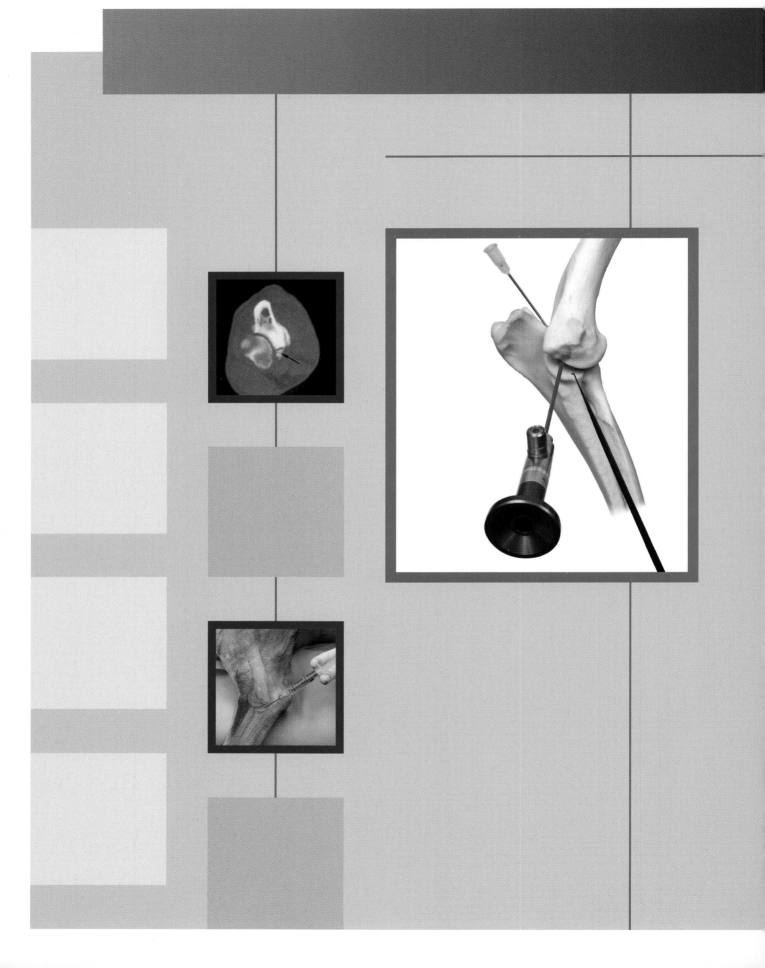

Arthroscopically Assisted Surgery of the Elbow Joint

Introduction

The canine elbow is potentially the simplest joint to examine arthroscopically. Usually there is only thin soft tissue, and there are clean anatomical landmarks, so insertion of the arthroscope is relatively easy. Arthroscopic treatment in the canine elbow can be straightforward or very complex, depending on the disease and its severity. Outcomes with canine elbow arthroscopy are not predictable and depend largely on the nature of the disease being treated. Canine elbow arthritis remains a disease of uncertain cause, and the associated osteoarthritis can involve substantial portions of the articular cartilage, making successful treatment difficult with any modality. In addition to its use in elbow dysplasia, arthroscopy is used in the canine elbow for management of septic arthritis, assistance in repair of condylar fractures, and incomplete fusion of the humeral condyle.

Arthroscopy of the Elbow Joint

Equipment and Instrumentation. The surgical table should be one that can be lowered and raised and should be adjusted to a position that allows the surgeon and assistants to hold the arms as close to the body as possible. The surgeon's shoulders should be in a neutral position, with the elbows close to 90 degrees. This position prevents fatigue and improves the efficiency of the operating team. The imaging tower is positioned at the back of the patient or opposite the surgeon for unilateral cases and at the head of the patient or at the end of the surgery table for bilateral procedures (Figs. 4–1 and 4–2).

Canine elbow arthroscopy was originally described using a 2.7-mm, 30-degree rigid arthroscope. A 1.9-mm, 30-degree short arthroscope is recommended (Fig. 4–3A). The smaller size significantly decreases cartilage trauma while allowing greater visualization and closer inspection of the joint. The 1.9-mm arthroscope also allows intervention into the elbows of smaller breeds, such as the Shetland sheepdog, Border collie, and Australian cattle dog. Appropriate fluid flow is necessary in arthroscopy. Large-joint arthroscopy may be performed routinely with gravity flow alone; however, smaller joints, such as the elbow, require higher fluid pressures and may have more tenuous outflow. The use of a fluid pump for canine elbow arthroscopy may increase the reliability of fluid flow. Most arthroscopy pumps have both pressure

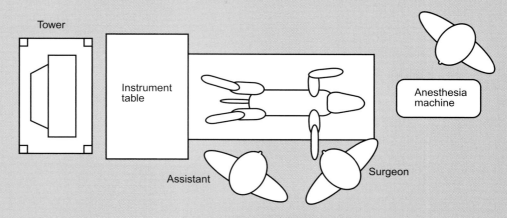

FIGURE 4–1 Arrangement of the operating room for bilateral elbow arthroscopy. For unilateral elbow arthroscopy, the tower may be placed on the side of the table opposite the limb that is being treated (see Fig. 3–1).

Tower

Instrument table

Anesthesia machine

Assistant

Surgeon

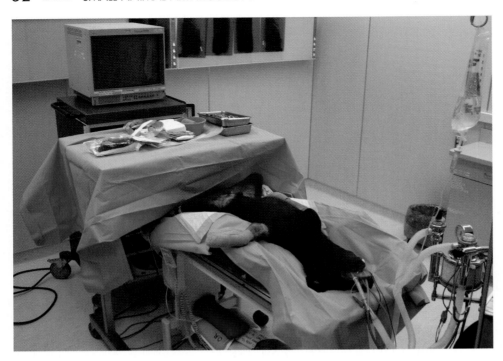

FIGURE 4–2 Positioning of the dog and surgical equipment used for bilateral elbow arthroscopy before draping is performed. The left elbow joint is positioned over an elbow brace that is used as a fulcrum point.

and flow control. Pressure is the priority setting. For smaller joints, such as the canine elbow, pressure between 60 and 70 mm Hg is preferred and flow is kept relatively low (10% to 20%) to avoid sudden surges of fluid. If a fluid pump is not available, a pressure bag can be used to deliver an adequate volume of pressurized fluids.

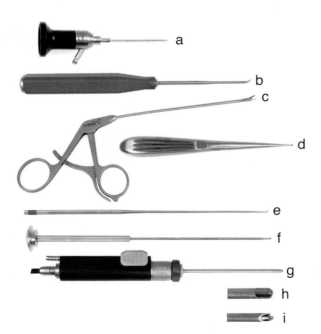

FIGURE 4–3 Instrumentation for elbow arthroscopy. A 1.9-mm, 30-degree short arthroscope (a); arthroscopic micropick (b); small-joint graspers (c); 5–0 curette (d); right-angle probe (e); hand burr (f); power shaver (g); aggressive cutter tip for a power shaver (h); burr tip for a power shaver (i).

A simple instrumentation pack (see Chapter 2) is all that is necessary for elbow arthroscopy. The pack should include small, high-quality arthroscopic hand tools that are specified for canine arthroscopy. Basic hand tools used for canine elbow arthroscopy include a curette, right-angle probe, and grasper (see Fig. 4–3). Other helpful instruments include a manual or power hand shaver, hand biter, cannulas, and switching sticks. The curette is used to débride damaged cartilage and diseased bone. Standard small surgical curettes are suitable for elbow arthroscopy. The most appropriate size is 5–0 and smaller. Angled curettes also may be useful, but are more difficult to insert into the portal or cannula. A small-joint, right-angle probe is used to palpate joint surfaces and manipulate fragments. Some probes have measuring marks that aid in determining lesion size. A high-quality small-joint grasper is another necessary tool (see Fig. 4–3C). It should be very small in diameter (2.5 to 2.9 mm) and have a smooth, enclosed locking mechanism. A delicate grasper must be used carefully. Overaggressive use can damage the grasping mechanism and may lead to the need for costly repair or replacement. A second, larger grasper is often useful to grasp and remove larger fragments. Traditional small alligator forceps can be used, but are more difficult to manipulate because the unenclosed mechanism may not operate correctly in small portals and joints and also because the jaws cannot be locked. Additional hand instruments that may be helpful include a hand burr to destroy fragments and perform abrasion arthroplasty and a small-joint biter to perform soft tissue excision and biopsy.

Many elbow arthroscopy procedures in dogs can be completed without the aid of power instruments. However, some procedures, such as fragment removal and bone or cartilage débridement, can be performed more quickly and with less trauma with the aid of a power shaver (see Fig. 4–3G to I). The small size of the canine elbow necessitates the use of small-joint shaving equipment. The most useful power shavers in this setting are an aggressive cutter and a burr. The cutter is most useful for débridement of diseased cartilage, and the burr is used to remove cartilage or bone. Most hand shavers have suction attachments to help evacuate debris. Arthroscopic cautery units and radiofrequency instruments are rarely necessary in elbow arthroscopy and may pose a risk to the nearby median and ulnar nerves.

Anesthetic Considerations and Perioperative Pain Management. Most dogs that undergo elbow arthroscopy are younger than 2 years of age and have minimal medical problems. For this reason, little diagnostic testing is normally required. Additional blood tests, urinalysis, and radiography may be indicated for older patients undergoing anesthesia and arthroscopy, particularly if neoplasia, infection, or immune-mediated joint disease is suspected.

In most cases, preoperative pain management during hospitalization is not a concern, although many patients may have had recent administration of NSAIDs, including carprofen, aspirin, and etodolac. The effect of aspirin on platelets and the heparin-like action of etodolac may increase the risk of operative hemorrhage. For this reason, these medications are usually discontinued approximately 2 weeks before surgery. A standard anesthetic protocol, including preemptive pain medication, is shown in Table 3–1. There are no specific anesthetic requirements for elbow arthroscopy. Most patients are comfortable and fully ambulatory shortly after recovery, and in many cases, they are discharged from the hospital the same day. For this reason, short-acting anesthetic regimens with rapid recovery rates are recommended (see Table 3–1). Perioperative pain management usually includes general anesthesia and local analgesia (Fig. 4–4). Brachial plexus blocks may be used, but their effectiveness requires expertise and accuracy in administration. In addition, many cases of elbow arthroscopy are bilateral and require bilateral blocking. Because local blocks may last for 5 to 6 hours, an animal that has a brachial plexus block may have difficulty ambulating for several hours after anesthetic recovery.

Alternatively, infusion of the joint with bupivacaine is simple and effective (see Fig. 4–4). Bupivacaine may be administered either preoperatively, after clipping and scrubbing are complete, or at the end of the procedure. The maximum recommended dosage is 2 mg/kg, which is divided between the two elbows if bilateral arthroscopy is performed. Preoperatively, bupivacaine is injected either medially or laterally. The needle is inserted as for arthrocentesis; it is placed just aside the olecranon and directed distally and axially into the joint (see Fig. 4–4). The joint is aspirated before injection to observe for joint fluid and confirm proper needle location. Bupivacaine usually requires approximately 20 minutes to take effect, and when it is injected preoperatively, the bupivacaine is diluted or flushed out of the joint at the initiation of

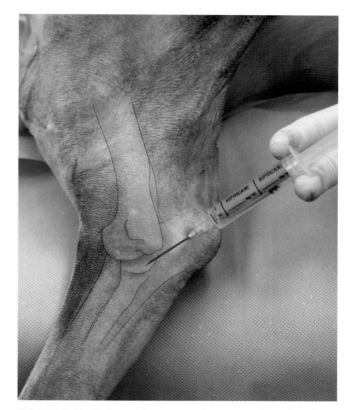

FIGURE 4–4 Technique for intra-articular injection of local analgesic for the canine elbow. The needle is placed adjacent or just proximal to the anconeal process. Joint fluid is aspirated before injection to ensure proper location.

surgery. Alternatively, the joint may be infused with the bupivacaine through one of the portals at the end of the procedure. This practice allows greater absorption of the drug, although the late timing of delivery is not ideal and some drug may leak out through the portals and into the periarticular space.

Most patients require minimal postoperative pain management. Administration of NSAIDs usually suffices. Cold therapy may be applied to the elbows during recovery to reduce pain and swelling. This treatment is administered by alternating 15 minutes on and 10 minutes off for two applications. Commercial cold packs or ice wrapped in a towel can be used. At home, the owner continues cold therapy for the first 2 days after surgery. When the dog is dismissed from the hospital, nonsteroidal anti-inflammatory drugs (NSAIDs) and oral butorphanol (see Table 3–1) are dispensed for administration at home. NSAIDs are continued for 5 days, and butorphanol is discontinued after 48 hours. If the dog remains in the hospital overnight, buprenorphine is administered in the evening. NSAIDs and butorphanol are prescribed for home administration. Fentanyl transdermal patches also are used for postoperative pain management.

Antibiotic Treatment. The risk of infection with routine arthroscopic surgery is probably less than that associated with open surgery; however, the use of prophylactic perioperative antibiotics is recommended. In most cases, administration of cefazolin 22 mg/kg at the time of induction and every 2 hours during the procedure is adequate.

Patient Preparation and Positioning. The patient is clipped and prepared for an open elbow arthrotomy in case the arthroscopy procedure needs to be aborted for technical reasons and an open arthrotomy performed. This situation is more common when the surgeon is beginning to learn arthroscopy. The dog is positioned in dorsal recumbency, and the fur is clipped from the midantebrachium to the level of the shoulder joint (see Fig. 4–2). The remaining fur on the lower portion of the legs is wrapped. As the surgeon becomes more experienced and adept at elbow arthroscopy, less maneuverability is needed and a medial limb preparation can be done for each limb.

In the operating room, dorsal recumbency is the standard position for both unilateral and bilateral elbow arthroscopy. Another option is positioning the dog in lateral recumbency with the affected limb downward. This position allows the use of the surgery table edge as a fulcrum for distraction of the joint. For positioning with dorsal recumbency, sandbags may be used as a fulcrum or elbow braces may be constructed and placed under each elbow to provide a fulcrum for joint distraction (Fig. 4–5).

The patient is draped according to the standard technique for open arthrotomy. Stockinet or sterile adhesive draping may be used at the discretion of the surgeon (Fig. 4–6). After the patient is fully draped, the limb is rotated down until it is parallel to the floor. The limb is placed in a normal standing position relative to the joint angles, with the elbow joint positioned over the fulcrum device or table edge. The assistant places moderate downward (lateral) pressure to open the medial com-

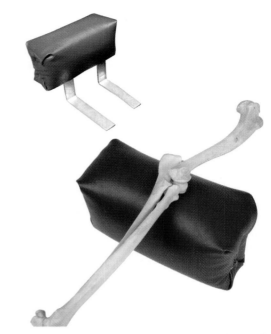

FIGURE 4–5 Use of custom-made braces as a fulcrum for elbow arthroscopy. Braces are manufactured from wood blocks that are covered with foam and vinyl and attached to right-angle brackets.

partment of the elbow joint (see Fig. 4–6). Additional internal rotation of the limb also enlarges the joint space for instrumentation. The relative positions of the surgeon and assistant, cranial or caudal to the limb, depend on the handedness of the surgeon, the specific procedure being performed, and the surgeon's preference (see Fig. 4–1).

Portal Sites. Two or three portal sites are used for elbow arthroscopy, depending on the purpose of the procedure. If visual exploration of the elbow joint is all

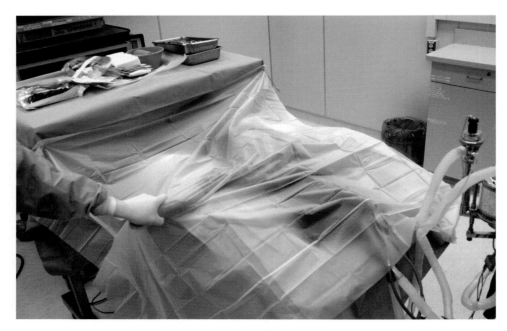

FIGURE 4–6 Patient prepared for elbow arthroscopy with plastic adhesive drapes. The use of plastic drapes helps to keep the patient drier and warmer than standard draping methods.

that is required, an egress portal and an arthroscope portal are necessary. However, an additional instrument portal is required for tissue biopsy or treatment of joint pathology.

The egress site is established first (Figs. 4–7 to 4–9). With the joint in a standing position and the medial compartment forced open with moderate downward pressure, a needle (25- to 18-gauge) is inserted in a craniodistal and slight lateral direction, beginning just proximal or adjacent to the anconeus. The needle is directed to place the tip in the joint pouch just proximal to the anconeus.

To ensure placement within the joint, a syringe is attached to the needle and used to aspirate synovial fluid. In most cases, when the egress portal is properly placed, synovial fluid is easily aspirated. If synovial fluid is not aspirated and the surgeon believes that the joint has been entered, lactated Ringer's solution can be instilled into the joint. If the needle is located in the joint, fluid is easily instilled. Also, as the joint cavity fills with fluid, reverse pressure is felt on the syringe plunger. This sensation ensures that the needle is placed properly. If the needle is placed incorrectly, fluid may be injected around the joint instead of into the joint, making the procedure much more difficult. In some cases, even when the needle is positioned properly, it may be impossible to aspirate any joint fluid. Joint infusion and lavage are performed with lactated Ringer's solution, which may

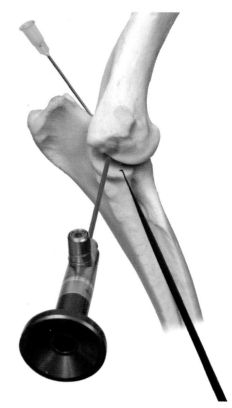

FIGURE 4–8 Bone model showing a medial view of the positioning of instruments for joint arthroscopy of the canine elbow.

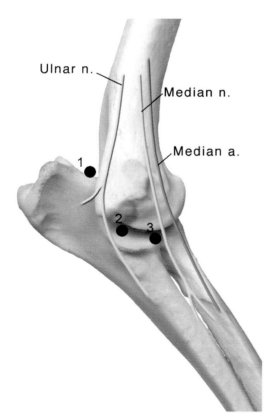

FIGURE 4–7 Medial view of portal locations and pertinent anatomy for canine elbow arthroscopy. *1*, Infusion and egress portal; *2*, arthroscope portal; *3*, instrument portal.

cause less damage to cartilage than saline. The joint is filled until moderate pressure is felt against the plunger. Underfilling makes establishment of the arthroscope portal more difficult and traumatic, and overfilling may lead to rupture of the joint cavity and loss of fluid into the periarticular soft tissues. The volume of fluid that is needed may vary tremendously between joints. Normal or mildly pathologic joints may require only several milliliters of lactated Ringer's solution, whereas more diseased joints may require as much as 20 mL fluid. After adequate pressure is reached, an assistant should hold the syringe under pressure or cap off the needle to maintain joint pressurization during insertion of the arthroscope portal.

The arthroscope portal is established next. The arthroscope cannula with the attached blunt obturator is inserted first. The standard arthroscope insertion site is based on localization of the medial epicondyle and approximation of the location of the joint surface. The beginning arthroscopist should be careful to localize the medial epicondyle before the joint is infused because joint distension may make palpation more difficult. A finger should be placed on the medial epicondyle and drawn down distally until the approximate level of the joint is reached. This level is estimated by evaluating the lateral radiographic view. Next, the finger is drawn approximately 5 mm caudal to this point for arthroscope insertion (see Figs. 4–7 to 4–9). The exact location of

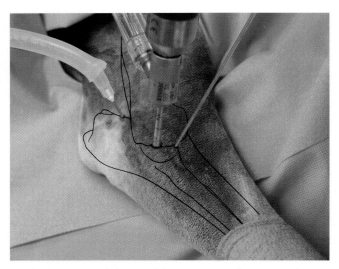

FIGURE 4–9 Medial view of the positioning of instruments for joint arthroscopy of the canine elbow.

this insertion may be modified according to the disease being treated. For example, the arthroscope portal may need to be moved further caudal to allow visualization of an entire humeral osteochondrosis dissecans (OCD) lesion. An 18- to 25-gauge needle may be inserted at the location of the proposed port to ensure that the level is correct. The needle should pass easily into the joint with a minimum of proximodistal angulation. To insert the arthroscope, a small blade (no. 15 or no. 11) is used to make a short (2- to 3-mm) proximodistal incision through the skin and superficial soft tissues. The incision should not be continued through the entire joint capsule, or the joint distension will be eliminated and excessive extravasation of fluid will occur into the surrounding soft tissues. The assistant should maintain a valgus force (downward pressure) to the foot to open the medial compartment of the joint. The arthroscope cannula is fitted with a blunt obturator and inserted through the incision and into the joint. The ideal angle of insertion, perpendicular to the limb, permits maximum manipulation and visualization, with minimal trauma. When a blunt conical obturator is used, pressure is applied to penetrate the joint capsule. The cannula and blunt obturator are inserted with the fingers braced against the limb to avoid overpenetration, which can damage the cartilage. With experience, the surgeon will learn to feel when the joint is entered. After entry is confirmed, the obturator is removed from the cannula. If the cannula is placed correctly, fluid flows freely from the cannula. The fluid ingress line is attached to the cannula, and the arthroscope is inserted.

If gravity flow is used, a 10-drop/mL administration set is used wide open. If a fluid pump is used, relatively high pressures (60 to 75 mm Hg) and low flow (10% to 20%) are recommended. The egress needle is uncapped at this point. Sterile extension tubing can be attached to the outflow needle to scavenge fluid into a canister (see Fig. 4–9); however, in low-flow situations, particularly with gravity flow, the tubing may establish a siphon

effect and draw air bubbles into the joint. Alternatively, the fluid can be allowed to flow onto the floor for removal with a floor scavenging system or towels.

The instrument portal is established if a biopsy specimen of intra-articular tissue is needed or if treatment of joint pathology is required. Instrumentation portals are used to insert a variety of instruments, including small-joint graspers, right-angle probes, small-joint shavers, and curettes. Less often, a radiofrequency probe, biopsy punch, or soft tissue biter is used. After the joint is thoroughly explored, the arthroscope is positioned to visualize the craniomedial portion of the joint (Fig. 4–10A). The field of view should include the cranial aspect of the medial coronoid, An 18- to 20-gauge needle is inserted into the joint in the region of the medial collateral ligament (see Figs. 4–7 to 4–9). Successful visualization and manipulation of the needle by the arthroscope is referred to as *triangulation*. The most common reason for failure to triangulate is inadvertent crossing of the needle and arthroscope within the joint. It is surprising how relatively parallel in the transverse plane the arthroscope and instrument need to be. When attempting to triangulate the position for the ports, the surgeon should observe the location and direction of the actual instruments instead of watching the monitor. The needle is inserted at the same proximodistal level and proximodistal angle as the arthroscope (see Fig. 4–9). The needle should be inserted nearly parallel to the arthroscope in the craniocaudal plane. Insertion of the needle at too oblique an angle to the arthroscope causes crossing of the needle under the arthroscope. In this situation, it is impossible to visualize the needle with the arthroscope, although the surgeon may be able to feel the two rub against each other. Ideally, the arthroscope and needle are both perpendicular to the long axis of the limb. The specific craniocaudal position of entry on the limb varies with the size of the dog and the disease being treated. The surgeon's hands should be positioned a comfortable distance apart to permit ease of manipulation. This ease of manipulation occurs with proper portal sites, but should not be the determining factor in portal placement. After the needle is inserted into the joint, the surgeon should look at the monitor to determine whether the needle tip is in view (see Fig. 4–10B). If the needle tip cannot be seen, in most cases, it is not productive for the surgeon to manipulate the arthroscope to look for the needle tip. Typically, it will not be visible, and if it is, it will usually be in an inappropriate position. In other words, the surgeon should keep the arthroscope view constant and reinsert the needle correctly.

After the needle is visualized and the internal and external positioning is satisfactory, a no. 15 or no. 11 blade is used to make a 3- to 5-mm longitudinal incision directly adjacent to the needle. An assistant should remove the needle so that the surgeon may immediately insert a small blunt trocar at a similar angle to the needle (see Fig. 4–8). If an instrument cannula is needed, it is inserted at this time. Once inserted, the trocar is gently manipulated to further enlarge the portal while avoiding damage to the articular cartilage. The portal is

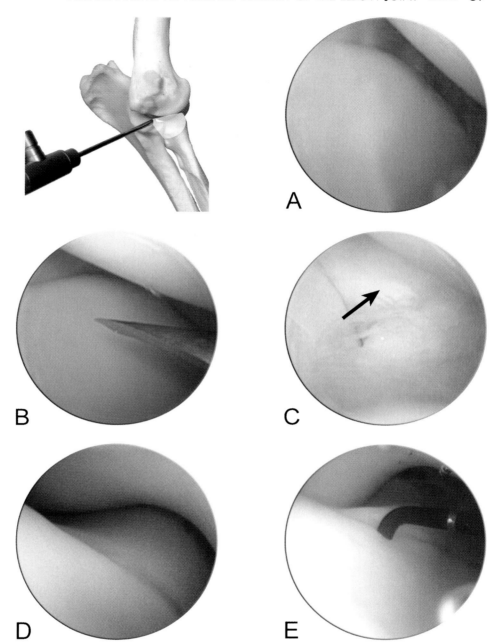

FIGURE 4-10 Positioning and normal joint findings for arthroscopic evaluation of the medial portion of the coronoid process, radial head, and distal trochlear notch; *A,* Cranial aspect of the normal medial coronoid process. *B,* Visualization of q needle over the cranial aspect of a normal medial coronoid process. *C,* Normal annular ligament *(arrow).* The collateral ligament is behind the fat, to the right of the annular ligament. *D,* Commissure of the coronoid process and caudal aspect of the radial head. *E,* Use of a right-angle probe to palpate the commissure and lateral aspect of the medial coronoid process.

now ready for use. A cleanly created, large portal allows easy insertion of all necessary instruments without the need for a cannula. A larger portal also allows more effective drainage of egress fluid, with less extravasation into the subcutaneous tissues. The ease of insertion through the instrument portal usually improves as the surgery progresses, unless the portal is handled roughly and fluid extravasates into the adjacent tissues.

The decision to use a cannula in small animal arthroscopy is based on the individual surgeon's preference. A cannula allows instruments to be inserted easily and avoids extravasation of periportal fluid. However, many instruments used in elbow arthroscopy are too large for a cannula that can be easily inserted into the

joint. The surgeon also may use both a cannula portal and an open portal, depending on the procedure.

Surgical Anatomy. The initial step in elbow joint arthroscopy is thorough exploration of the joint. It is important to apply downward pressure to maintain adequate opening of the medial joint to allow maximum manipulation of the arthroscope with minimal trauma to the cartilage. The surgeon also should feel comfortable in manipulating the light post of the arthroscope to rotate the bevel and maximize visualization. As the arthroscope is manipulated and the light post is rotated, the camera is maintained in an upright position so that the proximal aspect of the joint is always at the top of

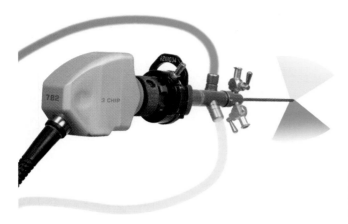

FIGURE 4-11 Arthroscopic manipulation of the camera and arthroscope. The camera is always maintained in an upright position so that the top of the image on the screen is always dorsal. The arthroscope is twisted relative to the camera by rotating the light and fluid posts.

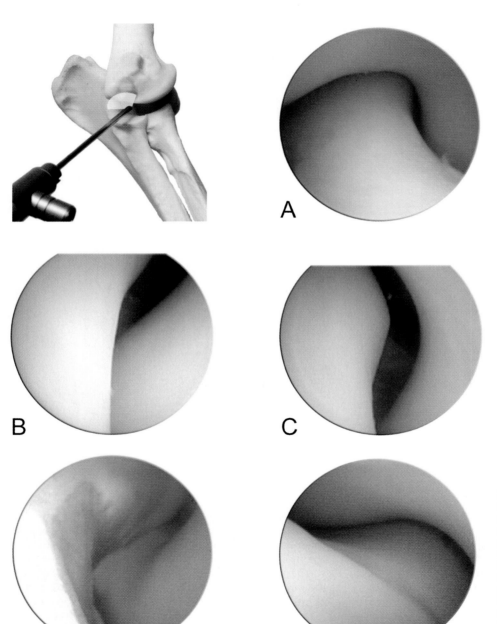

A

B

C

D

E

FIGURE 4-12 Positioning and normal joint findings for arthroscopic evaluation of the anconeus and trochlear notch. *A,* Normal anconeal process and trochlear notch with full cartilage coverage. *B,* Normal central trochlear notch with full cartilage coverage. *C,* Extreme proximal aspect of the anconeus. The elbow is mildly flexed to bring the proximal tip into view. *D,* Normal trochlear notch with absence of cartilage in the central notch. *E,* Distal trochlear notch and caudal radial head.

the screen (Fig. 4–11). This position aids significantly in maintaining orientation. Developing a standard pattern for examination of the joint helps the surgeon to improve arthroscopic skills and also ensures that all accessible areas of the joint are examined. Standard images of specific regions are routinely obtained, even when these areas are normal. In addition to documenting the type, severity, and location of lesions, imaging and reporting these findings aids in determining the degree of iatrogenic trauma to the cartilage at the conclusion of the primary surgery and aids in conducting assessments of healing or progression during second-look arthroscopy. An example of standard examination of the medial elbow joint is to visualize and image each area of the medial joint as follows:

1. Anconeus
2. Trochlear notch
3. Lateral coronoid
4. Central medial coronoid
5. Cranial medial coronoid
6. Radial head
7. Cranial medial humeral condyle
8. Central medial humeral condyle
9. Caudal medial humeral condyle
10. Lateral condyle (axial region)

When the arthroscope enters the joint, the camera is positioned to provide proper spatial orientation on the monitor. The light post is rotated craniodistally (with the bevel directed caudodorsally) and the camera head is moved craniodistally to view the anconeus (Fig. 4–12A and B). The camera head is moved slightly proximally and the light post is rotated cranially to observe the medial and axial portions of the central trochlear notch (see Fig. 4–12C and D). In normal joints, this area is often devoid of cartilage. The underlying subchondral bone is smooth and different in color than the bone that is exposed during osteoarthritis. The area around the exposed bone is free of fibrillation, which is also unlike the appearance of diseased cartilage.

The light post is rotated proximally and the camera head is moved slightly proximally to visualize the distal trochlear notch (see Fig. 4–12E). In this view, the caudomedial edge of the radial head and the medial coronoid also become apparent. Advancing the arthroscope slightly deeper allows the lateral coronoid and lateral humeral condyle to be visualized (Fig. 4–13). External rotation of the elbow may aid advancement of the arthroscope.

The articular surface of the medial coronoid is examined by moving the camera head caudally and keeping the light post proximal (see Fig. 4–10). The area is closely examined for cartilage damage, including fibrillation, excoriation, and full-thickness injury. The central and cranial aspects of the medial coronoid are examined next by advancing the arthroscope further into the joint and moving the camera head further caudal. The area is

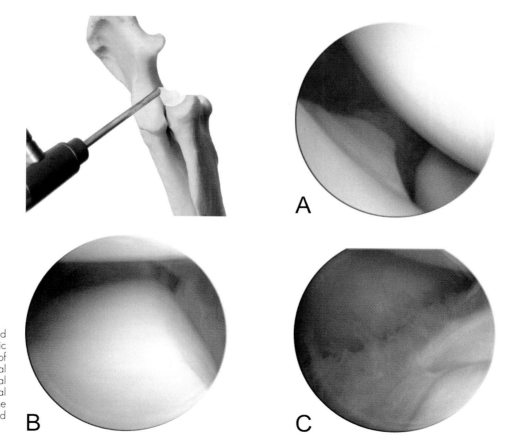

FIGURE 4–13 Positioning and normal joint findings for arthroscopic evaluation of the lateral portion of the coronoid process. *A,* Normal lateral coronoid process; *B,* normal lateral coronoid process showing the radial articular surface; *C,* insertion of the annular ligament on the lateral coronoid process.

examined again for cartilage damage and fragmentation of the craniolateral aspect of the medial coronoid. In a normal joint, the radial head is also visible at this point. In some cases of fragmentation of the medial coronoid process (FCP), the elevated or large fragment obscures the radial head.

The entire visible aspect of the humerus is examined for osteoarthritic lesions and OCD (Fig. 4–14). The light post is rotated distally to allow observation of the inter-condylar region (see Fig. 4–14A). The camera head is progressively tilted cranially to view the central and caudal portions of the humeral condyle (see Fig. 4–14B). Then the light post is rotated caudally and the camera head is moved distally to view the most proximal portion

(see Fig. 4–14B and C). Careful attention must be paid to the region that articulates with the medial coronoid of the ulna. The central portion of the area is a common site for partial- or full-thickness cartilage defects, and the medial aspect is a common site for osteochondrosis (see Fig. 4–14D and E). The surgeon must be careful not to pull the arthroscope out of the joint when evaluating this region. Other structures that may be examined in the medial compartment of the elbow joint include the synovium, medial collateral ligament, and annular and oblique ligaments (see Fig. 4–10C). The synovium is seen most easily cranial to the medial coronoid and radial head. The light post is faced caudally and the camera head is moved caudally. Rotating the light post

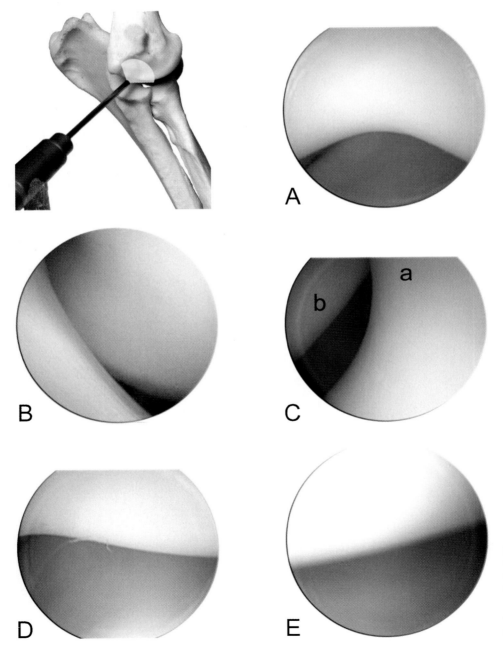

FIGURE 4-14 Positioning and normal joint findings for arthroscopic evaluation of the humeral condyle. A, Craniodistal area; B, central area; C, proximal aspect (a, anconeus; b, humerus); D and E, medial aspect, in the region typical for osteochondrosis dissecans.

slightly proximally allows the annular and oblique ligaments to be visualized as they cross between the radial head and the medial coronoid (see Fig. 4–10C). Pulling the arthroscope out slightly may allow the cranial branch of the collateral ligament to be visualized.

Joint Lavage and Closure. The conclusion of elbow arthroscopy includes joint lavage, surgical wound closure, and injection of local analgesic. If an instrument cannula is used, the joint can be lavaged with inflow through the arthroscope cannula and outflow through the instrument cannula. If the surgeon does not use an instrument cannula, lavage can be achieved by connecting the fluid line to the egress needle and removing the arthroscope from its cannula, leaving the cannula in the joint. Suction can be held at the end of the arthroscope cannula during lavage. This method is recommended when an instrument cannula is not used because the large diameter of the arthroscope cannula allows more efficient lavage and the removal of larger debris than is possible through the egress needle. After the joint is thoroughly lavaged, the arthroscope cannula is removed and the arthroscope and instrument portals are sutured with nylon in a cruciate pattern through the skin if needed. Closure of deeper layers usually is not necessary. Bupivacaine may be injected into the joint through the egress cannula or needle, which is then removed. Postoperatively, a bandage is placed on the limb for 24 hours if there is significant swelling around the joint as a result of fluid extravasation.

Indications for Arthroscopic Surgery of the Elbow Joint

Indications for elbow arthroscopy in dogs and cats include the diagnosis and therapy of infectious, neoplastic, traumatic, developmental, and degenerative diseases. Arthroscopy provides a means of minimally invasive synovial biopsy in cases of immune-mediated arthritis or neoplasia. Biopsy specimens of the synovium are usually obtained with a small or medium biter (see Chapter 2). The sharp biting action on these instruments permits several biopsy specimens to be obtained rapidly and in a single step. Cartilage or soft bone biopsy may be performed with very small trephines or a meniscal vascular punch. Biopsy specimens are easiest to obtain at the periphery of the joint surface, and the portal for the biopsy instrument may need to be modified to provide a proper angle for the instrument. After the area for biopsy is identified, a needle is inserted into the joint to identify a portal that allows the instrument to contact the area at an angle that is as close to perpendicular as possible.

The most common application of elbow arthroscopy in small animal surgery is to diagnose and treat developmental and degenerative diseases, specifically OCD, FCP, ununited anconeal process (UAP), and osteoarthritis. These diseases are often grouped together as *canine elbow dysplasia.*

Fragmentation of the Medial Coronoid Process

This condition is characterized by fragmentation of the cartilage and subchondral bone in the lateral aspect of the medial coronoid and grade II to grade IV erosion of the cartilage over the center of the medial coronoid (Table 4–1). Its pathophysiology is not well defined, but may include joint incongruity that leads to increased transarticular pressure. A well-accepted hypothesis is that developmental incongruity of the elbow predisposes certain areas of the joint to degeneration under physiologic loads. Two potential types of incongruity are proposed. Radioulnar incongruity is a step defect between the proximal articular surfaces of the radius and ulna. Humeroulnar incongruity is an imperfect match between the curvature of the trochlear notch of the ulna and the trochlea of the humerus. Significant incongruity of either type may cause fragmentation of the subchondral bone and erosion of the adjacent articular cartilage by significantly increasing the articular load on the coronoid process. The lesions of FCP are varied and complex. Although the common name for this disease might suggest that the loose fragment is the source of pain, the associated osteoarthritis and joint capsular distension is more likely to be the cause of chronic disability. Arthroscopy of the canine elbow has dramatically increased the ability to evaluate most joint surfaces. Through these evaluations, surgeons can observe the severe degradation of cartilage that often accompanies FCP. Although loose bodies of FCP can be removed simply and rapidly, the challenge to the surgeon is the lifelong management of the associated osteoarthritis.

History and Signalment. FCP is reported in many purebred and mixed-breed dogs; however, it is most common in Labrador retrievers, rottweilers, Bernese

TABLE 4–1
Proposed Grading of Articular Cartilage Lesion with Arthroscopy

GRADE	FINDING
0	Normal cartilage
I	Chondromalacia (softening and swelling)
II	Fibrillation
	Superficial fissures with a velvet-like appearance
	Superficial erosion with pitting or a "cobblestone" appearance
	Lesions that do not reach the subchondral bone
III	Deep fissures that reach the subchondral bone
	Deep ulceration that does not reach the subchondral bone
IV	Exposure of the subchondral bone, with or without bone cavitation
V	Eburnated bone

mountain dogs, and golden retrievers, and has been identified with increasing frequency in Shetland sheepdogs. Clinical signs may become apparent as early as 4 or 5 months of age, but patients may present at any time after this age. The history usually includes unilateral or bilateral lameness and exercise intolerance. In mild cases, lameness is apparent only after extensive exercise.

Physical Examination Findings. Physical examination usually shows generalized muscle atrophy of the affected limbs that is most apparent over the scapular spine and acromion process. Manipulation of the elbows elicits pain and decreased range of motion, primarily in flexion. Palpation of the elbow joint may show mild to severe effusion. As the disease progresses, the effusion changes to fibrosis and then to bony proliferation, which can be differentiated by palpation. In mild cases, minimal abnormal findings are noted on orthopedic examination.

Differential Diagnosis. The differential diagnosis includes osteochondrosis, UAP, osteoarthritis, panosteitis, septic arthritis, and immune-mediated joint disease.

Diagnosis. Diagnostic tests for elbow dysplasia include radiography, arthrocentesis, nuclear scintigraphy, and computed tomography (CT). Radiographic findings vary dramatically with the severity of disease. In the mildest cases, only sclerosis of the ulna in the region of the medial coronoid process is visible (Fig. 4–15). This finding is best seen on a lateral radiograph and is often the earliest radiographic sign of disease. More advanced findings include blunting of the region of the coronoid and osteophytosis. The initial site of osteophyte production is the proximal aspect of the anconeal process, which is best visualized on a flexed lateral view (Fig. 4–16). Craniocaudal views show lipping and osteophytosis in the region of the medial coronoid process and epicondyles. Arthrocentesis usually shows cell counts of 2000 to 5000/µl and differentials typical

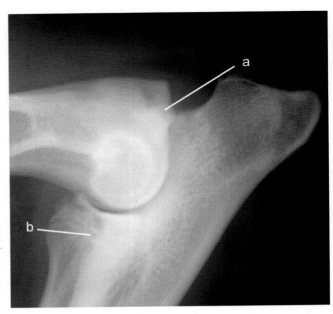

FIGURE 4–16 Flexed lateral view of a canine elbow with moderate osteoarthritis and a fragmented medial coronoid process, showing early osteophytosis on the anconeus (a) and lack of clarity in the region of the medial coronoid process (b).

of osteoarthritis, with a predominance of mature mononuclear cells.

CT allows visualization of the fragment that usually is not possible with plain films (Figs. 4–17 and 4–18). CT also may show an abnormally shaped medial coronoid or an alteration in bone density. A high degree of suspicion of FCP may be based on radiographs alone because of the development of characteristic secondary changes. Therefore, CT is not necessary to justify arthroscopic exploration. In most, but not all, cases, CT and arthroscopy findings concur. In a few cases, however, CT shows fissuring of the medial coronoid process that is not visible or palpable arthroscopically. This discrepancy in findings is most likely the result of incomplete fragmentation of the coronoid. Computerized tomography findings may include partial fragmentation, a full nondisplaced fragment, migrated fragments, a misshapen medial coronoid, abnormal bone density, or incongruity of the articular surfaces of the humerus, ulna, and radius.

Treatment. Medical treatment of FCP consists of anti-inflammatory medication and control of activity and body weight.

Anesthetic Considerations and Perioperative Pain Management. In general, juvenile dogs with FCP are young, healthy patients requiring minimal preoperative laboratory screening. A standard anesthetic protocol including preemptive pain medication is used. Postoperative pain is controlled with cold therapy, opioids, and NSAIDs.

Surgical Intervention. Arthroscopy allows a much greater appreciation of the variety of lesions that occur

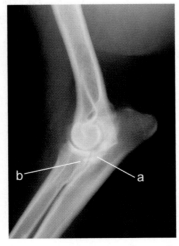

FIGURE 4–15 Lateral view of a canine elbow with mild osteoarthritis and a fragmented medial coronoid process, showing mild sclerosis (a) and lack of clarity in the region of the medial coronoid process (b).

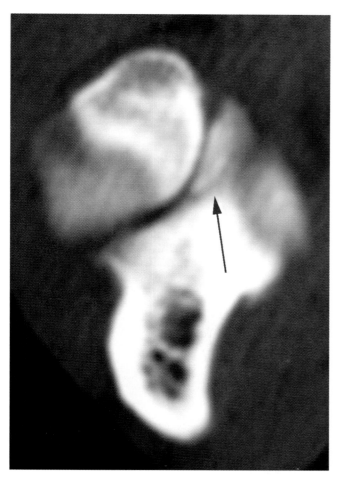

FIGURE 4–17 Computed tomography of a canine elbow with mild fragmentation of the medial coronoid process. A line of fragmentation (*arrow*) is visible on the craniolateral extent of the medial coronoid process.

condyle is also seen in many cases, and its arthroscopic management is described later. These accompanying lesions adversely affect the prognosis. In fact, osteoarthritis probably has a much greater effect than fragmentation on the prognosis of elbow dysplasia.

FCP may involve only the most craniolateral portion or a much larger section. Numerous variations occur in the appearance of the fragmentation. Variations in disease of the medial coronoid process include the following (see Figs. 4–19 and 4–20):

Chondromalacia
Avascularity of bone
Incomplete fragmentation
Fragment in situ
Minimally migrated fragment
Fully migrated fragment

In most cases, the radiographic findings cannot be correlated with the type of coronoid disease. Direct visualization of the region of fragmentation is difficult, and other factors may affect radiographic changes. CT aids in differentiation of the type of coronoid disease in many cases, but is not as conclusive as direct arthroscopic visualization.

Portal sites and surgical anatomy were discussed earlier. With the advent of arthroscopy, in bilateral cases, both elbows are treated simultaneously. FCP is often bilateral, and radiographic and clinical changes may be

in association with FCP than does open arthrotomy. Although the definitive benefit of surgical management over medical management is not known, arthroscopic management of FCP is growing in popularity. The use of arthroscopy to manage FCP is justified based on its ability to provide minimally invasive assessment of disease, remove fragments, and débride diseased cartilage.

A tremendous variation of combinations of lesions may be identified in cases of FCP. The major categories of lesions identified are as follows (Figs. 4–19 and 4–20):

Fragmentation of the medial coronoid process
Osteochondrosis of the humeral condyle
Osteoarthritis of the humeral condyle
Osteoarthritis of the medial coronoid

Osteochondrosis of the humeral condyle is identified in a significant percentage of cases, and management of this lesion is described later. Osteoarthritis of the medial coronoid process or the medial portion of the humeral

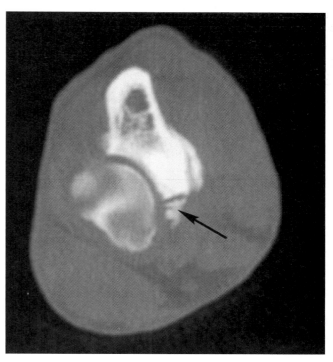

FIGURE 4–18 Computed tomography of a canine elbow with moderate to severe fragmentation of the medial coronoid process. A large fragment (*arrow*) is visible on the cranial extent of the medial coronoid process.

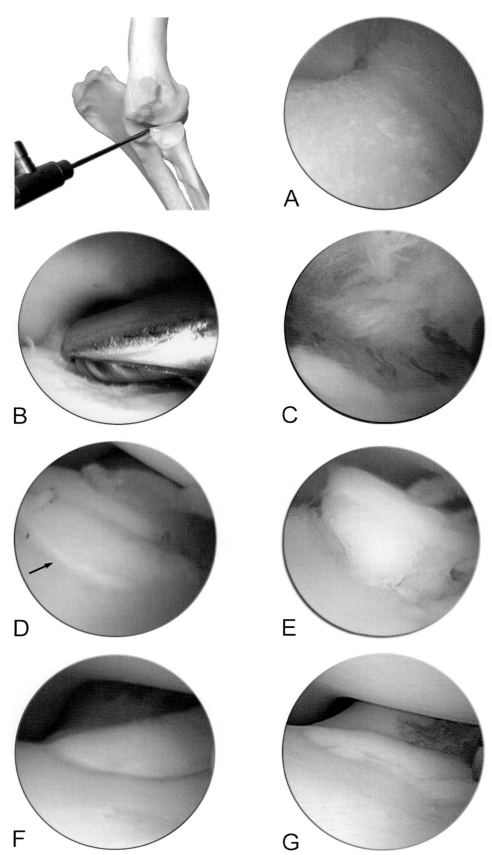

FIGURE 4-19 Positioning for arthroscopic evaluation of the medial coronoid process. Abnormal joint findings are shown. *A*, Grade II to III fibrillation of the medial coronoid process. *B*, Abrasion arthroplasty of the medial coronoid process with a power burr. *C*, Bleeding of the subchondral bone after abrasion arthroplasty of the medial coronoid process. Strands of the annular ligament are shown at the top. *D*, Line of fragmentation (*arrow*) of the medial coronoid process seen below intact articular cartilage. *E*, Elevated fragment of the medial coronoid process showing the typical yellow discoloration of avascular bone. *F* and *G*, In situ fragment of the medial coronoid process.

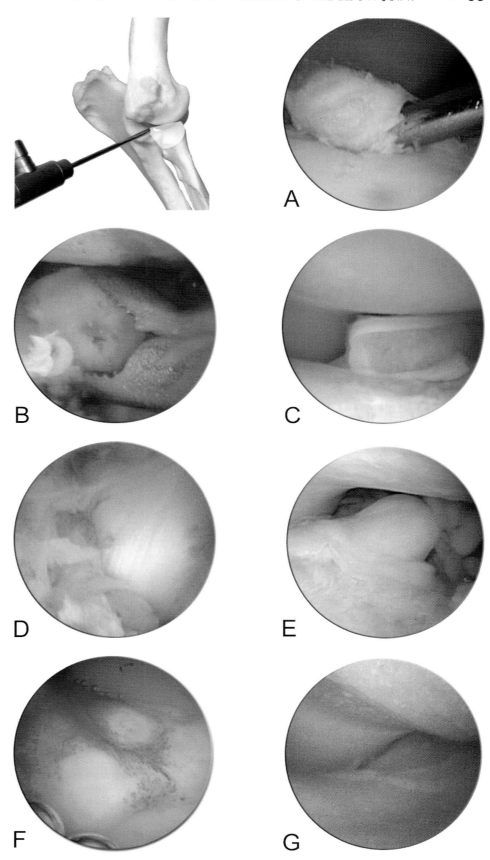

FIGURE 4-20 Positioning for arthroscopic evaluation of the medial coronoid process. Abnormal joint findings are shown. *A,* Elevation of a fragment from cranial to caudal with an arthroscopic curette. *B,* Retrieval of a fragment with grasping forceps. *C,* Minimally migrated fragment of the medial coronoid process showing both the cartilage and underlying bone. *D,* Annular and collateral ligaments after the removal of a migrated osteochondral fragment of the medial coronoid process. *E,* Fully migrated osteochondral fragment of the medial coronoid process. The radial head is obscured from view by the large fragment. *F,* Second-look arthroscopy showing fibrocartilaginous healing of a lesion of the medial coronoid process. *G,* Second-look arthroscopy showing failure of healing of the medial coronoid and a humeral grade IV cartilage lesion.

subtle, so after achieving proficiency with arthroscopic techniques, the surgeon may choose to routinely examine both elbows. The operative sites are clipped and prepared as described above. A hanging limb preparation provides the greatest degree of freedom for manipulating limb position. Liberal clipping and thorough sterile preparation are recommended because an open arthrotomy may be required. A 1.9-mm, 30-degree fore-oblique arthroscope is used in most cases. Basic instrumentation includes probes to inspect the cartilage surface or help raise a fragment, graspers to remove the fragment, and a hand curette or hand burr to prepare the lesion bed (see Fig. 4–3). A hand burr or power burr can be used to grind down large fragments. If the surgeon works through an instrument cannula, different-sized cannulas and switching sticks facilitate the surgery. The dog is positioned in dorsal recumbency, and the first limb to be operated on is placed over a sandbag or an elbow brace (see Fig. 4–6).

Egress is established with a needle or cannula (see Figs. 4–7 to 4–9), lactated Ringer's solution is instilled to distend the joint, and the arthroscope site is established. The arthroscope is inserted, and ingress flow is established through the arthroscope cannula. The caudoproximal portion of the joint, including the anconeus, trochlear notch, and caudal aspect of the humeral condyle, is inspected for evidence of inflammation or cartilage disease. The region of the lateral coronoid is inspected for cartilage damage (see Fig. 4–13). The light post is rotated distally, and the medial portion of the humeral condyle is inspected for OCD or osteoarthritic lesions. The camera head and the light post are positioned caudally to visualize the craniomedial portion of the joint. If the radial head is visible, the size and location of fragmentation must be evaluated. If no fragment is visible, the most cranial aspect of the medial coronoid is inspected for evidence of cartilage disease or avascular bone (see Fig. 4–19). Avascular bone appears as a slight yellow discoloration visualized through the articular cartilage. The condition of this region of the joint is documented with still or video imaging.

The arthroscope is positioned such that the craniomedial region of the joint is clearly visible. With the guide needle, the surgeon triangulates the position for the instrument port (see Figs. 4–7 to 4–9). The most common reason for not visualizing the guide needle in the joint is crossing the arthroscope. After the position for the instrument portal is established, the surgeon must decide whether to work through an open instrument portal, an instrument cannula, or a combination. If the surgeon chooses to work through an open portal site, a no. 11 Bard-Parker scalpel blade is used to make a 3- to 7-mm soft tissue tunnel adjacent to the guide needle. A blunt obturator is inserted through the portal to dilate the soft tissue tunnel. Alternatively, the obturator and instrument cannula may be inserted at this time.

In the mildest cases of FCP, no lesion is visible arthroscopically, although CT shows a minor fissure, hypodense bone, and adjacent regions of hyperdense bone. A right-angle probe is inserted to palpate the medial coronoid surface. Palpation of the cartilage may show normal texture, mild chondromalacia, or mild fissuring (see Fig. 4–19A and Table 4–1). If chondromalacia is present, the cartilage is soft and fragile when carefully palpated with a right-angle probe. If the cartilage is obviously diseased, it is débrided, and yellowed avascular bone may be visible beneath the cartilage. In these cases, the bone is removed with the burr attachment of a small-joint shaver, a hand curette, or hand burr (see Fig. 4–19B). A 5–0 curette is inserted into the joint, and the malacic or fibrillated cartilage is gently scraped to expose the underlying avascular bone. The avascular bone is removed until the remaining bone is pale red or bleeding is apparent (see Fig. 4–19C). When this type of procedure is performed in a small joint, such as the elbow, the egress needle may become clogged with debris and may need to be flushed. Alternatively, the fluid flow may be switched intermittently (in through the egress needle and out through the arthroscope cannula) and the arthroscope removed from the cannula to thoroughly flush the joint.

Fluid flow to the joint is stopped intermittently to allow the surgeon to evaluate the vascularity of the bone without the positive pressure created by the irrigation fluid. It is important to preserve as much normal bone and cartilage as possible. The efficacy of removing avascular bone in this disease has not been determined, but removing this material may allow revascularization and healing with bone and fibrocartilage. Because of the mild and presumably early nature of these lesions, joints usually have minimal preoperative effusion and are arthroscopically tight. For this reason, insertion of the arthroscope and instrumentation is difficult and much more likely to damage the cartilage. The surgeon must minimize further cartilage damage during arthroscopy. In tight joints, this goal is best achieved by slowly fatiguing the joint with valgus pressure and using the smallest possible instruments with gentle, precise movements.

In another variation of FCP, avascular bone is visible through the cartilage. The CT and arthroscopic findings are similar to those described earlier, but arthroscopy shows a fine, yellowed line of avascular bone that is visible through the thinned but intact articular cartilage (see Fig. 4–19D). In some cases, the entire fragment region appears avascular, but is palpably stable. In these cases, the lesion is likely to progress, and removal of the avascular bone is recommended. In most of these cases and those described earlier, additional arthritic lesions are rare, presumably because the underlying abnormality is mild. A small curette is carefully inserted into the joint to remove the cartilage and avascular bone (see Fig. 4–19E). If the surgeon is unsure whether the bone is vascular or avascular, it is best left alone and medical treatment instituted. If lameness worsens or persists, the region is reassessed with second-look arthroscopy.

In FCP, when a fragment initially separates, it may remain in its original location (in situ) (see Fig. 4–19F and G). A small (5–0) curette is inserted into the joint, and the tip is placed cranial to the tip of the coronoid in the region of fragmentation (see Fig. 4–20A). The curette is used in front of and below the fragment to push it toward the arthroscope. This approach is usually easier and safer than pushing the fragment from caudal to cranial, is less likely to cause iatrogenic damage to the cartilage, and places the fragment in a location that allows easy retrieval (see Fig. 4–20B). The curette is removed, and a small-joint grasper is inserted to retrieve the fragment in whole or in parts. During the retrieval process, fluid flow may cause fragment pieces to float into other portions of the joint. This problem can be diminished by slowing or stopping the fluid flow for a short time during fragment retrieval or by reversing the direction of flow (in through the egress portal) to push the fragments back toward the working space. Twisting the small-joint grasper during retrieval of the fragment can free it from small areas of synovial attachment if present.

Partially migrated fragments are usually small and easily retrieved (see Fig. 4–20C). However, they may have soft tissue attachments, particularly to the annular ligament. The surgeon inserts a small-joint grasper, grasps the fragment, and locks the grasper. The grasper and fragment are rotated several times to tear any soft tissue attachments (alligator roll), and the fragment is removed. When using and rotating a grasper, the surgeon must be careful to avoid damaging adjacent cartilage. The serrated jaws of a grasper can be particularly damaging to articular cartilage, and can leave partial-thickness linear abrasions that will not heal and may contribute to long-term morbidity.

Larger, more chronically migrated fragments are more difficult to remove because of their size, location, and soft tissue attachments (see Fig. 4–20D). Once migrated, fragments may continue to grow and may become very large (see Fig. 4–20E). To remove these fragments with a grasper alone, the surgeon inserts a locking grasper and removes the fragment in one piece. Alternatively, the grasper is used to break the fragment into smaller parts, being careful to avoid damage to adjacent cartilage. Alternatively, the surgeon can insert a small-joint shaver with a shielded burr and suction. With the shield protecting the radial head, humerus, and remaining coronoid, the surgeon burrs the fragment down to a size that can be removed or burrs away the entire fragment (see Fig. 4–19B). Fragments may migrate cranially to a point where they cannot be reached with a burr or grasper. In this case, a 5–0 curette is inserted, and the tip is passed medial and cranial to the fragment. The tip of the curette is used to push parts of the fragment or the entire fragment back into the working space. This technique can be difficult at first, but once mastered, permits retrieval of most cranially migrated fragments.

After the fragments are completely removed, joint lavage is performed to remove remaining bone debris. If OCD or additional cartilage damage is identified, treatment is provided as described in the following sections. At the conclusion of the procedure, the surgeon injects bupivacaine, if desired, and closes the skin wounds.

Postoperative Care. Cold therapy is applied to the elbow during recovery to relieve pain and reduce swelling. Cold therapy is applied by alternating 15 minutes on and 10 minutes off for two applications. Commercial cold packs or a commercial circulating cold water pack can be used. Alternatively, ice wrapped in a towel or packs of frozen vegetables can be used. If the dog is dismissed from the hospital the day of surgery, NSAIDs and oral butorphanol (see Table 3–1) are dispensed for administration at home. If the dog remains in the hospital overnight, buprenorphine is administered in the evening. NSAIDs and butorphanol are dispensed for administration at home. NSAIDs are continued for 5 days, whereas butorphanol is discontinued after 48 hours. At home, the owner continues cold therapy for the first 2 days after surgery. A high-quality chondroprotective complex (glucosamine/chondroitin) may be used for additional anti-inflammatory effects and to promote the healing of cartilage lesions. After the surgical swelling is gone (48 to 72 hours), the owner should begin heat therapy and passive motion and stretch exercises. First, the owner applies moist heat to the elbow region with a commercial heat pack or moistened warm towel. The owner should hold the warm pack against the inside of his own elbow for 30 seconds to ensure that it is not too hot. Then the warm pack is placed over the patient's elbow area for 10 minutes. Afterward, the owner removes the warm pack and begins gentle flexion and extension movements of the elbow joint, starting with small movements and gradually increasing to the limit of comfort over a period of 1 to 2 minutes. At the limit of comfort, the joint is held in position for 10 seconds. The motion and stretch exercises are repeated five times two to three times daily. The client should examine the portal sites daily for signs of irritation or drainage.

Exercise is limited to controlled walking on a leash for the first 4 weeks. Dogs undergoing arthroscopy use the legs immediately after surgery. To increase the weightbearing load on the limbs, walking at a slow pace is recommended. As postoperative time increases, the pace can be hastened. To increase the range of motion in the elbow when walking, the client should walk the dog in high grass (e.g., weeds), shallow water, or sand, which forces the dog to pick up the feet and step high with the legs. After 4 weeks, the owner should introduce limited amounts of free activity with controlled walking, starting with 5 minutes of free activity and increasing to 30 minutes over the next 2 weeks. After 6 to 8 weeks, free activity is gradually increased to normal levels. If during any exercise period (controlled or free activity), the dog becomes sore or is sore the next day, the owner should decrease the pace and return to controlled activity for 2 to 3 days. Swimming is encouraged if the dog can enter and exit the water without causing stress to the joints. Enrollment in a professional physical therapy program also may be of benefit.

Patients are routinely examined 12 weeks postoperatively and should undergo evaluation by palpation and force plate analysis. Continued deterioration or lack of improvement at this time is an indication for second-look arthroscopy to evaluate healing, for repeated débridement of any unhealed lesions, and for potential corrective or modifying osteotomies to alter loads on the areas of diseased cartilage (see Fig. 4–20F and G).

Complications. Complications are rare and usually minimally significant. A relatively common complication is extravasation of fluid into the soft tissues surrounding the joint. This situation is managed by postoperative bandaging and usually resolves within 24 hours. As with all surgical cases, the owners are warned of the risk of infection, although the incidence in elbow arthroscopy appears low. Nerve damage is reported secondary to human arthroscopy, but the risk of this complication in canine elbow arthroscopy appears low. The most common complication is likely iatrogenic damage to the articular cartilage as a result of the insertion and manipulation of instruments. Some degree of cartilage damage is unavoidable. The magnification provided by arthroscopy shows cartilage damage that likely occurs similarly with routine arthrocentesis and open surgery. It is the surgeon's responsibility to minimize this damage and thus to avoid significant contribution to the progression of osteoarthritis. This goal is achieved through the use of appropriately sized instruments, adequate joint distension and positioning, and gentle manipulation within the joint.

Prognosis. The prognosis after arthroscopic management of FCP is not known and likely varies tremendously with the severity of disease, the function of the animal, postoperative management, and the patient's temperament. Although many dogs with mild disease return to normal function without analgesic therapy, some show progressive lameness. Similarly, although the most severely affected dogs typically are given the worst prognosis, especially dogs with moderate to severe elbow effusion, many of these dogs also show the greatest improvement after arthroscopy. Owners who are considering arthroscopic treatment for FCP should be given the following information:

1. Elbow arthroscopy is minimally invasive and has minimal risk of morbidity.
2. The outcome cannot be predicted, particularly without arthroscopic visualization of the severity of cartilage defects.
3. In clinically and radiographically mild cases, arthroscopy offers at least a 50% chance of improvement, and in some cases, the signs resolve without the need for analgesic therapy.
4. In clinically and radiographically severe cases, the prognosis for complete resolution of signs is poor. However, arthroscopy provides important information about the severity of disease and is part of the long-term management of elbow osteoarthritis.
5. Elbow osteoarthritis may require lifelong management that may include additional arthroscopy, corrective or modifying osteotomies, physical therapy, and medical management.
6. It is advisable to address osteoarthritis as early as possible, and given the minimal morbidity associated with arthroscopy, it plays an important role in the management of this disease.

OSTEOCHONDROSIS OF THE HUMERAL CONDYLE

Osteochondrosis is a common disease of the canine elbow that occurs alone or in combination with FCP. In affected dogs, a region of abnormally thickened cartilage at the most medial and distal region of the humeral condyle separates partially or completely from the subchondral bone. Potential mechanisms of this disease include abnormal maturation of cartilage, compromised vascular supply to the region, trauma, nutrition, and genetic predisposition.

History and Signalment. Like FCP, the most commonly affected breeds include Labrador retrievers, rottweilers, Bernese mountain dogs, and golden retrievers. Affected dogs may have a history of unilateral or bilateral lameness and exercise intolerance starting as early as 3 to 4 months of age, although most dogs are presented for treatment several months later.

Differential Diagnosis. The differential diagnosis includes fragmented coronoid process, UAP, osteoarthritis, panosteitis, and septic arthritis.

Diagnostic Findings. Physical examination findings include generalized forelimb muscle atrophy, pain and decreased range of motion of the elbow joints, and mild to severe lameness. OCD can cause complete recumbency, especially when multiple joints are affected. Diagnostic tests include radiography, arthrocentesis, and CT. Radiographic findings vary dramatically with the severity of disease. The typical finding is a region of subchondral bone loss on the distal and medial portion of the humeral condyle (Fig. 4–21) that is best appreciated on a craniocaudal radiograph. More advanced findings include sclerosis around the affected region and osteophytosis. The initial site of osteophyte production is the proximal aspect of the anconeal process, which is best visualized on a flexed lateral view. Arthrocentesis usually shows cell counts of 2000 to 5000/µl and differentials typical of osteoarthritis, with a predominance of mature mononuclear cells. CT confirms the area of subchondral bone loss and sclerosis.

Treatment. Medical treatment of OCD consists of anti-inflammatory medication and control of activity and body weight.

Anesthetic Considerations and Perioperative Pain Management. In general, juvenile dogs with OCD are young, healthy patients requiring minimal preoperative laboratory screening. A standard anesthetic protocol including preemptive pain medication is used. Postoperative pain is controlled with cold therapy, opioids, and NSAIDs.

Surgical Intervention. Portal sites and surgical anatomy were discussed earlier. With the advent of arthroscopy, both elbows are treated simultaneously if the condition is bilateral. The condition is often bilateral,

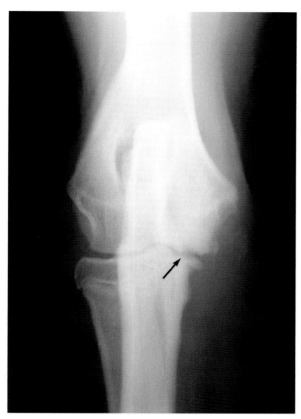

FIGURE 4–21 Craniocaudal radiograph of a canine elbow with mild osteoarthritis and osteochondrosis dissecans (*arrow*).

and radiographic and clinical changes may be subtle, so once proficiency with the technique is achieved, the surgeon may choose to perform arthroscopy routinely on both elbows. The operative site is clipped and prepared as described earlier. A hanging limb preparation provides the greatest degree of freedom for manipulating limb position. Liberal clipping and thorough sterile preparation are necessary because an open arthrotomy may be required. A 1.9-mm, 30-degree fore-oblique arthroscope is used in most cases. Basic instrumentation includes probes to inspect the cartilage surface or help raise a fragment, graspers to remove the fragment, and a hand curette or hand burr to prepare the lesion bed. If the surgeon works through an instrument cannula, different-sized cannulas and switching sticks facilitate the surgery. The dog is positioned in dorsal recumbency, and the first limb to be operated on is abducted over a sandbag or an elbow brace.

Egress is established with a needle or cannula, lactated Ringer's solution is instilled to distend the joint, and the arthroscope portal is established (see Figs. 4–7 to 4–9). The arthroscope is inserted, and ingress flow is established through the arthroscope cannula. When a standard medial portal is used, OCD of the humeral condyle is most commonly seen directly adjacent to the site of insertion of the arthroscope. Because of the location and size of these lesions, the arthroscope portal should be placed further caudal in the joint to permit

complete visualization of the caudal portion of the flap. With the aid of switching sticks, the instrument and arthroscope portals can be reversed to permit visualization of the caudal area of the lesion.

The surgeon inspects the caudoproximal portion of the joint, including the anconeus, trochlear notch, and caudal aspect of the humeral condyle for evidence of inflammation or cartilage disease. The camera head is moved caudally and the light post is rotated distally to bring the most distal portion of the humeral condyle into view (Fig. 4–22). The lesion may appear as soft, proliferative cartilage at the medial extent of the joint or as an obvious flap of cartilage at the medial extent of the joint (see Fig. 4–22A and B). The lesion may be as large as 15 mm long and 5 mm or more wide. The rest of the joint is explored for additional lesions, including FCP and cartilage damage.

After the joint is thoroughly explored and the extent of the lesion defined, an instrument portal is created with or without a cannula. If the lesion is partially detached, graspers are inserted to grip the flap (see Fig. 4–22C). With the graspers locked on the flap, the surgeon peels the flap from the underlying bone, working around the periphery of the lesion. Because normal cartilage does not peel off, there is little risk of additional cartilage damage with this technique. The flap may be removed in one piece or in multiple smaller pieces. After the flap is removed, the difference between an OCD lesion and other types of cartilage damage is obvious. A crater is caused by the absence of normal subchondral bone thickness. This crater does not occur with most other types of cartilage disease (see Fig. 4–22D and E). The surgeon palpates the edges of the lesion with a right-angle probe or a small curette, removes any remaining loose cartilage, and creates edges that are relatively perpendicular to the joint surface (see Fig. 4–22F). If bleeding of the subchondral bone bed is not apparent when fluid inflow is stopped, then microfracture or abrasion with a burr or curette is indicated. This technique is described later (see Fig. 4–22G).

After the fragments are removed, the joint is lavaged to remove remaining bone debris. If FCP or additional cartilage damage is identified, treatment is instituted as described later. At the conclusion of the procedure, bupivacaine is injected if desired, and the skin wounds are closed.

Postoperative Care. Postoperative management is identical to that of FCP.

Complications. Complications associated with elbow OCD arthroscopy are rare and usually of little significance. A relatively common complication is extravasation of fluid into the soft tissues surrounding the joint. This may be managed by postoperative bandaging and usually resolves within 24 hours. The most common complication associated with elbow arthroscopy is iatrogenic damage to the articular cartilage. This damage occurs with insertion of needles and cannulas and manipulation of instruments. It is the surgeon's responsibility to ensure minimization of this damage to avoid significant

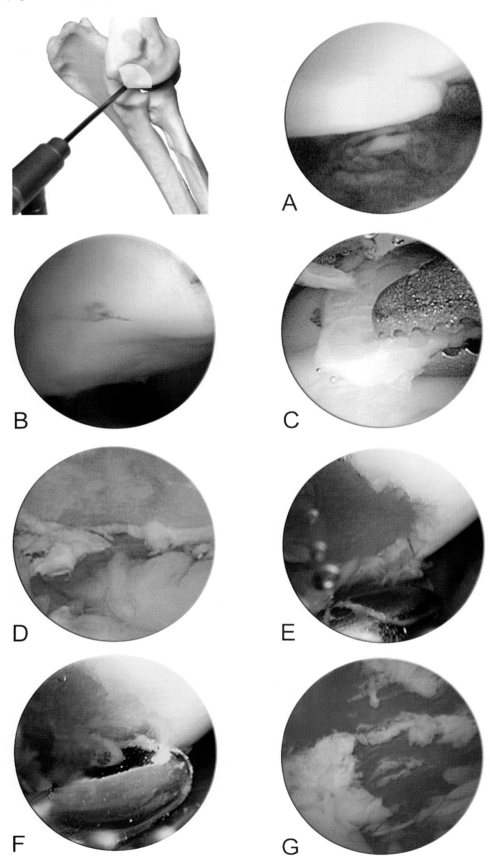

FIGURE 4–22 Positioning for arthroscopic evaluation of the medial portion of the humeral condyle. Abnormal joint findings are shown. *A*, osteochondrosis dissecans (OCD) flap. The edges are easily visible through the arthroscope. *B*, OCD flap. In the elbow, the flap often appears as an irregular surface of cartilage directly above the arthroscope tip. *C*, The use of grasping forceps in the canine elbow for removal of an OCD flap. *D*, Subchondral bone bed after removal of an OCD flap. *E*, Subchondral bone bed after removal of an OCD flap. The obvious margins of the lesions are not as apparent with osteoarthritic cartilage disease. *F*, Use of a curette to leave the edges of the OCD bed at right angles to the bone surface. *G*, Bleeding of the ODC bed after curettage and discontinuation of fluid inflow.

contribution to the progression of osteoarthritis. This is achieved through the use of appropriately sized instruments, adequate joint distension and positioning, and gentle manipulation within the joint.

Prognosis. The extent of cartilage damage in elbow OCD may be more severe than that seen in FCP; however, the quality of bleeding of the subchondral bone bed is often better. Second-look arthroscopy confirms that these lesions tend to fill with fibrocartilage, although no data are available from long-term second-look studies to demonstrate the durability of this healing. Like FCP, the prognosis is variable. Some dogs show continued deterioration, whereas others show significant improvement. Early clinical findings are often related to the size of the lesion. Management of these cases must be considered a lifelong process, and reevaluation is indicated to determine whether the patient needs second-look arthroscopy or osteotomies to alter the loads on the healing regions of cartilage.

UNUNITED ANCONEAL PROCESS

Little anecdotal or published information is available on the use of arthroscopy to manage UAP in dogs, although arthroscopy provides visual access to the lesion and theoretically may play a role in treatment.

History and Signalment. UAP is primarily a disease of German shepherds. The center of ossification of the anconeus should unite with the proximal ulna at approximately 20 weeks of age, although it may occur later in German shepherds and greyhounds. Failure of unification can be definitively diagnosed after 5 months of age and may be caused by failure of endochondral ossification or joint incongruence that places excessive pressure on the process. Dogs often present between 6 and 18 months of age with unilateral or bilateral forelimb lameness. Other clinical signs include elbow joint pain, effusion, and decreased range of motion as well as generalized forelimb muscle atrophy. The diagnosis is usually easily confirmed by a lateral or flexed radiograph of the elbow that shows the failure of unification (Fig. 4–23A).

Differential Diagnosis. The differential diagnosis includes fragmented coronoid process, UAP, osteoarthritis, panosteitis, septic arthritis, and immune-mediated joint disease.

Diagnostic Findings. Physical examination findings include generalized forelimb muscle atrophy, pain, and decreased range of motion of the elbow joints as well as mild to severe lameness. Radiography is the diagnostic method of choice. The primary finding on a lateral radiograph is a radiolucent line between the anconeal process and the olecranon (see Fig. 4–23A). Additional radiographic findings include generalized osteophytosis and sclerosis. Arthrocentesis usually shows cell counts of 2000 to 5000/μl and differentials typical of osteo-

arthritis, with a predominance of mature mononuclear cells. CT confirms the area of subchondral bone loss and sclerosis.

Treatment. Medical treatment of OCD consists of anti-inflammatory medication, and control of athletic activity and body weight.

Anesthetic Considerations and Perioperative Pain Management. In general, juvenile dogs with UAP are young, healthy patients requiring minimal preoperative laboratory screening. A standard anesthetic protocol including preemptive pain medication is used. Postoperative pain is controlled with cold therapy, opioids, and NSAIDs.

Surgical Intervention. Reported surgical therapies include fragment removal, screw-and-pin fixation, and ulnar osteotomy to reduce pressure on the process and encourage healing. None of these approaches alone has provided satisfactory results in a substantial case series, and dogs with UAP often progress to severe elbow osteoarthritis with variable degrees of disability. An ulnar osteotomy in combination with an anconeal compression screw provided successful results in two clinical studies. This method is currently the treatment of choice. Arthroscopy may be used in conjunction with this treatment to visualize the fragment during screw fixation and decrease the risk of damage to the articular surface.

Portal sites and surgical anatomy were discussed earlier. The operative site is clipped and prepared as described earlier. A hanging limb preparation provides the greatest degree of freedom for manipulating limb position. Liberal clipping and thorough sterile preparation are necessary because an open arthrotomy may be required. A 1.9-mm, 30-degree fore-oblique arthroscope is used in most cases. In larger dogs, a 2.7-mm arthroscope may be used. The dog is positioned in dorsal recumbency and the limb to be operated on is abducted over a sandbag or an elbow brace.

Egress is established with a needle or cannula (see Figs. 4–7 to 4–9), lactated Ringer's solution is instilled to distend the joint, and the arthroscope site is established. The arthroscope is inserted, and ingress flow is established through the arthroscope cannula.

The cranial portion of the joint is inspected for OCD, FCP, and other cartilage disease. The camera head is moved caudodistally, and the light post is rotated distally to bring the anconeal process into view. The UAP lesion appears as a line of fibrous tissue and irregular cartilage between the anconeus and the remainder of the ulna (see Fig. 4–23B). A small Kirschner wire is inserted, beginning at the caudal aspect of the ulna. The pin is directed perpendicular to the line between the ulna and the anconeal process. Through the arthroscope, the surgeon can observe the pin passing between the ulna and the anconeus (see Fig. 4–23C). A second Kirschner wire is inserted parallel to the first, but 5 to 10 mm distally. If a cannulated drill system is available, a 2.5-mm cannulated drill bit is used over the Kirschner wire to drill a hole to the tip of the anconeus. Alternatively,

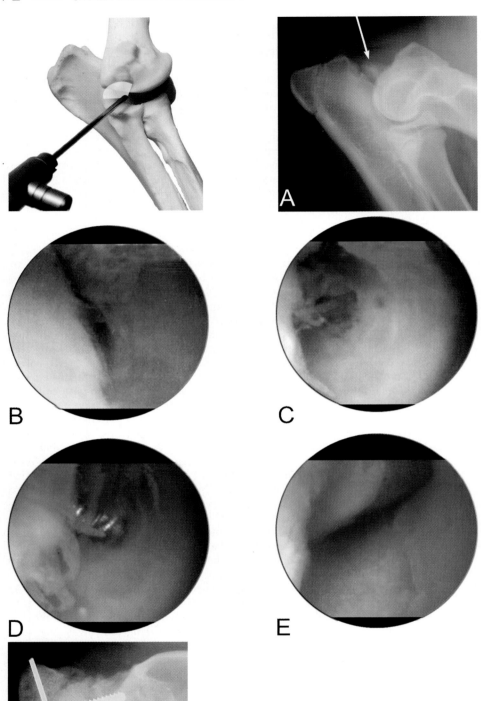

FIGURE 4-23 Radiographic and arthroscopic findings and treatment of a canine elbow with ununited anconeal process. *A,* lateral view showing the fissure line (*arrow*) between the anconeus and the remainder of the ulna; *B,* arthroscopic view of the fissure line of an ununited anconeal process; *C,* arthroscopic view of a orthopedic pin placed across the fissure line; *D,* arthroscopic view of a bone screw crossing the fissure line; *E,* arthroscopic view after the bone screw is tightened and the fissure line is no longer visible; *F,* lateral view of early healing of lag screw fixation and ulnar osteotomy.

the Kirschner wire is removed and a standard 2.5-mm drill bit is used to make the hole. The depth of the hole is measured, and if a partially threaded 3.5-mm cancellous bone screw has appropriate thread length, it is used to compress the nonunion site. Alternatively, the proximal segment is overdrilled with a 4.0-mm drill and a fully threaded cancellous bone screw is inserted in lag fashion. The drill and screw are observed through the arthroscope to avoid additional articular injury (see Fig. 4–23D).

The skin is incised along the caudolateral aspect of the joint, beginning at the level of the coronoid process and ending at the junction of the proximal and middle thirds of the ulna. The muscles are dissected off of the ulnar diaphysis at a level approximately 2 to 3 cm distal to the level of the coronoid process, and the ulna is isolated with small Hohman retractors. A power oscillating saw is used to cut the ulnar diaphysis in a caudo-proximal to craniodistal direction. The proximal segment is gently levered dorsally with an osteotome or periosteal elevator. A small (5/64-inch) Steinmann pin is inserted down the ulnar shaft to avoid rotation of the proximal segment. Bending over the proximal aspect of the pin prevents migration of the distal pin and allows easier removal after the osteotomy heals (see Fig. 4–23F).

Postoperative Care. A bandage may be placed on the limbs for 24 hours to decrease swelling. Cold therapy is applied to the elbow during recovery to relieve pain and reduce swelling. The rest of the immediate postoperative protocol is identical to that for FCP.

Exercise is limited to controlled walking on a leash for the first 6 weeks. Radiographs of the elbow are obtained at this time to evaluate for healing of the osteotomy and union of the UAP. If healing of the osteotomy has occurred, the intramedullary pin is removed. After 6 weeks, the owner should begin limited amounts of free activity with controlled walking, starting with 5 minutes of free activity and increasing to 30 minutes over the next 2 weeks. After 8 weeks, free activity is gradually increased to normal levels. If during any exercise period (controlled or free activity), the dog becomes sore or is sore the next day, the owner should decrease the pace and return to controlled activity for 2 to 3 days. Swimming may be encouraged if the dog can enter and exit the water without causing stress to the joints. Enrollment in a professional physical therapy program may be of significant benefit.

Complications. Complications are similar to those described for elbow arthroscopy. In addition, there may be significant complications associated with the stabilization technique and osteotomy. These include nonunion and infected nonunion. Other complications are implant failure or migration, particularly of the intramedullary pin.

Prognosis. Early treatment with ulnar osteotomy combined with lag screw fixation appears to provide the best prognosis. In one study of 26 dogs, 87% had an excellent outcome. Three dogs were free of lameness but had some impairment after heavy exercise. Their outcome was considered good. In a second study of four cases, clinical outcome as assessed by the owner and veterinarian was excellent in all cases.

Osteoarthritis of the Elbow

In many cases of FCP and some cases of OCD, osteoarthritic lesions are identified on the medial portion of the humeral condyle and the medial coronoid process. These lesions are the likely source of chronic disability. Their cause remains unknown, but they are typical of lesions associated with increased transarticular pressure as a result of joint incongruence or malalignment. Intra-articular arthroscopic management of these lesions is routinely recommended in the treatment of arthritis in humans, although the long-term benefits are not known. If the underlying cause is eliminated (e.g., acute trauma, loose body abrasion), then arthroscopic treatment of the arthritic lesions may aid in reformation of a low-friction surface of fibrocartilage. If the underlying cause of damage to bone and cartilage is not eliminated, however, the disease process will be perpetuated and the lesions are less likely to heal adequately. The primary cause of these lesions in canine FCP is unknown, and it is not known whether the underlying cause manifests only during skeletal development or persists after skeletal growth is complete.

Numerous scales are used to grade gross arthritic lesions (Figs. 4–24 and 4–25). One recommended scale is shown in Table 4–1. The surgeon must assess the lesions and decide whether arthroscopic débridement and treatment will contribute to the healing of the joint or potentially contribute to degeneration. Partial-thickness cartilage lesions that do not penetrate the tidemark do not heal as readily as those that penetrate this mark. The surgeon may remove partial-thickness lesions in an effort to promote healing by temporarily increasing the severity of the defect.

Management of articular cartilage lesions is based on the idea that healing, through the formation of fibrocartilage, is promoted when the lesion is exposed to blood that contains mesenchymal stem cell precursors. Several methods are used. Abrasion arthroplasty involves the uniform removal of subchondral bone until bleeding is achieved (see Fig. 4–24A). In the canine elbow, either a curette or a burr attachment on a small-joint shaver is used. The shaver is usually more rapid and efficient and just as accurate. Another method used to treat grade IV lesions is microfracture. Numerous microcracks are created in the subchondral bone plate to allow bleeding at the lesion surface (see Fig. 4–24B). Microfracture awls are available for use in small-joint arthroscopy. Alternatively, a small microfracture pick may be created by bending the end of a 0.035- or 0.045-inch K-wire to approximately a 45-degree angle. The wire is then secured into a Jacobs chuck. A final technique used to manage these lesions is forage, in which small holes are drilled in the subchondral bone. In humans and horses, this technique leads to the formation of cystic lesions.

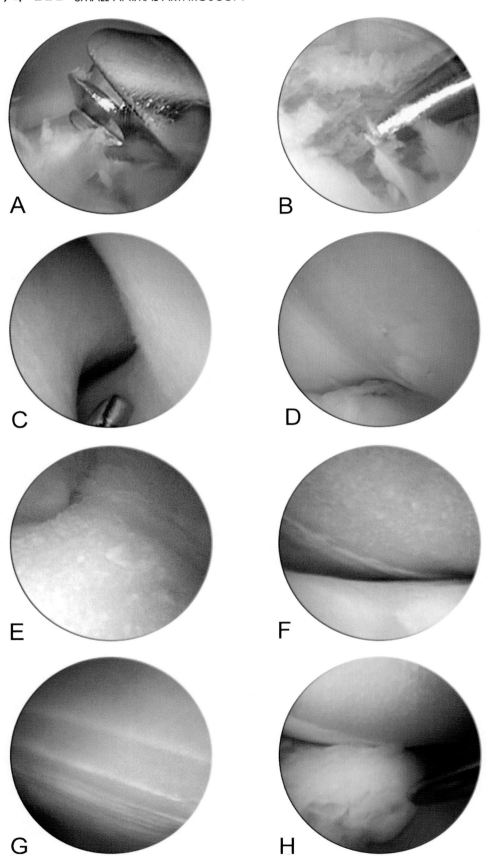

FIGURE 4–24 Arthroscopic findings and treatment of canine elbows with osteoarthritis. *A,* Use of a power burr on a grade IV osteoarthritic lesion; *B,* use of a micropick on a grade IV osteoarthritic lesion; *C,* grade II osteoarthritis showing fine fibrillation of the cartilage surface; *D,* grade II osteoarthritis showing partial-thickness cartilage loss and the "cobblestone" appearance of the cartilage; *E,* grade III osteoarthritis showing gross fibrillation that continues to the depth of the subchondral bone; *F,* grade IV osteoarthritis showing a large area of subchondral bone adjacent to normal cartilage; *G,* grade IV osteoarthritis showing full-thickness linear excoriations with some cartilage remaining; *H,* grade IV osteoarthritis showing subchondral bone adjacent to the hyalin cartilage and a large osteochondral fragment.

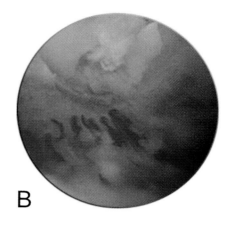

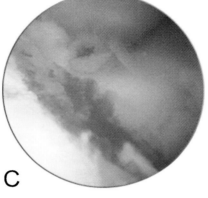

FIGURE 4–25 Arthroscopic findings and treatment of canine elbows with osteoarthritis. *A,* Grade IV osteoarthritis showing subchondral bone on both the humeral condyle and the opposing coronoid process; *B,* bleeding after abrasion arthroplasty or microfracture and cessation of fluid flow; *C,* clot formation in the subchondral bone bed after abrasion arthroplasty or microfracture.

History and Signalment. Osteoarthritis of the elbow joint may occur in any dog as a result of traumatic, infectious, immune-mediated, or developmental causes. Treatment is most often indicated in dogs that have developmental diseases of the elbow (FCP, OCD, UAP). Clinical signs may become apparent as early as 4 or 5 months of age, but patients may present at any time after this age. The history usually includes unilateral or bilateral lameness and exercise intolerance. In mild cases, lameness may be apparent only after aggressive exercise.

Physical Examination Findings. Dogs with elbow arthritis usually have generalized muscle atrophy of the affected limbs. The atrophy is usually most apparent over the scapular spine and acromion process. Manipulation of the elbows causes pain and decreased range of motion, primarily in flexion. Palpation of the elbow joint may show mild to severe effusion. As the disease progresses, the effusion changes to fibrosis and then to bony proliferation, which can be differentiated by palpation. In mild cases, minimal abnormal findings may be noted on orthopedic examination.

Differential Diagnosis. The differential diagnosis includes osteochondrosis, fragmented coronoid process, UAP, neoplasia, immune-mediated arthritis, panosteitis, and septic arthritis.

Diagnosis. Diagnostic tests include radiography and arthrocentesis. Radiographic findings vary dramatically with the severity of disease. In the mildest cases, only sclerosis of the ulna in the region of the medial coronoid process is visible. This finding is best appreciated on a lateral radiograph and is often the earliest radiographic sign of disease. As the osteoarthritis progresses, osteophytosis, sclerosis, and radiolucency increase. Arthrocentesis usually shows cell counts of 2000 to 5000/μl, with a predominance of mature mononuclear cells.

Treatment. Medical treatment of elbow osteoarthritis consists of anti-inflammatory medication and control of activity and body weight.

Anesthetic Considerations and Perioperative Pain Management. A standard anesthetic protocol including preemptive pain medication is used. Postoperative pain is controlled with cold therapy, opioids, and NSAIDs.

Surgical Intervention. Portal sites and surgical anatomy were discussed earlier. With the advent of arthroscopy, both elbows may be treated simultaneously if the condition is bilateral. However, in severe cases, the surgeon may elect to stage the joints to limit postoperative weightbearing on the treated limb. A hanging limb preparation provides the greatest degree of freedom for manipulating limb position. In most cases, a 1.9-mm,

30-degree fore-oblique arthroscope is used. Basic instrumentation includes probes to inspect the cartilage surface or help raise cartilage fragments, graspers to remove fragments, a hand burr or power burr to perform abrasion arthroplasty, and a micropick set and mallet to perform microfracture. The dog is positioned in dorsal recumbency, and the first limb to be operated on is abducted over a sandbag or an elbow brace.

Egress is established with a needle or cannula, lactated Ringer's solution is instilled to distend the joint, and the arthroscope site is established. The arthroscope is inserted, and ingress flow is established through the arthroscope cannula. The caudoproximal portion of the joint, including the anconeus, trochlear notch, and caudal aspect of the humeral condyle, is inspected for evidence of inflammation or cartilage disease. The camera head is moved caudally, and the light post is rotated distally to bring the most distal portion of the humeral condyle into view. This area of the canine elbow is a common site for cartilage disease. The camera head and the light post are positioned caudally to visualize the craniomedial portion of the joint. The medial coronoid process will be in view and is the other major site of cartilage damage in the canine elbow.

After the joint is thoroughly explored and the extent of the lesion defined, an instrument portal is created with or without a cannula. Palpation of lesions with a right-angle probe may be performed through an instrument cannula; however, most power shavers and micropicks do not fit easily through a small-joint cannula. The surgeon should visually evaluate and palpate areas of cartilage damage and note the size and severity of the lesion based on the scale shown in Table 4–1.

The surgeon must decide whether to débride grade I lesions with chondromalacia. Small areas of grade II fibrillation in the absence of other lesions also may be left undisturbed (see Fig. 4–24C and D). Larger areas of grade II cartilage disease can be treated similarly to grade III lesions, at the discretion of the surgeon. Grade III lesions are areas of full-thickness fibrillation (see Fig. 4–24E). A curette or burr is used to remove the diseased cartilage, with care taken to avoid damaging the more normal surrounding cartilage. The resulting subchondral bone bed is treated in the same way as grade IV lesions. Grade IV cartilage damage is full-thickness loss of cartilage in addition to exposure and, in some cases, eburnation of the subchondral bone (see Figs. 4–24F to H and 4–25A). These lesions are treated with abrasion or microfracture until adequate bleeding occurs (see Fig. 4–25B and C).

To perform abrasion arthroplasty, the surgeon inserts a hand burr or, preferably, a power shaver burr through the instrument portal. Because either method produces significant bone debris that can clog the egress portal and impede visualization, it is important to monitor and maintain fluid flow through the joint during this procedure. The surgeon should spin the burr to remove subchondral bone over the area of the lesion (see Fig. 4–24A). In addition, the surgeon should check for resulting bleeding frequently by stopping the inflow of fluid and ensuring that outflow is adequate to decrease the pressure in the joint. When bleeding is observed diffusely from the lesion bed, the joint is lavaged to remove the remaining bone debris, and then it is closed routinely (see Fig. 4–25B and C).

To perform microfracture, an appropriately angled micropick is inserted into the joint, and the tip is pressed against the subchondral bone surface. An assistant should tap the pick handle once or twice (see Fig. 4–24B). The pick should be held securely to avoid gouging the surface and adjacent healthy cartilage. The surgeon applies the micropick diffusely across the diseased area and checks for resulting bleeding frequently by stopping the inflow of fluid and ensuring that outflow is adequate. When bleeding is observed diffusely from the lesion bed, the surgeon lavages the joint to remove the remaining bone debris and then performs routine closure (see Fig. 4–25B and C).

The production of diffuse effective bleeding is more difficult in some joints than in others. Combining abrasion and microfracture may increase subchondral bleeding. However, in cases of eburnation, it may be difficult or impossible to obtain significant bleeding with these techniques.

Postoperative Care.   Postoperative management and complications are identical to those of FCP. In most cases, osteoarthritis requires lifelong medical management. Treatment includes control of body weight, exercise and physical therapy, and NSAIDs and chondroprotective medications.

Complications.   Complications of arthroscopic management of osteoarthritis are similar to those described for management of FCP. Controversy remains in the human and veterinary fields as to the success of these treatment modalities. Additional potential complications include the formation of subchondral bone cysts and the acceleration of cartilage disease and joint space collapse.

Prognosis.   The efficacy of arthroscopic treatment to manage osteoarthritis of the elbow is unknown; however, this treatment is likely to be much more effective when it is combined with medical management, physical therapy, and weight control. Severe cases may be unresponsive, and many patients may require additional surgical intervention, including corrective osteotomies, arthrodesis, or joint replacement.

Articular Pressure and Osteotomies in the Management of FCP, OCD, and Elbow Osteoarthritis

Osteotomies are used to treat joint diseases by altering joint congruency, transarticular load, or both. Healing of subchondral bone and cartilage defects depends on the loads experienced by the healing tissues. Fibrocartilage and hyalin cartilage do not heal under supraphysiologic loads, and arthritic lesions and angular joint deformity

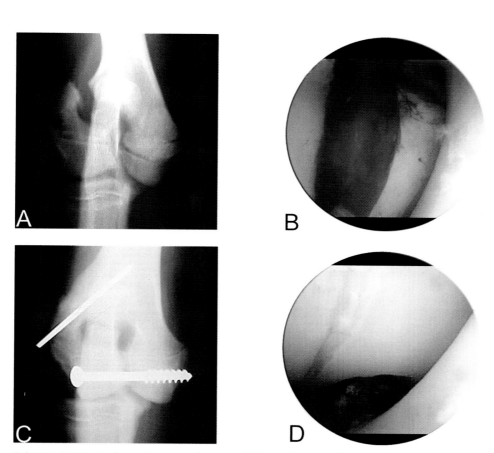

FIGURE 4-26 Radiographic and arthroscopic findings of canine elbows with a humeral condylar fracture and incomplete ossification of the humeral condyle. *A,* Preoperative radiograph showing fracture of the lateral portion of the humeral condyle; *B,* arthroscopic view of the fracture line; *C,* postoperative radiograph showing arthroscopically assisted repair of a fracture of the lateral portion of the humeral condyle; *D,* arthroscopic appearance of incomplete fusion of the humeral condyle.

continue to progress. Excessive articular loads establish a destructive cycle whereby increased load leads to articular cartilage degeneration, which leads to collapse of the joint at the site of the lesion and subsequently to further increased articular loads. Therefore, a basic principle in the management of articular cartilage lesions is the normalization of loads at the site of healing cartilage. Numerous osteotomies are used to manage diseases of the canine elbow.

Ulnar osteotomy is used to treat FCP, both alone and in combination with fragment removal. This surgery is based on the theory that radioulnar incongruence leads to FCP and degradation of the adjacent cartilage. Shortening the ulna decreases pressure on the medial coronoid, thereby permitting healing of the lesions or minimization of progression. If this type of incongruence exists at the time of surgery and adequate congruence can be restored, the procedure may be of benefit. However, few studies have evaluated the outcome of this procedure, and this technique may inadvertently increase articular pressures in the medial compartment of the joint, thereby hindering the healing of the arthritic lesions. A study of joint surface contact that simulated radioulnar incongruence showed that regions of normal contact can be restored by proximal ulnar osteotomy in an in vitro model. However, removal of a segment of the ulna may lead to varus deformity at the elbow joint. This deformity would shift the axis of loading medially and increase pressure in the medial compartment.

Proximal ulnar ostectomy is performed with a caudal approach to the ulna. The incision is centered over the distal aspect of the elbow joint and extends several centimeters in either direction. Subperiosteal elevation of muscles is performed on either side to provide access to the cranial aspect of the bone. Small Hohman retractors may be placed on either side of the bone to protect muscle from the saw blade. An oblique cut is made with an oscillating saw, beginning at the distal level of the elbow joint caudally on the ulna and ending several centimeters distally on the cranial extent of the elbow joint. In mild cases, the kerf of the blade may allow for adequate distal movement of the proximal segment. In more severe cases, a thin section of bone may be removed. The oblique nature of the cut eliminates the risk of failure associated with the pull of the triceps. An intramedullary pin may be placed down the ulna to increase stability, but the pin increases the risk of implant complications. However, in vitro studies showed that the proximal segment was displaced laterally when an intramedullary pin was not used. Nonunion and infected nonunion can occur with this procedure, and the definitive benefit of ulnar osteotomy is not known.

Alternatively, an ostectomy may be performed on the distal segmental of the ulna. This procedure involves removing a small segment of bone in the distal third of the diaphysis and avoids many of the potential complications of proximal ulnar osteotomy. However, the interosseous ligament may limit significant movement of the proximal segment. In vitro studies confirm the limitations of movement with the distal ostectomy in the acute setting, although in the live animal, gradual fatigue of the interosseous ligament may permit greater movement.

Lengthening of the radius is used to treat premature closure of the radial growth plates. In this traumatic disease, the medial coronoid process is fragmented, supporting theories of radioulnar incongruence in elbow dysplasia. The lengthening treatment appears to be successful in the management of subluxation of the elbow joint. Radial lengthening may have a role in the management of canine elbow dysplasia, but degradation of cartilage in traumatic cases has not been described, and overlengthening of the radius would contribute to varus deformity and overload of the medial compartment.

Future Applications of Elbow Arthroscopy

Arthroscopy is used to manage articular fractures in humans and may have a role in closed management of canine humeral condylar fractures (Fig. 4–26A to C). In these cases, arthroscopy may be used to aid in alignment of the articular surface in combination with closed implant placement, as was described in the dog. Arthroscopy is also used to diagnose incomplete ossification of the humeral condyle (see Fig. 4–26D). Humeral condylar fractures are one of the most common fractures of the canine forelimb. Methods of repair include open reduction and fixation and closed fluoroscopically guided reduction and fixation. Despite the obvious benefits of closed reduction and fixation, accurate reduction with fluoroscopic guidance is difficult and fluoroscopy is not readily available. Arthroscopy may improve the outcome of the closed technique by allowing direct visualization of the fracture surfaces.

Suggested Readings

Bardet JF: Arthroscopy of the elbow in clinically normal dogs using the caudal portals. Vet Comp Orthop Traum 13:87, 2000.

Bouck GR, Miller CW, Tares CL: A comparison of surgical and medical treatment of fragmented coronoid process and osteochondritis dissecans of the canine elbow. Vet Comp Orthop Traum 8:177–183, 1995.

Boulay JP: Fragmented medial coronoid process of the ulna in the dog. Vet Clin N Am 28:51, 1998.

Fox SM, Burbridge HM, Bray JC: Ununited anconeal process: lag-screw fixation. J Am Anim Hosp Assoc 32:52–56, 1996.

Hornof WJ, Wind AP, Wallack ST: Canine elbow dysplasia: the early radiographic detection of fragmentation of the coronoid process. Vet Clin N Am 30:257–266, 2000.

Krotscheck U, Hulse DA, Bahr A: Ununited anconeal process: lag screw fixation with proximal ulnar osteotomy. Vet Comp Orthop Traum 13:212–216, 2000.

Nap RC: Pathophysiology and clinical aspects of canine elbow dysplasia. Vet Comp Orthop Traum 9:58, 1996.

Ness MG: Treatment of fragmented coronoid process in young dogs by proximal ulnar osteotomy. J Small Anim Pract 39:15, 1998.

Roy RG, Wallace LJ, Johnston GR: A retrospective long-term evaluation of ununited anconeal process excision on the canine elbow. Vet Comp Orthop Traum 7:94–97, 1994.

Mason D, Schulz KS, Samii V: Sensitivity of radiography to radio-ulnar incongruence. Vet Surg 31:125–132, 2002.

Sjostrom L, Kasstrom H, Kallberg M: Ununited anconeal process in the dog. Pathogenesis and treatment by osteotomy of the ulna. Vet Comp Orthop Traum 8:170–176, 1995.

Thomson, M. J. and Robins, G. M. Osteochondrosis of the elbow, a review of the pathogenesis and a new approach to treatment. Aust Vet J 72: 375–378. 1995.

Turner BM, Abercromby RH, Innes J: Dynamic proximal ulnar osteotomy for the treatment of ununited anconeal process in 17 dogs. Vet Comp Orthop Traum 11:76–79, 1998.

Van Ryssen B, van Bree H: Arthroscopic findings in 100 dogs with elbow lameness. Vet Rec 140:360, 1997.

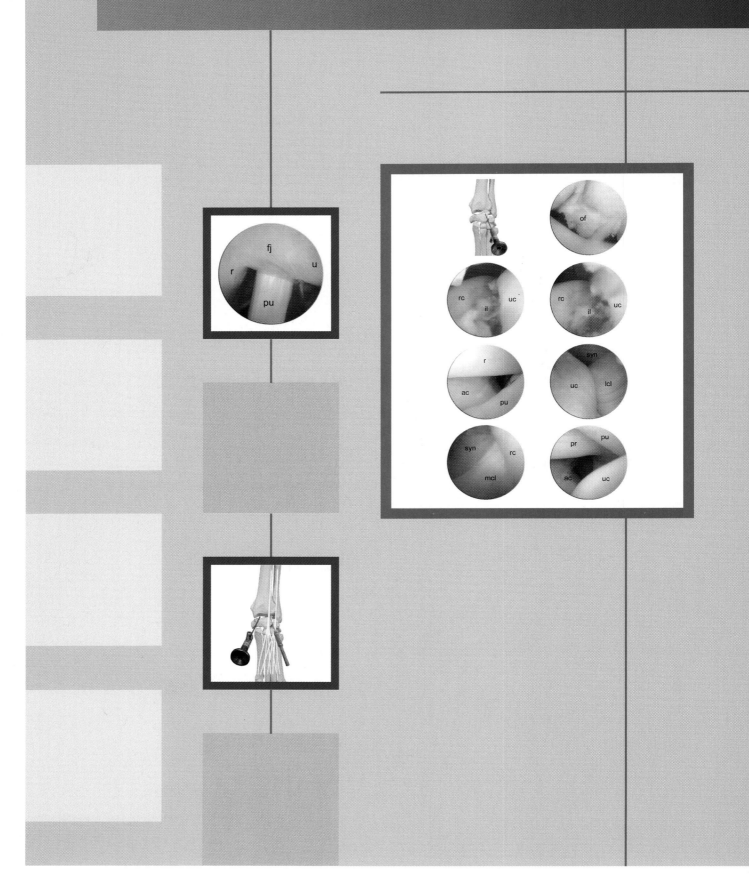

Arthroscopically Assisted Surgery of the Carpal Joint

Introduction

Carpal arthroscopy is a new treatment modality in small animal surgery. Potential indications for carpal arthroscopy include evaluation of ligamentous damage, intra-articular fractures, septic arthritis, and removal of small bone chips. Technically, carpal arthroscopy is relatively easy to perform, and little special instrumentation is required. Arthroscopic exploration of the carpus allows a thorough evaluation of the radiocarpal joint for evaluation of the distal radius, distal ulna, radiocarpal, ulnar carpal, and accessory carpal bones. Ligamentous structures can also be evaluated and synovial biopsies obtained.

Arthroscopy of the Carpal Joint

Equipment and Instrumentation. The surgical table should be one that can be lowered, raised, and tilted in at least one direction. For carpal arthroscopy, the surgery table should be adjusted to a position that allows the surgeon and assistants to hold their arms as close to the body as possible. The surgeon's shoulders should be in neutral position, with the elbows close to 90 degrees. This position prevents fatigue and improves the efficiency of the operating team. The imaging tower is placed at the back of the patient or opposite the surgeon (Fig. 5–1). Fluid ingress is achieved with a pressurized gravity bag or an infusion fluid pump administered through the arthroscope cannula. Fluid can be evacuated by allowing it to flow freely through the egress needle (or cannula) or through a working cannula; evacuation of fluid can be assisted with suction attached to the egress needle (or cannula). If suction is used, it must be set at a low level or bubbles will be produced that obscure the surgeon's view.

A 30-degree fore-oblique arthroscope is commonly used in the carpal joint. In most dogs, a 1.9-mm arthroscope is the best choice for the small radiocarpal joint

space (Fig. 5–2). In large breeds, a 2.4- to 2.7-mm arthroscope may be used. In general, a smaller scope is suggested to prevent iatrogenic damage to cartilage during insertion or manipulation of cartilage during surgery. In choosing which arthroscope to use, the surgeon must consider the outside diameter of the arthroscope cannula because it too must enter the joint. Each arthroscope cannula is fitted with a blunt obturator and a sharp trocar. In most cases, it is not necessary to use the sharp trocar to enter the joint. If the surgeon chooses to use the sharp trocar, caution must be exercised when entering the joint to prevent iatrogenic damage to cartilage. A blunt conical obturator is the recommended instrument for use in entering the joint. If the surgeon experiences difficulty in entering the joint,

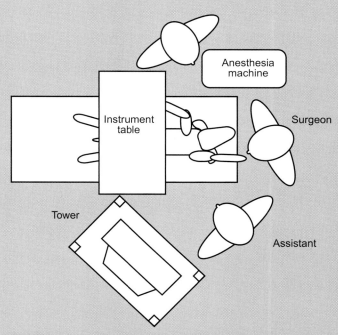

FIGURE 5–1   Arrangement of the operating room for carpal arthroscopy.

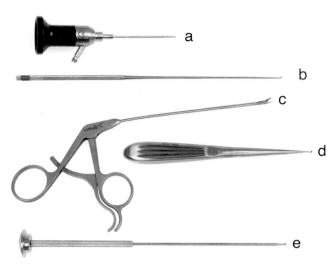

FIGURE 5–2 Instrumentation for carpal arthroscopy. A 1.9-mm arthroscope is ideal for most patients (*a*). A blunt probe is used to evaluate the articular cartilage and ligaments (*b*). Grasping forceps are used to remove small osteochondral fragments or synovium (*c*). A curette is used for débridement of cartilage and curettage of eburnated bone (*d*). A hand burr is used for débridement of articular cartilage and eburnated bone (*e*).

a no. 11 scalpel blade can be used to make a small stab incision in the joint capsule to ease placement of the obturator and cannula.

An assortment of hand instruments is necessary for carpal arthroscopy. Recommended are instruments to assist in the inspection of intra-articular structures (probes), grasping forceps for removal of free bodies, biopsy forceps, and instruments for surface abrasion and synovectomy (see Fig. 5–2). Instruments can be inserted into the joint through an open instrument port,

instrument cannulas, or a combination of the two. If the surgeon works through an instrument cannula, different-size cannulas and switching sticks are necessary.

Anesthetic Considerations and Perioperative Pain Management. Preoperative laboratory workup is based on the patient's physical status and surgical risk. Most dogs undergoing carpal arthroscopy are young, healthy patients with no underlying systemic problems. These cases require minimal laboratory workup. Older dogs should undergo a complete blood screen, urinalysis, chest radiographs, and electrocardiogram. Table 3–1 shows a standard anesthetic protocol, including preemptive pain medication. Postoperative pain is usually minimal but can be controlled with opioids and nonsteroidal anti-inflammatory drugs (NSAIDs) as needed. If arthroscopy is completed early in the day, the patient may be dismissed from the hospital that same afternoon unless a surgical procedure is performed and requires hospitalization. If arthroscopy is completed later in the afternoon, the patient is discharged the next day.

All patients receive preemptive analgesic drugs as part of their premedication protocol. Buprenorphine is preferred because of its effectiveness in patients that experience mild to moderate postoperative pain and its prolonged mode of action (6 to 8 hours). When the dog is dismissed from the hospital, NSAIDs and oral butorphanol (see Table 3–1) can be dispensed for administration at home as needed. NSAIDs are continued for 5 days, and butorphanol is discontinued after 48 hours. If the dog remains in the hospital overnight, a second dose of buprenorphine is administered in the evening. NSAIDs and butorphanol are prescribed for home administration. Fentanyl transdermal patches can also be considered for postoperative pain management.

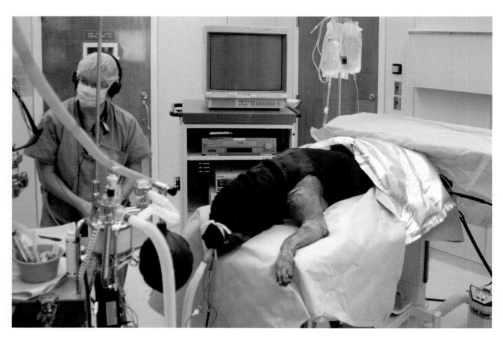

FIGURE 5–3 Positioning of the dog for carpal arthroscopy before draping.

Patient Preparation and Positioning. The patient is clipped and prepared for open arthrotomy in case the arthroscopy procedure needs to be aborted for technical reasons and an open arthrotomy performed. This situation is more common when the surgeon is beginning to learn arthroscopy. The surgeon must accurately identify the region of the articular surface that is damaged by thoroughly assessing the joint radiographically before surgery. The radiocarpal joint is the only joint within the carpus that can be readily evaluated with the arthroscope. The patient should be positioned in ventral recumbency, with the carpus and foot protruding off the end of the table (Fig. 5–3). This position allows adjustment of the carpus position and permits greater manipulation of the scope by avoiding interference of the scope with the surgical table. The carpus can be draped in a similar fashion to that used for open surgery (Fig. 5–4). Some surgeons prefer translucent drapes because of their water-repellant properties (Fig. 5–5).

Portal Sites. Two portal sites are typically used for carpal arthroscopy, but three can be used if the surgeon prefers. If visual joint exploration of the carpal joint is all that is required, an egress portal and an arthroscope portal are necessary. However, if tissue biopsy or treatment of joint pathology is undertaken, then an additional instrument portal is required. Alternatively, the egress portal may be converted into an instrument portal. When a cannula system is used, the egress of fluid and instrumentation can be accomplished through a single portal.

The egress portal is usually established first, followed by the scope portal. The two commonly used scope portals are the dorsolateral and dorsomedial (Figs. 5–6 to 5–9). The scope portal is usually located lateral if the lateral aspect of the joint is to be viewed and medial if

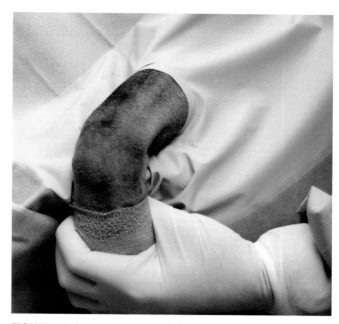

FIGURE 5–4 Patient prepared for carpal arthroscopy with four quadrant towels and a sterile drape. This method of preparation permits good manipulation of the limb during arthroscopy and allows the surgeon to convert the procedure to an open arthrotomy if needed. This positioning is ideal for arthroscopy of the carpus and subsequent carpal arthrodesis.

the medial aspect of the joint is to be viewed. The extensor tendons should be avoided because they course over the dorsal aspect of the carpus. Many surgeons start with one scope portal and switch to the opposite portal to thoroughly evaluate the radiocarpal joint. In this situation, the scope and egress portals are simply interchanged.

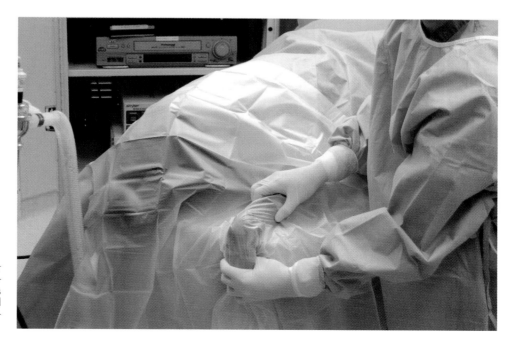

FIGURE 5–5 Patient prepared for carpal arthroscopy with a clear adhesive sterile drape. This drape repels water, keeping the patient dry and reducing the opportunity for contamination from wet towels and drapes.

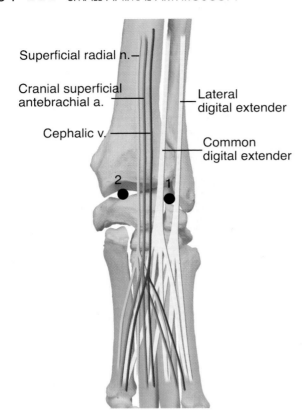

Superficial radial n.—

Cranial superficial
antebrachial a.

Cephalic v.

Lateral
digital extender

Common
digital extender

2   1

FIGURE 5-6 Portal locations and pertinent anatomy for canine carpal arthroscopy. *1*, Dorsolateral portal location; *2*, dorsomedial portal location.

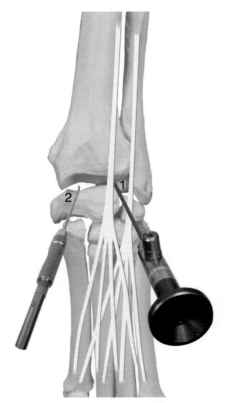

2   1

FIGURE 5-7 Portal locations and pertinent anatomy for canine carpal arthroscopy. *1*, Dorsolateral arthroscope portal location; *2*, dorsomedial instrument portal location.

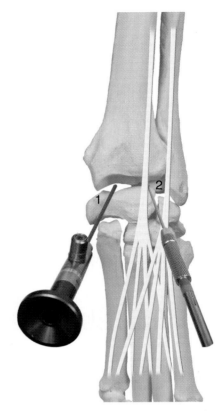

1   2

FIGURE 5-8 Portal locations and pertinent anatomy for canine carpal arthroscopy. *1*, Dorsomedial arthroscope portal location; *2*, dorsolateral instrument portal location.

Dorsolateral Scope Portal. If an instrument portal is needed, the egress portal should be located adjacent to the instrument portal. If necessary, the egress portal can be relocated to a more convenient location. Alternatively, the egress portal and the instrument portal can function through a single portal, as described earlier. The arthroscope cannula and blunt obturator are introduced lateral to the common extensor tendons (see Figs. 5–6 and 5–7). The cannula is directed toward the radiocarpal joint in a palmaromedial direction (see Figs. 5–7 and 5–9). The tip of the cannula and scope can be carefully moved to view the central and lateral aspects of the joint. The post cable is rotated to increase the total viewing angle (see Fig. 5–9). The dorsolateral scope portal is commonly used to assess the dorsolateral joint compartment, the synovium, the ulnar carpal bone, the distal ulna, the accessory carpal bone, a portion of the radiocarpal bone, the ligaments to the accessory carpal bone, the palmar radiocarpal ligament, and the palmar ulnocarpal ligament (Figs. 5–10 and 5–11). The synovial reflection at the level of the proximal intercarpal joint also can be visualized. The basic technique for establishing portals was described earlier.

Dorsomedial Scope Portal. The egress portal is established first. If an instrument portal will be used, the egress portal should be located adjacent to the instrument portal. The egress portal can be relocated to a more convenient location as needed. Alternatively, the egress

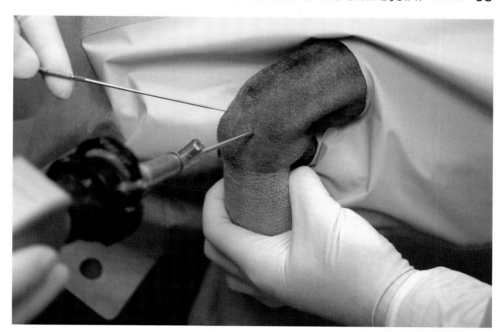

FIGURE 5–9 Dorsolateral arthroscope portal and dorsomedial instrument portals for canine carpal arthroscopy.

portal and the instrument portal can function through a single portal, as described earlier. The arthroscope cannula and blunt obturator are introduced medial to the extensor tendons (see Figs. 5–6 and 5–8). The cannula is directed in a palmarolateral direction toward the radiocarpal joint. The tip of the cannula and scope can be carefully moved to view the central and medial aspects of the joint. The post cable is rotated as needed to increase the total viewing angle. The dorsomedial scope portal is commonly used to assess the dorsomedial joint compartment, the synovium, the radiocarpal bone, the distal radius, a portion of the ulnar carpal bone, the palmar radiocarpal ligament, the palmar ulnocarpal ligament, and the accessory carpal bone (Fig. 5–12). The basic technique for establishing portals was described earlier.

General Surgical Procedure. An 18- to 20-gauge spinal needle (1.5-inch) is used to distend the joint with saline and function as an egress cannula. This needle is positioned on the opposite side of the joint from the intended location of the scope portal. For instance, if the scope portal is dorsomedial, the egress portal would be dorsolateral. If the need for an instrument portal is anticipated, the egress cannula can be located in an alternative position to allow three functional portals. In this case, the egress needle is located adjacent to the instrument portal.

The surgeon palpates the radiocarpal joint while flexing the carpus and inserts the needle into the joint, perpendicular to the surface of the skin. The surgeon often feels a popping sensation when entering the joint. To ensure placement within the joint, the surgeon attaches a syringe to the needle and aspirates synovial fluid. In most cases, when the needle is properly placed, synovial fluid is easily aspirated. If synovial fluid is not aspirated and the surgeon believes that the joint has been entered,

lactated Ringer's solution can be instilled into the joint. If the needle is located in the joint, fluid is easily instilled. As the joint cavity is filled with fluid, reverse pressure is felt on the syringe plunger from the instilled fluid. This sensation ensures that the needle is placed properly into the joint. The joint cavity should be distended with 3 to 6 mL lactated Ringer's solution. Joint distension is maintained by leaving the syringe attached to the needle (the assistant needs to keep pressure on the plunger). The fluid ingress line can be temporarily attached to the egress needle (replacing the syringe) to sustain joint distension while the scope cannula is being inserted. The needle should be maintained as the egress cannula. Evacuation of fluid maintains fluid flow through the joint and enhances visualization. Intravenous or suction tubing can be attached to the needle to capture fluid as it leaves the joint. Alternatively, fluid can be allowed to spill onto the floor for capture by a floor suction unit, basin, or towels.

A guide needle (20- to 22-gauge) is inserted at the intended site for the scope portal. If the needle is positioned correctly, fluid should leak from its hub. A no. 11 Bard-Parker blade is used to make a small entry wound through the skin and superficial soft tissues adjacent to the needle. It is not advisable to enter the joint with the scalpel blade because doing so may cause extravasation of fluid outside the joint cavity. The needle is removed, and the arthroscope cannula is inserted with the attached pointed, blunt obturator in the same direction as the needle. When a pointed, blunt obturator is used, pressure must be applied to penetrate the joint capsule. With experience, the surgeon will learn to feel when the joint is entered. After the joint is entered, the obturator is removed from the cannula. Fluid will flow freely from the cannula, confirming correct placement. The fluid ingress line is attached to the cannula, and the arthroscope is inserted.

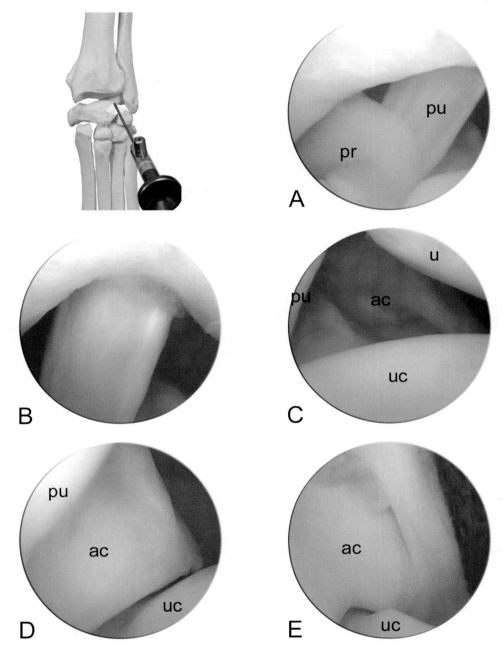

FIGURE 5-10 Positioning and normal joint findings for arthroscopic evaluation of the left radiocarpal joint using a dorsolateral arthroscope portal. *A*, Palmar radiocarpal (*pr*) and ulnocarpal ligaments (*pu*). *B*, Origin of the palmar ulnocarpal ligament arising from the distal ulna. *C*, Distal ulna (*u*), ulnar carpal bone (*uc*), accessory carpal bone (*ac*), and palmar ulnocarpal ligament (*pu*). *D*, The tip of the scope is advanced in a palmar direction to view the articulation between the accessory carpal bone (*ac*) and the ulnar carpal bone (*uc*). The edge of the palmar ulnocarpal ligament (*pu*) is visible. *E*, More palmar view of the accessory carpal bone (*ac*) showing a lateral ligament and the ulnar carpal bone (*uc*).

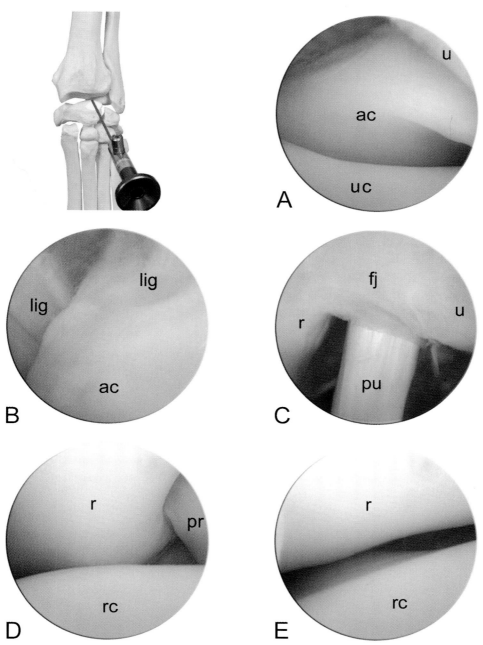

FIGURE 5-11   Positioning and normal joint findings for arthroscopic evaluation of the left radiocarpal joint using a dorsolateral arthroscope portal. *A,* Distal ulna (*u*), accessory carpal bone (*ac*), and ulnar carpal bone (*uc*). *B,* Proximal medial aspect of the accessory carpal bone (*ac*) with the medial and dorsal ligaments (*lig*). *C,* The fibrous junction (*fj*) between the distal radius (*r*) and ulna (*u*) near the origin of the palmar ulnocarpal ligament (*pu*) can be viewed by rotating the light post downward. *D,* Distal radius (*r*), radiocarpal bone (*rc*), and origin of the palmar radiocarpal ligament (*pr*). *E,* Distal radius (*r*) and radiocarpal bone (*rc*).

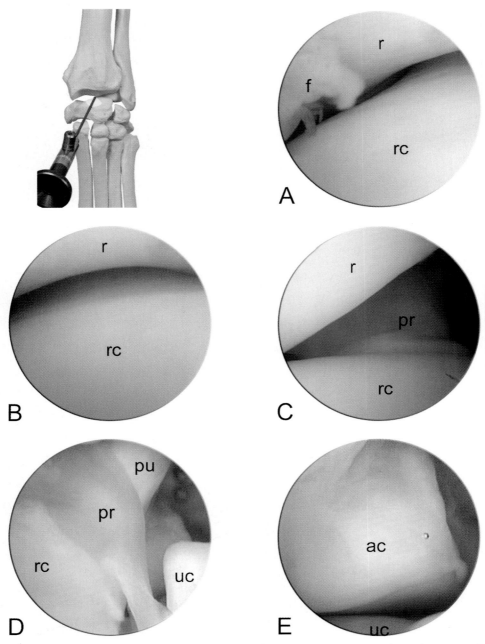

FIGURE 5-12 Positioning and normal joint findings for arthroscopic evaluation of the left radiocarpal joint using a dorsomedial arthroscope portal. *A*, Radius (*r*), radiocarpal bone (*rc*), and intra-articular fat (*f*). *B*, Radius (*r*) and radiocarpal bone (*rc*). *C*, Radius (*r*), radiocarpal bone (*rc*), and palmar radiocarpal ligament (*pr*). *D*, Radiocarpal bone (*rc*), insertion of the palmar radiocarpal ligament (*pr*), palmar ulnocarpal ligament (*pu*), and ulnar carpal bone (*uc*). *E*, Accessory carpal bone (*ac*) and ulnar carpal bone (*uc*).

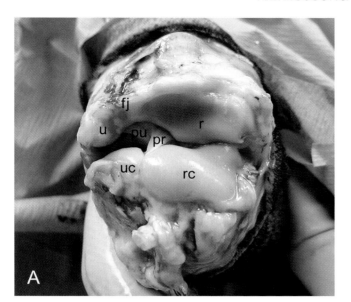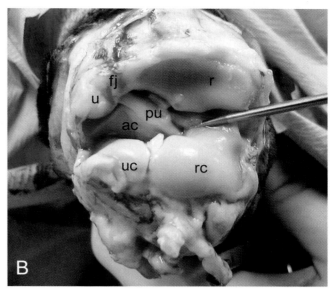

FIGURE 5–13 A, Gross anatomy of the right carpus. Radius (r), ulna (u), radiocarpal bone (rc), ulnar carpal bone (uc), palmar radiocarpal ligament (pr), palmar ulnocarpal ligament (pu), and fibrous junction between radius and ulna (fj). B, Gross anatomy of the right carpus with the palmar radiocarpal ligament removed. Radius (r), ulna (u), radiocarpal bone (rc), ulnar carpal bone (uc), accessory carpal bone (ac), palmar ulnocarpal ligament (pu), and fibrous junction between the radius and ulna (fj).

An instrument portal is established if a biopsy of intra-articular tissue is needed or if treatment of joint pathology is required. Like the egress portal, the instrument portal is usually placed on the side of the limb opposite the scope portal (e.g., a dorsomedial instrument portal would be used with a dorsolateral arthroscope portal). The instrument portal also may be placed directly adjacent to the arthroscope portal if this location will facilitate the needed manipulation. If three portals will be used, the position of the scope and instrument portals must be established to permit visualization and treatment of the lesion. The position of the egress needle can be shifted to a convenient location that provides egress drainage but does not interfere with the other two portals. The egress portal also can function as an instrument portal. This approach may be logistically easier in small dogs whose size may cause difficulty in establishing and maintaining three functional portals. A cannula system allows good egress while permitting the introduction of instruments into the joint. The surgeon must learn to triangulate the instrument relative to the position of the tip of the arthroscope within the joint. It is helpful to use a 20-gauge (1.5-inch) hypodermic needle as a guide needle to locate the appropriate site for the instrument portal. The guide needle must penetrate the skin surface at a 75- to 90-degree angle and maintain this orientation through the soft tissues. As the needle enters the joint and is seen on the monitor, it appears to be entering at a very oblique angle. However, this illusion is created by the 30-degree fore-oblique arthroscope and does not represent the actual angle of penetration. The most common reason for failing to locate the appropriate instrument portal site is entering the skin at too oblique an angle. When too oblique an angle is used, the trian-

gulation needle used to locate the instrument port crosses the arthroscope and cannot be visualized on the monitor. If the triangulation needle cannot be visualized, it should be inserted at a different location at a 75- to 90-degree angle to the skin surface.

Surgical Anatomy. The carpus is a complex hinge joint composed of many individual smaller joints. The carpus primarily moves in flexion and extension, and more than 95% of the range of motion occurs at the radiocarpal joint. The radiocarpal joint is usually amenable to arthroscopy, but the other joints are not. The joint capsule, the collateral ligaments, the intercarpal and carpometacarpal ligaments, and the strong palmar ligaments provide joint stability. Structures that usually can be evaluated arthroscopically include the distal ulna, distal radius, ulnar carpal bone, radiocarpal bone, accessory carpal bone, palmar radiocarpal ligament, palmar ulnocarpal ligament, and synovium (Fig. 5–13).

During arthroscopic evaluation of the carpus, the anatomic structures located on the same side of the joint as the scope portal can be viewed more easily and completely than those located on the opposite side. A portion of the anatomic structures on the opposite side of the joint also can be viewed, but a thorough examination of the joint may require multiple scope portals. When the arthroscope enters the joint, the camera should be positioned to provide correct spatial orientation when viewing the monitor. Typically, surgeons prefer the fore-oblique direction, but most prefer to begin the procedure with a view that is 30 degrees down. The correct spatial orientation with a fore-oblique view is obtained when the controls on the camera head are upright and the light post is in the upright position (see Fig. 5–8). With the camera and light post in this position, the articular surface of the radiocarpal bone is visible. If necessary, the scope can be carefully withdrawn a very small distance to increase the size of the field of view. Slight flexion and extension can improve visualization or vary the region of articular surface that is visible. The position of the camera head is maintained and the light post is rotated ventrally to provide a more complete view of the articular surface of the distal radius. The ulnar carpal bone, intercarpal ligaments, distal ulna, and accessory carpal bone can be evaluated by advancing the tip of the scope and adjusting the position of the post cable slightly. The medial and lateral collateral ligaments also may be visible.

Indications for Arthroscopic Surgery of the Carpal Joint

Carpal arthroscopy is a new treatment modality in small animal surgery. As small animal surgeons become more adept at arthroscopy, more conditions will be treated arthroscopically or with arthroscopic assistance. Potential indications for carpal arthroscopy include intra-articular fractures, osteoarthritis, joint instability, and diagnostic examination (biopsy or culture of bone, cartilage, or synovial membrane). The arthroscope also can be used to place a drain within the joint capsule to allow ingress and egress flushing in patients with septic arthritis. Another potential application is evaluation of the radiocarpal joint in patients with obvious carpometacarpal or intercarpal instability. If radiocarpal involvement is confirmed arthroscopically, pancarpal arthrodesis, rather than partial arthrodesis, may be the treatment of choice.

Fractures and Instability of the Carpus

History and Signalment. Dogs have acute lameness of the front leg; most exhibit non-weightbearing lameness. In most cases, lameness occurs after a traumatic incident and does not respond to anti-inflammatory medication. Any age or breed of dog may be affected.

Physical Examination Findings. Gait analysis shows visible lameness. Swelling is usually palpable in the carpal region. Manipulation of the carpus elicits discomfort in most dogs. Collateral instability is characterized by excessive valgus or varus deviation when the joint is stressed. To better evaluate the function of the short and long components of the collateral ligament complex, collateral instability should be assessed in extension and flexion. Injury to the palmar ligaments leads to hyperextension of the carpal joints. Subluxation or luxation of the affected joint may occur at any level of the carpus, depending on the location of ligament damage.

Differential Diagnosis. The differential diagnosis includes septic arthritis and immune-mediated arthritis.

Radiographic Findings. Lateral and anteroposterior radiographic views are often insufficient to yield a definitive diagnosis. Occasionally, these views suggest collateral ligament injury by the presence of soft tissue swelling or evidence of an avulsion fragment in the area of the collateral ligament. Stress radiographs may show collateral and palmar ligamentous instability. While an anteroposterior radiographic view is obtained, a valgus or varus stress can be applied to check for injury to the lateral and medial collateral ligaments, respectively (Fig. 5–14). A lateral view that is obtained while the joint is

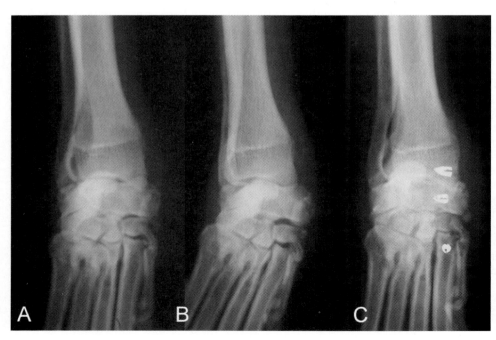

FIGURE 5–14 Radiograph from a dog with a tear of the medial collateral ligament of the carpus. *A,* Survey preoperative radiograph. *B,* A valgus stress is applied to the carpus, revealing instability of the medial side of the radiocarpal joint and presence of multiple avulsion bone fragments. *C,* A valgus stress is applied to the carpus following reconstructive restoration of the medial collateral ligament. Good stability has been achieved.

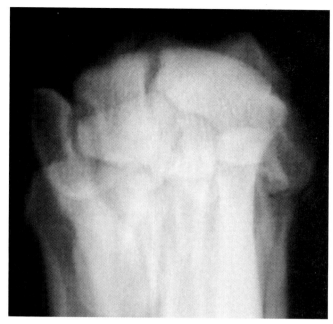

FIGURE 5–15 Some slab fractures of the carpus may best be visualized using a skyline view.

hyperextended may show palmar ligament injury. A lateral flexed view, skyline view, or oblique view may be helpful in assessing carpal slab or chip fractures (Fig. 5–15).

Diagnosis. Carpal instability and fractures are diagnosed based on the history, physical findings, and radiographic findings.

Treatment. Medical management can relieve pain, but definitive therapy requires coaptation or surgical stabilization, depending on the severity of the injury. Arthroscopic intervention can aid in visualizing the condition of the collateral ligaments, removing small avulsion fragments, reducing an avulsed fragment, and examining the articular surfaces of the radiocarpal joint. Arthroscopic evaluation of the palmar ligaments may aid in the assessment of patients with hyperextensional carpal injury. If these ligaments or other structures in the radiocarpal joint are injured, the surgeon may choose to perform pancarpal arthrodesis rather than partial arthrodesis.

Anesthetic Considerations and Perioperative Pain Management. Preoperative laboratory workup is based on the patient's physical status and surgical risk. Young, healthy patients with no underlying systemic problems require minimal laboratory workup. Older dogs should undergo a complete blood screen, chest radiographs, and electrocardiogram. A standard anesthetic protocol, including preemptive pain medication, is provided in Table 3–1. Postoperative pain is controlled with cold therapy, opioids, and NSAIDs.

Surgical Intervention. Carpal instability or fracture is usually treated with an open approach using arthrodesis or ligamentous reconstruction techniques. Many collateral ligament injuries are repaired with ligament reconstruction. Palmar ligament damage usually requires partial or pancarpal arthrodesis. These techniques are described in detail in veterinary surgical texts. Currently, arthroscopic intervention is used primarily for diagnostic and adjunctive purposes.

Portal sites and surgical anatomy were discussed earlier. The surgeon must decide whether to use a dorsolateral or dorsomedial scope portal. To improve visualization or access to the affected structures, the scope and egress portals can easily be exchanged during surgery. The operative site is clipped and prepared according to the amount of limb maneuverability desired during surgery. A hanging limb preparation provides the greatest degree of freedom for manipulating limb position and is recommended in most cases. Liberal clipping and thorough sterile preparation are necessary because an open arthrotomy may be required. In most cases, a 1.9-mm, 30-degree fore-oblique arthroscope is used. Basic instrumentation includes probes to inspect the joint capsule. If the surgeon works through an instrument cannula, different-sized cannulas and switching sticks facilitate the surgery. A motorized shaver is helpful to débride synovial proliferation but is not essential. The dog is positioned as described for the anticipated site of the lesion.

Egress is established as described earlier, and the joint is distended with saline. A guide needle is used to locate the joint space and the correct position for the arthroscope portal. The arthroscope is inserted, and ingress flow is established through the arthroscope cannula. The arthroscope and light post are positioned to visualize the articular surfaces of the radiocarpal bone, ulnar carpal bone, distal radius, distal ulna, accessory carpal bone, synovial membrane, palmar radiocarpal ligament, palmar radiocarpal cruciate ligaments, ligaments of the accessory carpal bone, intercarpal ligament, and collateral ligaments (see Figs. 5–10 to 5–13; Fig. 5–16). The light post is rotated 360 degrees to allow complete evaluation of the joint, and the scope is tipped in different directions and retracted or advanced to enhance the view of the structures. The medial and lateral collateral ligaments are examined in extension and partial flexion (see Fig. 5–16). The surgeon should look for avulsed fragments and assess the practicality of stabilization versus removal of the fragment (see Fig. 5–14). In addition, the surgeon should assess the condition of the articular cartilage and evaluate the fracture fragments to determine the degree of reduction or the need for removal.

If an instrument portal is needed, a guide needle is used to triangulate the position for its placement. The most common reason for failure to visualize the guide needle in the joint is crossing the arthroscope. To prevent crossing the arthroscope with the guide needle, the needle is inserted perpendicular to the skin surface and this orientation is maintained through the soft tissues. After the position for the instrument portal is

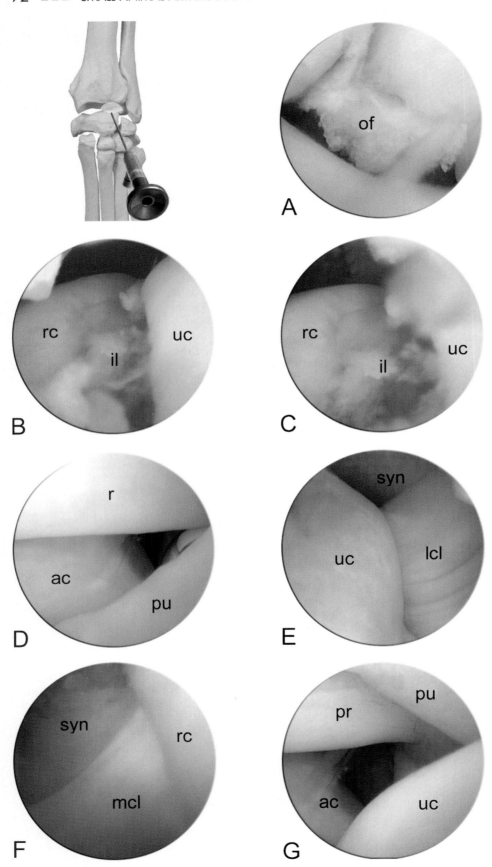

FIGURE 5-16 Positioning and abnormal joint findings for arthroscopic evaluation of the carpus using a dorsolateral arthroscope portal in a dog that had incidental trauma while playing. *A,* Free-floating osteochondral fragment (*of*), most likely originating from the site of an intercarpal ligament tear. *B,* Tear of the intercarpal ligament (*il*) between the radiocarpal (*rc*) and ulnar carpal (*uc*) bones. *C,* Because of instability caused by tearing of the intercarpal ligament (*il*), the space between the radiocarpal (*rc*) and ulnocarpal (*uc*) bones widens when stress is applied. *D,* Hyperemia at the craniolateral pole of the accessory carpal bone (*ac*) as a result of mild strain on an adjacent ligament. The radius (*r*) and palmar ulnocarpal (*pu*) ligament are visible. *E,* The lateral collateral ligament (*lcl*) is normal. The synovium (*syn*) and ulnar carpal bone (*uc*) are visible. *F,* The medial collateral ligament (*mcl*) is normal. The synovium (*syn*) and radial carpal bone (*rc*) are visible. *G,* The palmar radiocarpal (*pr*) and palmar ulnocarpal (*pu*) ligaments are normal. The accessory carpal (*ac*) and ulnar carpal (*uc*) bones are also visible.

established, a probe is inserted through a cannula or an open portal.

If the articular surfaces of the radiocarpal joint show excessive wear, arthrodesis rather than stabilization should be considered. If open reduction and stabilization are necessary, useful techniques include ligamentous reconstruction, transarticular fixation, and arthrodesis. These techniques are described in detail in various veterinary surgical textbooks and journals.

Postoperative Care. Cold therapy can be used during recovery to relieve pain and reduce swelling. Cold therapy is applied by alternating 15 minutes on and 10 minutes off for two applications. Commercial cold packs or a commercial circulating cold water pack can be used. Alternatively, ice wrapped in a towel or frozen packs of vegetables can be used. If the dog is dismissed from the hospital the day of surgery, NSAIDs and oral butorphanol (see Table 3–1) are dispensed for administration at home. If the dog remains in the hospital overnight, buprenorphine is administered in the evening. NSAIDs and butorphanol are dispensed for administration at home. NSAIDs are continued for 5 days, and butorphanol is discontinued after 48 hours. Adjunctive coaptation can be used for various lengths of time, depending on the severity of injury. If adjunctive coaptation is not performed, cold therapy can be continued by the owner at home for the first 2 days after surgery if needed. In addition, the owner should examine the portal sites daily for signs of irritation or drainage.

Leash walking is recommended for 4 to 8 weeks, followed by a progressive increase in activity. To increase the weightbearing load on the limb, walking at a slow pace is recommended. As postoperative time increases, the pace can be hastened. To increase the range of motion in the carpus when walking, the client should walk the dog in high grass (e.g., weeds), shallow water, or sand. Walking on this type of surface forces the dog to pick up the feet and step high with the legs. After 6 weeks, the owner should begin limited amounts of free activity with controlled walking, starting with 5 minutes of free activity and increasing to 30 minutes over the next 2 weeks. After 8 weeks, free activity is gradually increased to normal levels. If during any exercise period (controlled or free activity), the dog becomes sore or is sore the next day, the owner should decrease the pace and return to controlled activity for 2 to 3 days.

Complications. Complications are unusual. Occasionally, in the immediate postoperative period, excessive fluid extravasation occurs and causes swollen soft tissues around the carpus. This fluid resorbs within the first 24 hours. Residual mild swelling adjacent to portal sites may be noticeable for the first 48 hours.

Prognosis. Depending on the severity of injury and the surgical procedure required, the prognosis for satisfactory limb function after the treatment of ligamentous instability or carpal fracture is fair to excellent. Most dogs have a good outcome if collateral ligamentous reconstruction is performed satisfactorily. If good stability

cannot be achieved or if the dog has multiligamentous injury, arthrodesis may provide the best functional outcome. A good functional outcome is usually associated with arthrodesis of the carpus. The level of carpal instability should be assessed carefully to determine whether pancarpal or partial arthrodesis is indicated. A good prognosis is typical if fractures can be reduced anatomically and rigidly stabilized.

Inflammatory Arthritis

History and Signalment. Septic arthritis and immune-mediated arthritis are inflammatory arthropathies. Immune-mediated arthritis often presents as a polyarthritis, affecting more than one joint. Dogs present with lameness of one or more limbs. The lameness may be weightbearing or non-weightbearing and is often characterized as episodic or shifting from one leg to another. The lameness usually responds to antibiotics, corticosteroids, or NSAIDs, depending on its etiology and severity. Any age or breed of dog may be affected, but small breeds are more susceptible to immune-mediated polyarthritis.

Physical Examination Findings. Gait analysis shows visible lameness. Swelling is usually palpable in affected joints, and manipulation of affected joints elicits discomfort in most dogs. In addition, the joints may be warm to the touch.

Differential Diagnosis. The differential diagnosis includes traumatic joint injury.

Radiographic Findings. Radiographic evaluation usually shows soft tissue swelling of affected joints as a result of synovial effusion. A narrowed joint space may be evident in dogs that have septic arthritis or erosive immune-mediated arthritis as a result of articular cartilage erosion. If erosive immune-mediated arthritis becomes chronic, joint instability and luxation may occur.

Diagnosis. The history, physical findings, and radiographic findings may suggest the diagnosis of inflammatory arthritis. A definitive diagnosis usually requires synovial fluid analysis, culture, and sensitivity as well as a complete blood count, serum chemistry profile, urinalysis, and serologic evaluation for a variety of immune tests (rheumatoid factor, antinuclear antibody) and infectious agents (tickborne agents). Synovial biopsy is also helpful. Veterinary textbooks should be consulted for a comprehensive review of pathophysiology and diagnostic tests.

Treatment. Medical management is routinely used in the initial stages of treatment. Septic arthritis is treated with appropriate antibiotics, based on the results of culture and sensitivity tests, and with joint lavage and drainage where appropriate. Arthroscopy can be used to assess the condition of the articular cartilage, remove fibrinous debris, and lavage the joint. A closed-suction drain also can be inserted under arthroscopic visualization. Treatment of immune-mediated arthritis is usually initiated with immunosuppressive doses of corticosteroid drugs. Veterinary textbooks can be consulted for drug dosages and treatment protocols.

Anesthetic Considerations and Perioperative Pain Management.   Preoperative laboratory workup is based on the patient's physical status and surgical risk. Young, healthy patients with no underlying systemic problems require minimal laboratory workup. Older dogs should have a complete blood screen, chest radiographs, and electrocardiogram. Table 3–1 shows a standard anesthetic protocol, including preemptive pain medication. Postoperative pain is controlled with cold therapy, opioids, and NSAIDs.

Surgical Intervention.   Arthroscopic intervention is currently used primarily for diagnostic and adjunctive purposes. It can be used to evaluate the condition of articular cartilage and synovium (Fig. 5–17). Synovial biopsy specimens can be harvested arthroscopically for histopathologic evaluation (see Fig. 5–17).

Portal sites and surgical anatomy were described earlier. The surgeon must decide whether to use a dorsolateral or dorsomedial scope portal. If necessary, the scope and egress portals can be exchanged during surgery to improve visualization or access to the affected structures. The operative site is clipped and prepared according to the amount of limb maneuverability desired during surgery. A hanging limb preparation provides the greatest degree of freedom for manipulating limb position and is generally recommended. In most cases, a 1.9-mm, 30-degree fore-oblique arthroscope is used. Basic instrumentation includes probes to inspect the joint capsule and biopsy forceps. If the surgeon works through an instrument cannula, different-sized cannulas and switching sticks facilitate the surgery. A motorized shaver is helpful to débride synovial proliferation.

The egress needle is established as described earlier, and the joint is distended with saline. A guide needle is used to locate the joint space and the correct position for the arthroscope portal. The arthroscope is inserted, and ingress flow is established through the arthroscope cannula. The arthroscope and light post are positioned to visualize the articular surfaces of the radiocarpal bone, ulnar carpal bone, distal radius, distal ulna, accessory carpal bone, synovial membrane, palmar radiocarpal ligament, palmar radiocarpal cruciate ligaments, ligaments of the accessory carpal bone, intercarpal ligament, and collateral ligaments (see Fig. 5–16). The light post is rotated 360 degrees to allow thorough evaluation of the joint, and the scope is tipped in different directions and retracted or advanced to enhance the view.

If an instrument portal is needed, a guide needle is used to triangulate its position. The most common reason for failure to visualize the guide needle in the joint is crossing the arthroscope. To prevent crossing the

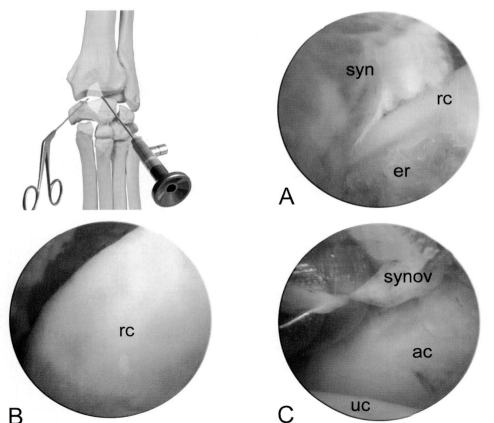

FIGURE 5–17 Positioning and abnormal joint findings for arthroscopic evaluation of the carpus using a dorsomedial arthroscope portal in a dog with immune-mediated polyarthritis. *A,* Erosion (*er*) of the peripheral articular cartilage of the radiocarpal bone (*rc*) at the edge of the synovial pannus (*syn*). *B,* Partial-thickness erosion of the articular cartilage of the radiocarpal bone (*rc*). *C,* Use of biopsy forceps to harvest synovium (*synov*) near the accessory carpal (*ac*) and ulnar carpal (*uc*) bones for histopathologic evaluation.

arthroscope with the guide needle, the needle is inserted perpendicular to the skin surface and this orientation is maintained through the soft tissues. After the position for the instrument portal is established, the instrument is inserted through a cannula or an open portal.

Postoperative Care. Cold therapy can be applied to the carpus during recovery to relieve pain and reduce swelling. Cold therapy is administered by alternating 15 minutes on and 10 minutes off for two applications. Commercial cold packs or a commercial circulating cold water pack can be used. Alternatively, ice wrapped in a towel or frozen packs of vegetables can be used. If the dog is dismissed from the hospital the day of surgery, oral butorphanol (see Table 3–1) is dispensed for administration at home. If the dog remains in the hospital overnight, buprenorphine is administered in the evening and butorphanol is dispensed for administration at home. If necessary, cold therapy can be continued by the owner at home for the first 2 days after surgery. In addition, the owner should examine the portal sites daily for signs of irritation or drainage.

Complications. Complications are unusual. In the immediate postoperative period, excessive fluid extravasation may occur and cause swelling of the soft tissues around the carpus. This fluid resorbs within the first 24 hours. Residual mild swelling adjacent to portal sites may be noticeable for the first 48 hours.

Prognosis. The prognosis depends on the underlying etiology, the response to treatment, and the condition of the articular cartilage at the time of initial therapy. If septic arthritis is treated early, the prognosis is usually good. Patients with immune-mediated arthritis may need long-term therapy with corticosteroids or cytotoxic drugs. Nonerosive forms of immune-mediated arthritis usually have a fair to good prognosis, whereas the prognosis for erosive forms is usually guarded to poor. Veterinary textbooks can be consulted for additional information.

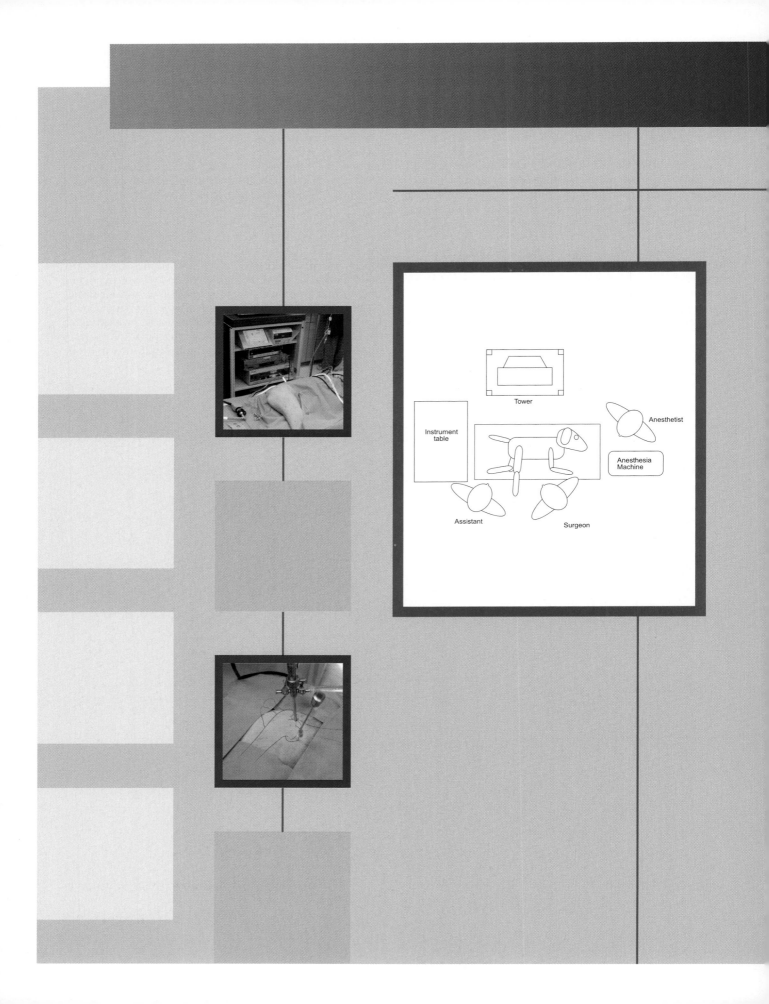

Tower

Instrument table

Anesthetist

Anesthesia Machine

Assistant

Surgeon

Arthroscopically Assisted Surgery of the Hip Joint

Introduction

The hip joint is difficult to examine arthroscopically in dogs that have thickened joint capsules as a result of chronic osteoarthritis. However, in young dogs with hip joint laxity, hip arthroscopy can be performed with minimal difficulty. Arthroscopy of the hip is in its infancy, and future applications will grow as surgeons gain expertise and experience.

Arthroscopic Surgery of the Hip Joint

Equipment and Instrumentation. The surgical table should be capable of being lowered, raised, and tilted in at least one direction. During hip arthroscopy, the surgery table should be adjusted to a position that allows the surgeon and assistants to hold the arms as close to the body as is possible. The surgeon's shoulders should be in neutral position, with the elbows close to 90 degrees. This position prevents fatigue and improves the efficiency of the operating team. The imaging tower is positioned at the back of the patient or opposite the surgeon (Fig. 6–1). Fluid ingress is achieved with a pressurized gravity bag or an infusion fluid pump and administered through the arthroscope cannula. Fluid can be evacuated by allowing it to flow freely through the egress needle (or cannula) or through a working cannula. Fluid evacuation can be assisted with suction attached to the egress needle (or cannula). If suction is used, it must be set at a low level or bubbles will be produced that obscure the surgeon's view.

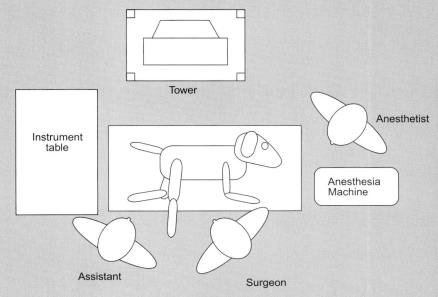

Tower

Instrument table

Anesthetist

Anesthesia Machine

Assistant

Surgeon

FIGURE 6–1 Arrangement of the operating room for hip arthroscopy.

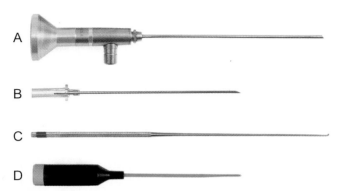

FIGURE 6–2 Instrumentation for hip arthroscopy. *A,* A 1.9- to 2.7-mm arthroscope is used, depending on the size of the patient. *B,* An 18- to 22-gauge spinal needle is used for an egress cannula. *C,* A blunt probe is useful for evaluating the round ligament, articular cartilage, and labrum. *D,* Radiofrequency units can be used to perform synovectomy, control bleeding, and shrink redundant joint capsule and round ligament.

A 30-degree fore-oblique arthroscope is commonly used in the hip joint. In most dogs, a 2.7-mm arthroscope is easily inserted into the joint space. In small breeds, the use of a 1.9- to 2.4-mm arthroscope is suggested to prevent iatrogenic damage to the cartilage during insertion or manipulation of the cartilage during surgery. Whichever size arthroscope is chosen, the outside diameter of the arthroscope cannula must be considered because it must enter the joint. Each arthroscope cannula is fitted with a blunt obturator and sharp trocar. In most cases, it is not necessary to use the sharp trocar to enter the joint. When the sharp trocar is used, caution must be exercised to prevent iatrogenic damage to the cartilage. The authors recommend entering the joint with a blunt conical obturator.

An assortment of hand instruments is necessary for hip arthroscopy. Recommended are instruments to assist in the inspection of intra-articular structures (probes), grasping forceps to remove free bodies, biopsy forceps, and instruments to perform surface abrasion and synovectomy (Fig. 6–2). Instruments can be inserted into the joint through an open instrument port, instrument cannulas, or a combination of the two. If the surgeon works through an instrument cannula, different-size cannulas and switching sticks are necessary.

Anesthetic Considerations and Perioperative Pain Management. Preoperative laboratory workup is based on the patient's physical status and surgical risk. Young, healthy patients with no underlying systemic problems require minimal laboratory workup. Older dogs require a complete blood screen, urinalysis, chest radiographs, and an electrocardiogram. Table 3-1 shows a standard anesthetic protocol, including preemptive pain medication. Depending on the procedure performed, perioperative pain is controlled with various combinations of intra-articular analgesics, epidural analgesia, opioids, and nonsteroidal anti-inflammatory drugs (NSAIDs). Intra-articular bupivicaine administered before the arthroscopic procedure is effective in controlling surgical pain (Fig. 6–3). Minimal analgesia is usually necessary for diagnostic arthroscopy alone. If arthroscopy is completed early in the day, the patient may be dismissed from the hospital the same afternoon unless a surgical procedure requires hospitalization. If arthroscopy is completed later in the afternoon, the patient is discharged the next day.

All patients receive preemptive analgesic drugs or epidural analgesia as part of the premedication protocol. Epidural analgesia is preferred if hip arthroscopy is coupled with a surgical procedure (e.g., triple pelvic osteotomy). Buprenorphine also can be used because it is effective in patients that have mild to moderate postoperative pain and it has a relatively long mode of action

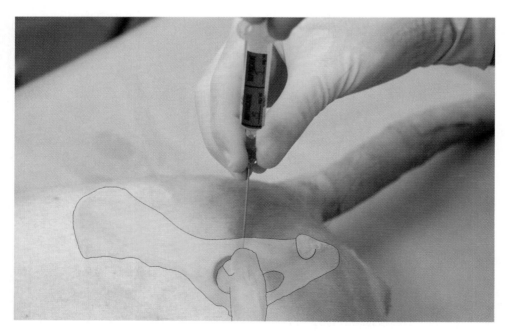

FIGURE 6–3 Technique for intra-articular injection of local analgesic for hip arthroscopy.

(6 to 8 hours). When the dog is dismissed from the hospital, NSAIDs and oral butorphenol (see Table 3–1) are dispensed for administration at home. NSAIDs are continued for 5 days, and butorphenol is discontinued after 48 hours. If the dog remains in the hospital overnight, a second dose of buprenorphine is administered in the evening. NSAIDs and butorphenol are prescribed for home administration. Fentanyl transdermal patches also can be used to manage postoperative pain.

Patient Preparation and Positioning. The patient is clipped and prepared for open craniolateral hip arthrotomy (Fig. 6–4) in case the arthroscopy procedure needs to be aborted for technical reasons and an open arthrotomy performed. Arthroscopy is most commonly used as a diagnostic or assessment tool in the hip and not as a definitive surgical treatment. The method of limb preparation used depends on the amount of limb maneuverability desired by the surgeon. If the surgeon wishes to have maximum maneuverability during the procedure or if a surgical procedure is to be performed at the time of arthroscopic examination, a hanging limb preparation is recommended (Fig. 6–5). The hanging limb preparation is the preferred method in most clinical patients. As the surgeon becomes more experienced and adept at hip arthroscopy or if only diagnostic arthroscopy is needed, less maneuverability is required and a lateral limb preparation can be used. A small area is clipped over the hip, and a sterile adhesive drape may be used. The lateral limb preparation also allows the surgeon to convert to an open procedure if needed. In either case, the dog is positioned in lateral recumbency

with the limb to be operated on positioned uppermost. The limb is supported in neutral position, with the femur parallel to the ground, or is slightly adducted (Fig. 6–5). It is also helpful to flex the hip to open the joint space. If both limbs need arthroscopic intervention, the dog is rolled over to the opposite side and the second side is prepared for sterile surgery. As the surgeon becomes more experienced, the area of clipped hair may be reduced to a small square area that is suitable for arthroscopy but unsuitable for arthrotomy. If a small area is clipped and the arthroscopic procedure must be converted to an arthrotomy, the dog can be prepared for an arthrotomy in routine fashion after the arthroscopic procedure is completed.

Portal Sites. Depending on the purpose of arthroscopic intervention, two or three portal sites are used (Fig. 6–6). If visual exploration of the hip joint is all that is required, an egress portal and an arthroscope portal are necessary. If tissue biopsy or treatment of joint pathology is undertaken, then an additional instrument portal is created. The egress and instrument portals can be converted to a single portal when a cannula system is used. A clock face analogy is helpful when planning the location of portals. For the right hip, the arthroscope portal is placed at 12 o'clock, the instrument portal at 2 o'clock, and the egress portal at 5 o'clock (Fig. 6–7). For the left hip, the arthroscope, instrument, and egress portals are placed at 12 o'clock, 10 o'clock, and 7 o'clock, respectively. The positions of the arthroscope and instrument portals can be switched with switching sticks to provide access to different parts of the joint. Landmarks

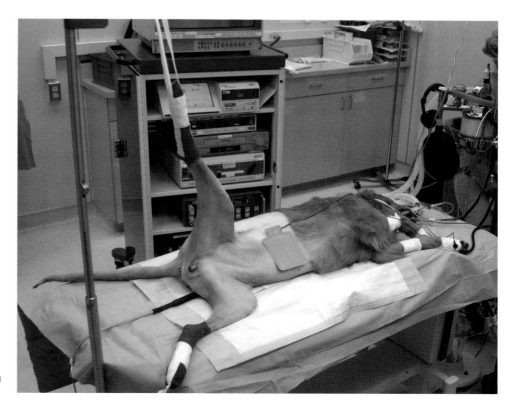

FIGURE 6–4 Positioning of the dog for hip arthroscopy before draping.

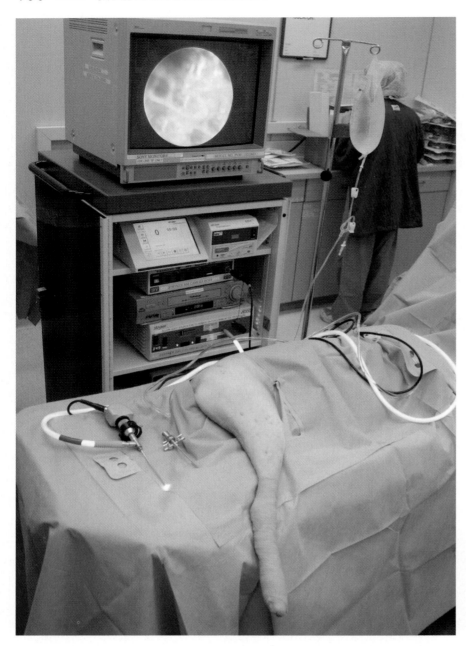

FIGURE 6-5 A patient prepared for hip arthroscopy with four quadrant towels and a sterile drape. This method of preparation permits good manipulation of the limb during arthroscopy and allows the surgeon to convert the procedure to an open arthrotomy if needed. This positioning is ideal for arthroscopy of the hip and subsequent triple pelvic osteotomy.

are intended to be used only as starting points; optimal instrument portal placement can be verified intra-articularly by visualization of a guide needle.

The scope portal is established first (Fig. 6–8). An 18- to 22-gauge spinal needle (2.5- to 3-inch) can be used as a guide to confirm the position for this portal. An assistant should apply traction to the leg while applying countertraction to the inguinal region to separate the joint surfaces and ease the insertion of the guide needle and arthroscope. The hip is flexed slightly, and the femur is positioned parallel to the table to maximize the width of the joint space. If the knee is flexed, the tibia can be used as a handle to place traction on the hip. A traction device has been developed that eliminates the need for

an assistant. Little manipulation of the limb is possible when the traction device is in use. The hip is palpated, and the needle is inserted at the midpoint of the proximal edge of the greater trochanter. The needle is inserted perpendicular to the skin surface, and this orientation is maintained through the soft tissues as the needle enters the joint. The surgeon may experience a popping sensation when the joint is entered. To ensure that the needle is placed within the joint, a syringe is attached to the needle and synovial fluid is aspirated. In most cases, when the needle is properly placed, synovial fluid is easily aspirated. If synovial fluid is not aspirated and the surgeon believes that the joint has been entered, lactated Ringer's solution can be instilled into the joint. If the

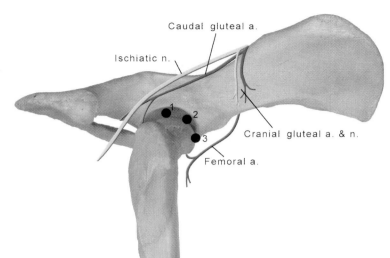

FIGURE 6–6 *Portal locations and pertinent anatomy for canine hip arthroscopy. 1, Arthroscope portal location; 2, instrument portal location (if no instrument portal is needed, this site is used as the egress portal); 3, egress portal location.*

needle is located in the joint, fluid is easily instilled. If joint fluid is not aspirated, the needle is withdrawn slightly and aspiration is repeated. Occasionally, during insertion, the needle is advanced into the ligament of the head of the femur, preventing fluid aspiration. Also, as the joint cavity fills with fluid, reverse pressure is felt on the syringe plunger from the instilled fluid. This sensation ensures proper placement of the needle into the joint. The joint cavity is distended with 5 to 10 mL lactated Ringer's solution. Joint distension is maintained by leaving the syringe attached to the needle (the assistant must keep pressure on the plunger). Distension aids in correct positioning of the arthroscope portal. A no. 11 Bard-Parker blade is used to make a small entry wound

through the skin and superficial soft tissues adjacent to the needle. A scalpel blade should not be used to enter the joint because it is likely to cause extravasation of fluid outside the joint cavity. Another concern is the prevention of iatrogenic injury to the sciatic nerve, which courses caudal to the joint in the ischiatic notch. Because of the location of this nerve, caudal portals to the hip are not recommended (see Fig. 6–6). To ease insertion of the arthroscope cannula in heavily muscled dogs, blunt dissection with small Metzenbaum scissors can be performed through the stab incision. This method avoids injury from traumatic insertion that may occur when excessive force must be applied. The needle is removed, and the arthroscope cannula with the attached blunt

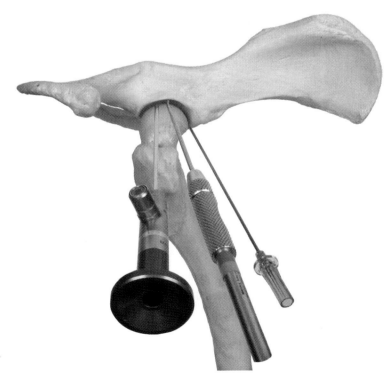

FIGURE 6–7 *Bone model showing the positioning of instruments for hip arthroscopy.*

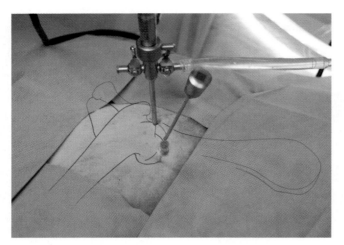

FIGURE 6-8 Instrument positioning for hip arthroscopy on a dog.

conical obturator is inserted in the same direction as the needle. The tip of the blunt obturator can be walked off the lateral edge of the dorsal acetabular rim to aid in localization of the joint space. When a blunt conical obturator is used, pressure is applied to penetrate the joint capsule. With experience, the surgeon will learn to determine by feel when the joint is entered. After the joint is entered, the obturator is removed from the cannula. Fluid flows freely from the cannula, confirming correct placement. The fluid ingress line is attached to the cannula, and the joint is lavaged for 10 to 15 seconds before the arthroscope is inserted to help obtain a clear fluid field.

The egress portal is established second (see Fig 6–8). A 18- to 22-gauge (2.5- to 3-inch) spinal needle is inserted approximately 2 cm cranial and 2 cm distal to the arthroscope portal. To avoid interfering with the light post, a needle that extends only slightly above the level of the skin is used. The needle is directed perpendicular to the limb. If the needle is placed properly, fluid flows from the needle hub. Evacuation of fluid maintains fluid flow through the joint and enhances visualization. Intravenous or suction tubing can be attached to the needle to capture fluid as it leaves the joint. Alternatively, fluid may be allowed to spill onto the floor for capture by a floor suction unit, a basin, or towels.

The instrument portal is established if a biopsy of intra-articular tissue is needed or if treatment of joint pathology is required (see Fig. 6–8). If a cannula system is used, the egress portal is converted to a portal that functions as both an instrument and an egress portal. If a cannula system is not used, a new egress portal is created slightly distal to the original portal and the instrument portal is placed at the site of the original egress portal. The craniocaudal and proximodistal position of the instrument portal relative to the greater trochanter can be estimated from the lateral radiograph. This site is often approximately 2 cm cranial to the scope portal. These numbers are only estimates, and the actual numbers will vary with the size of the dog. It is best to triangulate the instrument portal site relative to the position of the arthroscope tip.

Surgical Anatomy. Because the hip is a ball-and-socket joint, it is well suited for movement in all directions. However, although the hip can move in all directions, it primarily moves in flexion and extension. A combination of passive and active mechanisms provides joint stability. Passive mechanisms include the ligamentum teres, surrounding joint capsule, joint conformation, and synovial fluid cohesion. The ligamentum teres appears thick and courses from the fovea capitis of the femoral head to its origin in the acetabular fossa. The joint capsule originates from the periphery of the acetabulum, dorsal acetabular rim, and labrum. The labrum is a well-defined fibrocartilaginous band located between the acetabular rim and the joint capsule. The labrum continues as a free ligament (the transverse acetabular ligament) across the acetabular notch. The concavity of the acetabulum and the fit of the femoral head into the acetabulum provide joint stability. Contraction of the surrounding hip muscles provides dynamic active coxofemoral stability. These muscles include the gluteal, obturator, iliopsoas, and adductor muscles. Active contraction of the muscles of the hip causes compression across the hip joint and increases tension in the joint capsule.

When the arthroscope enters the joint, the camera should be positioned to provide correct spatial orientation when viewing the monitor. The proper spatial orientation and fore-oblique view is obtained when the controls on the camera head and the light post are upright (see Fig. 6–7). When the camera and light post are held in this position, the ligamentum teres and acetabular fossa are visible (Fig. 6–9). The articular cartilage of the medial and deep portions of the femoral head and acetabulum also can be seen (Fig. 6–10). The scope can be carefully withdrawn slightly to visualize the remaining surfaces of the articular cartilage on the proximal and lateral aspects of the femoral head and acetabulum. To improve visualization of the articular surfaces, the limb can be distracted to separate the joint surfaces and the hip can be adducted and rotated internally. The light post is positioned caudally to visualize the cranial compartment of the hip (Fig. 6–11). The surgeon should note the articular cartilage of the femoral head, the synovial membrane, and the recess of the joint capsule as it attaches to the femur cranially (see Fig. 6–11). The tip of the arthroscope is moved caudally and the light post is turned cranially to view the caudal joint compartment (Fig. 6–12). The surgeon should note the articular cartilage of the femoral head, the synovial membrane, and the recess of the joint capsule as it attaches to the femur caudally (see Fig. 6–12). The arthroscope and light post are returned to the original entry position to begin exploration of the acetabulum, the dorsal acetabular rim, the labrum, and the dorsal attachment of the synovial membrane (Figs. 6–13 and 6–14). The tip of the arthroscope is slowly and carefully retracted a small distance to avoid inadvertent displacement of the scope from the joint. Maintaining distraction of the limb can help to prevent displacement of the scope from the joint. The tip of the arthroscope is gently moved dorsally to view the dorsal compartment and joint capsule. The light

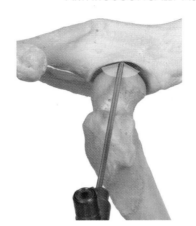

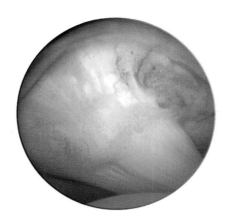

FIGURE 6-9 Positioning and normal joint findings for arthroscopic evaluation of the ligamentum teres (round ligament).

post is turned to view cranially or caudally. An example of a standard hip arthroscopic examination is to visualize and image each area of the joint as follows:

1. Ligamentum teres
2. Femoral head
3. Cranial joint pouch
4. Caudal joint pouch
5. Acetabulum
6. Acetabular labrum
7. Synovial membrane

Indications for Arthroscopic Surgery of the Hip Joint

Hip arthroscopy is a new treatment modality in small animal surgery. As small animal surgeons gain skill and experience, more conditions will be treated arthroscopically or with arthroscopic assistance. Potential indications include hip dysplasia, evaluation of the joint before triple pelvic osteotomy (TPO), osteoarthritis, hip dislocation, and diagnostic examination (biopsy or culture of bone, cartilage, or synovial membrane). In patients

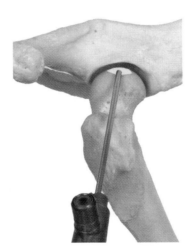

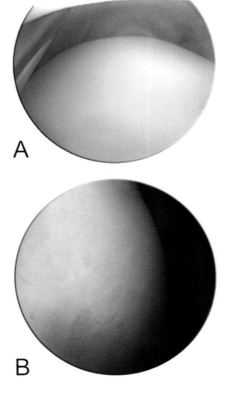

A

B

FIGURE 6-10 Positioning and normal joint findings for arthroscopic evaluation of the femoral head. *A,* Articular surface of the midportion of the femoral head; *B,* caudal aspect of the femoral head.

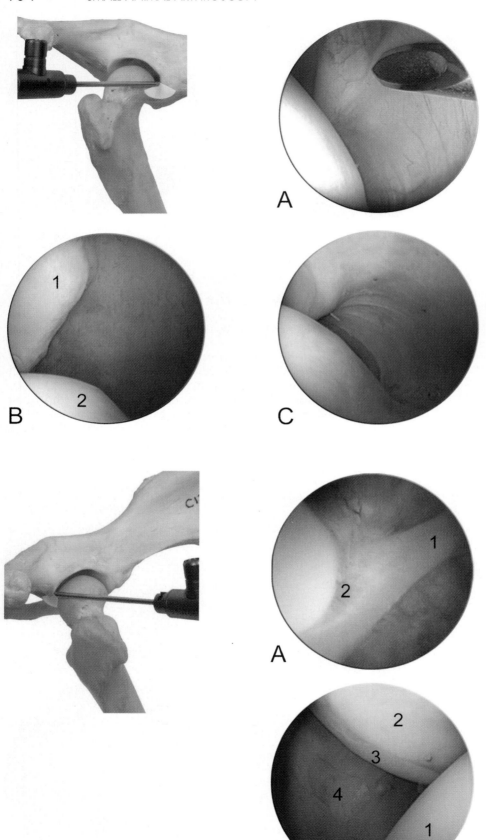

FIGURE 6-11 Positioning and normal joint findings for arthroscopic evaluation of the cranial joint pouch of the hip. *A,* Normal synovium and articular cartilage of the femoral head; *B,* normal appearance of the cranial aspect of the acetabulum (*1*) and femoral head (*2*); *C,* normal appearance of the cranial joint pouch and synovial attachments to the acetabulum and femoral head.

FIGURE 6-12 Positioning and normal joint findings for arthroscopic evaluation of the caudal joint pouch of the hip. *A,* Transverse acetabular ligament (*1*), extending from the cartilage labrum (*2*); *B,* normal appearance of the caudal femoral head (*1*), caudal acetabulum (*2*), cartilage labrum (*3*), and synovium (*4*).

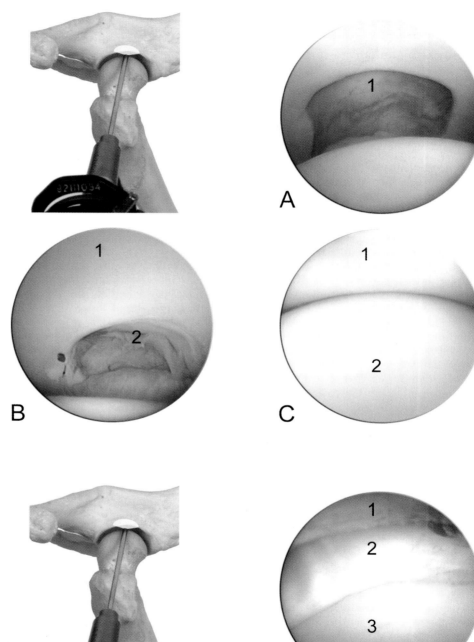

FIGURE 6–13 Positioning and normal joint findings for arthroscopic evaluation of the acetabulum. *A,* The origin of the round ligament in the acetabular fossa (*1*); *B,* normal appearance of the articular surface of the acetabulum (*1*) adjacent to the acetabular fossa (*2*); *C,* normal articulation of the acetabulum (*1*) and femoral head (*2*).

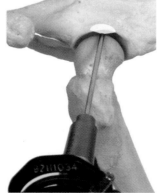

FIGURE 6–14 Positioning and normal joint findings for arthroscopic evaluation of the dorsal acetabular rim (*1*), the labrum (*2*), and femoral head (*3*).

with septic arthritis, arthroscopy also can be used to place a drain within the joint capsule to allow ingress and egress flushing.

Hip Dysplasia

History and Signalment. Dogs present with a wide variety of historical and clinical signs. Depending on the severity of hip instability and osteoarthritis, dogs may have symptoms that range from no known problem to marked lameness and difficulty rising. The condition is more common in large breeds, but any age or breed can be affected. Commonly affected breeds include the German shepherd, Labrador retriever, golden retriever, rottweiler, and chow chow. The owner typically reports a slow, progressive onset of clinical signs that may include difficulty rising, reluctance to play, decreased activity, reluctance to jump, hindlimb stiffness or lameness, pain, and a bunny-hopping gait.

Physical Examination Findings. Gait analysis may show obvious lameness; more often, however, lameness is difficult to detect during walking or trotting and is apparent only after exercise. Pain on extension of the hip and muscle atrophy are evident in most cases. Pain also may occur on abduction or rotation of the hip. An Ortolani test may show hip instability. The patient may assume an abnormal posture in the hindquarters, often standing with an arched low lumbar spine and the hind feet shifted cranially.

Differential Diagnosis. The differential diagnosis includes lumbosacral disease, rupture of the cranial cruciate ligament, discospondylitis, disease of the intervertebral disk, septic arthritis, sprain of the iliopsoas muscle, and strain of the ligamentum teres and joint capsule.

Radiographic Findings. Radiographic views include standard ventrodorsal and lateral projections of the pelvis. As the condition progresses, radiographic changes include coxofemoral subluxation and osteoarthritis. PENNHIP stress views, as described by Smith et al., can be used to evaluate the joint more completely and assist in prognostication. The condition of the dorsal acetabular rim can be evaluated with a skyline view (DAR view), as described by Slocum and Slocum.

Diagnosis. A complete orthopedic examination is essential to exclude other orthopedic problems. Hip stability should be assessed while the patient is adequately sedated or anesthetized. The hip should be assessed with an Ortolani test as well as by flexing, extending, abducting, and rotating the joint. The hip should be palpated to identify crepitus and estimate the depth of the acetabulum. The opposite hip also should be palpated because many cases are bilateral. Radiographic evaluation is used to confirm the diagnosis. Arthroscopic evaluation of the articular surfaces, dorsal acetabular rim, ligamentum teres, and joint capsule may be useful in assessing a patient with hip dysplasia,

especially if TPO is being considered (Figs. 6–15 through 6–21).

Treatment. Medical management provides symptomatic relief but cannot resolve hip dysplasia. Management includes NSAIDs, nutraceuticals, and other chondroprotectant agents. By improving joint congruity and stability, in many cases, TPO decreases the progression of osteoarthritis caused by hip dysplasia. Total hip replacement or femoral head and neck osteotomy may be performed in dogs that do not meet the criteria for TPO or those that have osteoarthritis that is not amenable to long-term medical treatment. Thermal contraction of a stretched ligamentum teres or joint capsule can be performed arthroscopically with a radiofrequency unit, but the clinical efficacy of this procedure is unknown (see Fig. 6–15G).

Anesthetic Considerations and Perioperative Pain Management. Preoperative laboratory workup is based on the patient's physical status and surgical risk. Young, healthy patients with no underlying systemic problems require minimal laboratory workup. Older dogs should undergo a complete blood screen, urinalysis, chest radiographs, and an electrocardiogram. Table 3–1 shows a standard anesthetic protocol, including preemptive pain medication. Postoperative pain is controlled with epidural analgesia, cold therapy, opioids, and NSAIDs.

Surgical Intervention. Portal sites and surgical anatomy were discussed earlier. The operative site is clipped and prepared according to the amount of limb maneuverability desired and the surgical procedure needed. A hanging limb preparation provides the greatest degree of freedom to manipulate the limb and is recommended. Liberal clipping and thorough sterile preparation are necessary because an open arthrotomy may be required. In most cases, a 2.7-mm, 30-degree fore-oblique arthroscope is used. Basic instrumentation includes probes to inspect the joint capsule. If the surgeon works through an instrument cannula, different-sized cannulas and switching sticks facilitate the surgery. A motorized shaver is helpful to débride synovial proliferation, but is not essential. If tissue ablation or thermal contracture is indicated, an electrothermal radiofrequency unit is necessary. The dog is positioned in lateral recumbency, with the leg to be operated on placed uppermost. The limb is supported in neutral position to prevent excessive adduction, which closes the joint space between the acetabulum and the femoral head. The limb also should be prepared in a manner that permits traction by an assistant or a traction device to separate the joint surfaces and allow easier insertion and manipulation of the arthroscope.

A guide needle is used to locate the joint space and the correct position for the arthroscope portal. Lactated Ringer's solution is instilled to distend the joint. The arthroscope is inserted, and ingress flow is established through the arthroscope cannula. The egress needle is established as described earlier. The arthroscope and light post are positioned to visualize the ligamentum

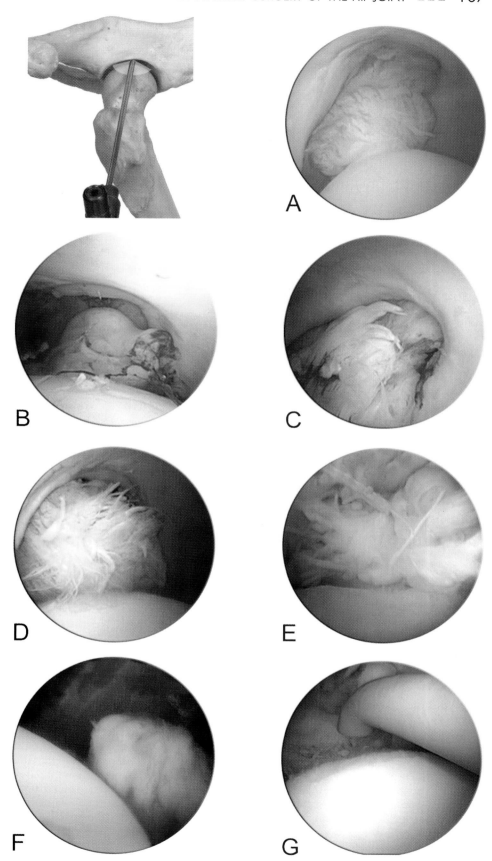

FIGURE 6–15 Positioning and abnormal joint findings for arthroscopic evaluation of the ligamentum teres in dogs with trauma and hip dysplasia. *A,* Swelling and neovascularization of the ligament; *B,* swelling and hemorrhage of the ligament; *C,* mild partial tear of the ligament; *D,* moderate partial tear of the ligament; *E,* severe partial tear of the ligament; *F,* complete tear of the ligament in a dog with a traumatic craniodorsal hip dislocation; *G,* shrinkage and débridement of the ligament with a radiofrequency probe.

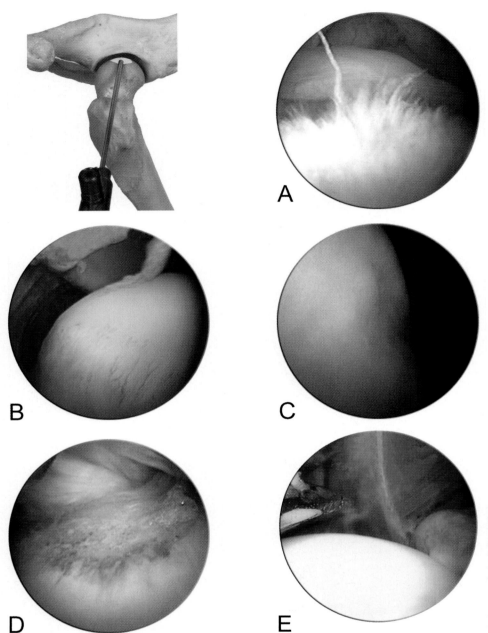

FIGURE 6–16 Positioning and abnormal joint findings for arthroscopic evaluation of the femoral head in dogs with trauma and hip dysplasia. *A,* Fibrillation of the articular cartilage (grade 2); *B,* neovascularization and early remodeling; *C,* partial-thickness cartilage erosion (grade 3); *D,* full-thickness cartilage erosion (grade 4); *E,* arthroscopic view of luxated coxofemoral joint.

teres and the articular surfaces of the medial compartment. The post cable is rotated cranially and the arthroscope tip is positioned caudally to allow the surgeon to examine the articular surfaces and joint capsule in the posterior compartment. The articular surfaces and joint capsule in the anterior compartment are examined by rotating the post cable caudally and positioning the scope tip cranially. The dorsal acetabular rim and joint capsule of the dorsal compartment are examined by withdrawing the scope slightly and positioning the tip dorsally. The post cable should be rotated in all directions to allow thorough evaluation of this region. If an instrument portal is required, a guide needle should be used to triangulate the position for the portal. The most common reason for failure to visualize the guide needle in the joint is crossing the arthroscope. To prevent crossing the arthroscope with the guide needle, the needle is inserted perpendicular to the skin surface. This orientation is maintained through the soft tissues. To verify the angle and the position for treatment with an instrument, the surgeon can simulate treatment with a guide needle. After the position for the instrument portal is established, a probe is inserted through a cannula or an open portal. Palpation and visualization may identify stretching of the ligamentum teres or joint capsule, but these conditions are not direct contraindications to TPO (see Fig. 6–15).

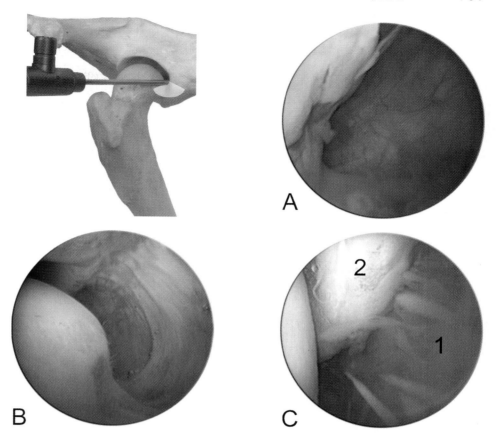

FIGURE 6-17 Positioning and abnormal joint findings for arthroscopic evaluation of the cranial joint pouch in dogs with hip dysplasia. *A*, Mild synovitis and femoral head remodeling; *B*, mild cartilage wear (grade 1) and remodeling; *C*, mild synovitis (*1*) and wear of the cranial margin of the acetabulum (*2*).

If the articular surfaces of the acetabulum or femoral head show excessive wear (see Figs. 6–16 to 6–21), the surgeon should consider abandoning a planned TPO. Other potential contraindications include tearing of the cartilaginous labrum, joint capsular tears, and wear of the dorsal acetabular rim (see Fig. 6–20). A radiofrequency unit may be used to contract the stretched connective tissue structures (see Fig. 6–15).

Postoperative Care. Cold therapy can be applied to the hip during recovery to relieve pain and reduce swelling. Cold therapy is applied by alternating 15 minutes on and 10 minutes off for two applications. Commercial cold packs or a commercial circulating cold water pack can be used. Alternatively, ice wrapped in a towel or frozen packs of vegetables can be used. If the dog is dismissed from the hospital on the day of surgery, NSAIDs and oral butorphenol (see Table 3–1) are dispensed for administration at home. If the dog remains in the hospital overnight, buprenorphine is administered in the evening as needed. Epidural administration is especially helpful for patients that undergo TPO. NSAIDs and butorphenol are dispensed for administration at home. NSAIDs are continued for 5 days, and butorphenol is discontinued after 48 hours. Cold therapy is continued by the client at home for the first 2 days after surgery if needed. In addition, the client should examine the portal sites daily for signs of irritation or drainage. Dogs under-

going arthroscopy use the leg immediately after surgery. Leash walking is recommended for 10 to 14 days before the patient resumes normal activity.

After TPO, activity is restricted to leash walking for 6 to 8 weeks. If the joint capsule is treated with thermal contracture, activity is restricted for 6 weeks to prevent overloading and stretching of the contracted collagen fibers during healing. Dogs that undergo arthroscopy use the leg immediately after surgery. Those that undergo TPO may be unable to bear weight initially, but usually can bear partial weight. To increase the weightbearing load on the limbs, walking at a slow pace is recommended. As postoperative time increases, the pace can be hastened. To increase the range of motion in the hip, the owner should walk the dog in high grass (e.g., weeds), shallow water, or sand, which forces the dog to pick up the feet and step high with the legs. After 6 weeks, the owner should begin limited amounts of free activity with controlled walking, starting with 5 minutes of free activity and increasing to 30 minutes over the next 2 weeks. After 8 to 10 weeks, free activity is gradually increased to normal levels. If during any exercise period (controlled or free activity), the dog becomes sore or is sore the next day, the owner should decrease the pace and return to controlled activity for 2 to 3 days.

Complications. Complications after hip arthroscopy are unusual. Occasionally, in the immediate postoperative

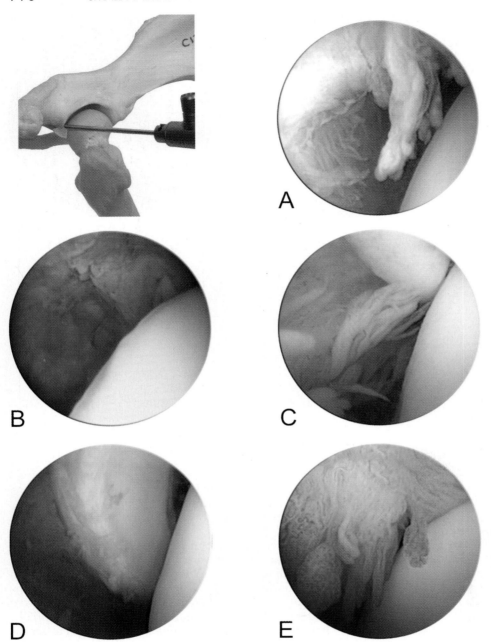

FIGURE 6-18 Positioning and abnormal joint findings for arthroscopic evaluation of the caudal joint pouch in dogs with hip dysplasia. *A,* Chronic synovitis; *B,* mild synovitis and wear of the cartilage of the femoral head; *C,* mild synovitis and normal cartilage; *D,* mild tear of the labrum, synovitis, and acetabular cartilage wear; *E,* marked synovitis and normal cartilage.

period, excessive fluid extravasation occurs and results in swollen soft tissues around the hip. The use of instrument cannulas can reduce this complication. This fluid resorbs within the first 24 hours. Residual mild swelling adjacent to the portal sites may be noticeable for the first 48 hours. Complications after TPO are uncommon as well. Occasionally, seromas occur and screws loosen prematurely. These conditions are treated conservatively by restricting activity in most patients.

Prognosis. The prognosis for satisfactory limb function after TPO is good in patients that are good candidates for the procedure. In patients with more extensive soft tissue injury, the prognosis is fair to good. If substantial wear of the articular cartilage of the acetabulum or femoral head is noted, the prognosis is guarded. The prognosis after total hip replacement and femoral head and neck excision is good.

Hip Dislocation

History and Signalment. Dogs present with acute hindlimb lameness. Most dogs cannot bear weight. Lameness is usually associated with a traumatic incident and is not responsive to anti-inflammatory medication. Any age or breed of dog can be affected.

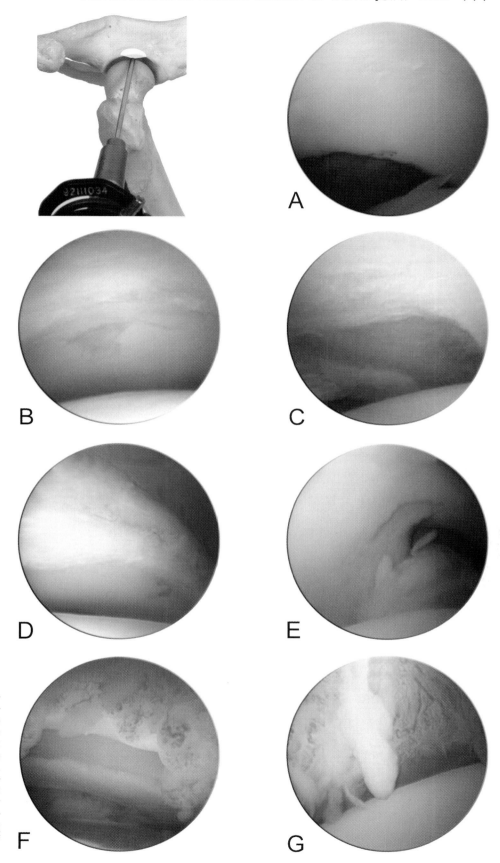

FIGURE 6–19 Positioning and abnormal joint findings for arthroscopic evaluation of the acetabulum in dogs with hip dysplasia. *A*, Mild cartilage wear (grade 1); *B*, mild cartilage wear (grade 2); *C*, severe cartilage wear with fissures and fibrillation (grade 4); *D*, synovitis, mild tear of the labrum, and mild cartilage wear of the acetabulum (grade 2); *E*, partial-thickness erosion of the articular cartilage (grade 3); *F*, full-thickness cartilage erosion (grade 4); *G*, extensive synovitis adjacent to the dorsal rim of the acetabulum.

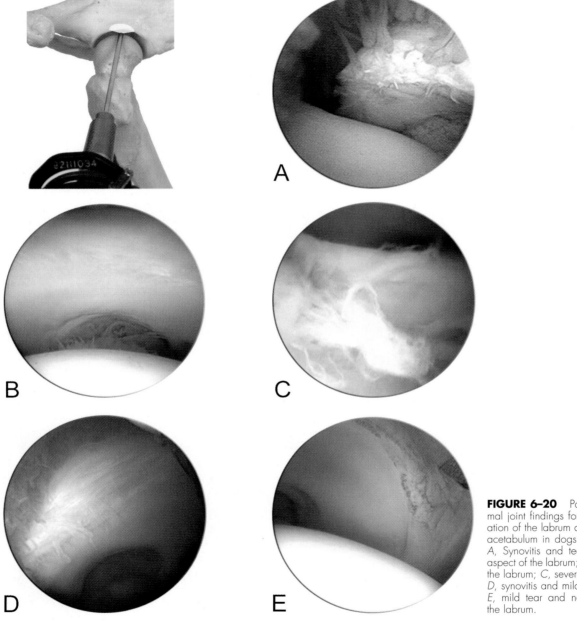

FIGURE 6–20 Positioning and abnormal joint findings for arthroscopic evaluation of the labrum and dorsal rim of the acetabulum in dogs with hip dysplasia. *A*, Synovitis and tearing of the cranial aspect of the labrum; *B*, early mild tear of the labrum; *C*, severe tear of the labrum; *D*, synovitis and mild tear of the labrum; *E*, mild tear and neovascularization of the labrum.

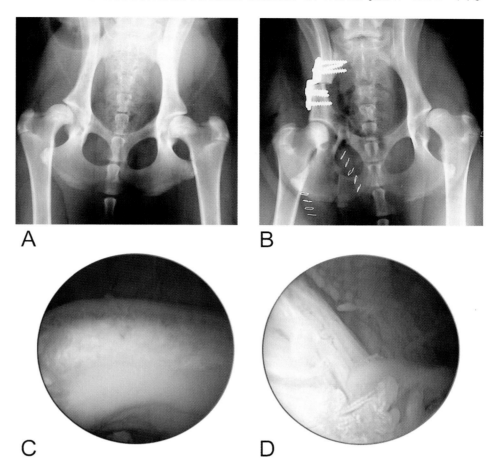

FIGURE 6-21 Arthroscopic evaluation of the hip can be used to help determine whether a patient is a candidate for triple pelvic osteotomy (TPO). *A,* Preoperative radiograph of a dog with bilateral hip dysplasia. *B,* Postoperative radiograph after TPO of the right hip; the left hip was not considered a candidate because the cartilage labrum and articular cartilage were damaged (see *D*). *C,* Arthroscopic image of the right hip showing only mild wear of the cartilage labrum; this hip is considered an acceptable candidate for TPO surgery. *D,* Arthroscopic image of the left hip showing extensive tearing of the labrum and erosion of the acetabular cartilage; this hip is considered an unacceptable candidate for TPO surgery.

Physical Examination Findings. Gait analysis shows visible lameness. Swelling is usually palpable in the hip region. Manipulation of the hip elicits discomfort in most dogs. Most dislocations are craniodorsal. The greater trochanter can be palpated in a more craniodorsal position when its position is compared with the wing of the ilium and the ischiatic tuberosity. The limb is usually held slightly abducted and externally rotated. The limb appears shortened as a result of dorsal displacement of the femoral head. Ventral hip dislocations are much less common. The limb is usually abducted and the greater trochanter is displaced slightly medially.

Differential Diagnosis. The differential diagnosis includes hip dysplasia, pelvic or femoral fracture, and sacroiliac luxation.

Radiographic Findings. A lateral radiographic view is usually diagnostic. A displaced femoral head can be seen in the craniodorsal or ventral position. A ventrodorsal radiograph clearly shows the dislocation but may be painful to acquire if the patient is not anesthetized or heavily sedated.

Diagnosis. The diagnosis is based on the history, physical findings, and radiographic findings. The patient should be carefully evaluated for preexisting hip dysplasia and osteoarthritis.

Treatment. Medical management can relieve pain, but definitive therapy with closed reduction or surgery is needed. Initially, closed reduction should be attempted in the anesthetized patient. Traction is applied while the limb is maintained in external rotation and adduction. Countertraction is placed on the inguinal region to facilitate hip reduction. As the femoral head is repositioned, the limb is rotated internally and abducted to reduce the femoral head within the acetabulum. If the reduction is secure, an Ehmer sling is applied for 10 to 14 days. Alternatively, an ilioischial pin (Devita pin) is placed in closed fashion. Currently, arthroscopic intervention is used on a limited basis to visualize the condition of the articular surfaces of the coxofemoral joint and remove avulsion fragments. This method may be used more extensively in the future (see Figs. 6–15 and 6–16).

Anesthetic Considerations and Perioperative Pain Management. Preoperative laboratory workup is based on the patient's physical status and surgical risk. Young, healthy patients with no underlying systemic problems require minimal laboratory workup. Older dogs should undergo a complete blood screen, chest radiographs, and an electrocardiogram. Table 3–1 shows a standard anesthetic protocol, including preemptive pain medication. Postoperative pain is controlled with epidural analgesia, cold therapy, opioids, and NSAIDs.

Surgical Intervention. Other comprehensive small animal surgery texts describe specific methods of surgical repair. Arthroscopy is not routinely used to manage hip dislocation. Early experience with arthroscopy in dogs with hip dislocation suggests that it is useful for evaluating the condition of the articular surfaces and removing avulsion fragments. Other applications may become available in the future.

Portal sites and surgical anatomy were discussed earlier. The operative site is clipped and prepared according to the amount of limb maneuverability required during surgery. A hanging limb preparation provides the greatest degree of freedom for manipulating limb position and is usually recommended. Liberal clipping and thorough sterile preparation are necessary because an open arthrotomy may be required. In most cases, a 2.7-mm, 30-degree fore-oblique arthroscope is used. Basic instrumentation includes probes to inspect the joint capsule. If the surgeon works through an instrument cannula, different-sized cannulas and switching sticks facilitate the surgery. The dog is positioned in lateral recumbency with the leg to be operated on placed uppermost. The limb is supported in neutral position to prevent excessive adduction, which closes the joint line between the acetabulum and the femoral head.

If possible, closed reduction is performed before arthroscopic evaluation is done. The femoral head and ligamentum teres can be evaluated in an extra-articular position (see Figs. 6–15 and 6–16). The scope is inserted after careful palpation of the dislocated hip. A guide needle is used to locate the joint space and the correct position for the arthroscope portal if reduction is accomplished. The arthroscope is inserted and ingress flow is established through the arthroscope cannula. The egress needle is established as described earlier. Extravasation of fluid is likely to occur if the joint capsule tears. Excessive extravasation can make surgical intervention more difficult. The arthroscope and light post are positioned to visualize the torn ligamentum teres and articular surfaces of the femoral head (see Figs. 6–15 and 6–16). The articular surfaces and joint capsule in the posterior compartment are examined by rotating the light post cranially and positioning the scope tip caudally. The articular surfaces and joint capsule in the anterior compartment are examined by rotating the light post caudally and positioning the scope tip cranially. The dorsal acetabular rim and joint capsule of the dorsal compartment are examined by withdrawing the scope slightly and positioning the scope tip dorsally. The light post should be rotated in all directions to allow the surgeon to evaluate this region thoroughly.

If closed reduction is not possible, the scope portal is established near the normal location. If the femoral head is located craniodorsally, the scope enters the acetabulum in a portal that is caudal to the greater trochanter. The femoral head is evaluated with a scope portal that is placed in the typical position in relation to the greater trochanter. Traction is applied to the limb to return the femoral head to as near a normal anatomic position as possible. The femoral head can be evaluated arthroscopically, but the acetabulum may be difficult to examine because of the malpositioned femoral head. If reduction is possible, routine arthroscopic evaluation can be performed to evaluate the condition of the articular surface. If reduction is not possible, a craniolateral approach to the hip should be performed to evaluate the condition of the articular surface.

If an instrument portal is required, a guide needle is used to triangulate the position for the instrument port. To prevent crossing the arthroscope with the guide needle, the needle is inserted perpendicular to the skin surface, and this orientation is maintained through the soft tissues. After the position for the instrument portal is established, a probe is inserted through a cannula or an open portal. If the articular surfaces of the acetabulum or femoral head show excessive wear, the surgeon should consider arthroplasty rather than reduction and stabilization.

If open reduction is necessary, the surgeon must decide whether to reduce and stabilize the hip or perform a total hip replacement, femoral head and neck excision, or TPO. The surgeon may use a variety of techniques to stabilize the hip joint after open reduction, including placement of a prosthetic joint capsule, imbrication of the joint capsule, placement of a toggle-pin, transposition of the greater trochanter, placement of an iliofemoral antirotational suture, and TPO. These techniques are described in detail in veterinary surgical textbooks and journals.

Postoperative Care. If an Ehmer sling is not used, cold therapy can be applied to the hip during recovery to relieve pain and reduce swelling. Cold therapy is applied by alternating 15 minutes on and 10 minutes off for two applications. Commercial cold packs or a commercial circulating cold water pack can be used. Alternatively, ice wrapped in a towel or frozen packs of vegetables can be used. If the dog is dismissed from the hospital the day of surgery, NSAIDs and oral butorphenol (see Table 3–1) are dispensed for administration at home. If the dog remains in the hospital overnight, buprenorphine is administered in the evening. NSAIDs and butorphenol are dispensed for administration at home. NSAIDs are continued for 5 days, and butorphenol is discontinued after 48 hours. Cold therapy is continued by the client at home for the initial 2 days after surgery if needed. The client also should examine the portal sites daily for signs of irritation or drainage. Leash walking is recommended for 4 weeks before the dog resumes a progressive increase in activity. To increase the weight-bearing load on the limbs, walking at a slow pace is recommended. As postoperative time increases, the pace can be hastened. To increase the range of motion in the hip when walking, the client should walk the dog in high grass (e.g., weeds), shallow water, or sand to force the dog to pick up the feet and step high with the legs. After 6 weeks, the owner should begin limited amounts of free activity with controlled walking, starting with 5 minutes of free activity and increasing to 30 minutes over the next 2 weeks. After 8 weeks, free activity is gradually increased to normal levels. If during any exercise period (controlled or free activity), the dog becomes sore or is sore the next day, the owner should decrease the pace and return to controlled activity for 2 to 3 days.

Complications. Complications are unusual. Occasionally, excessive fluid extravasation occurs and results in swollen soft tissues around the hip in the immediate postoperative period. This fluid resorbs within the first 24 hours. Residual mild swelling adjacent to portal sites may be noticeable for the first 48 hours. Complications with closed reduction of a traumatic dislocation are usually associated with recurrent dislocation or wounds associated with bandaging. Complications associated with open reduction and surgery vary with the technique used, but may include recurrent dislocation, implant failure, seroma, and infection.

Prognosis. Unless preexisting hip dysplasia is present, the prognosis for satisfactory limb function after reduction of a dislocated hip is good. If the hip remains reduced 1 month after closed or open reduction, recurrent dislocation is uncommon. If the articular cartilage of the acetabulum or femoral head shows substantial wear, the prognosis is guarded because of the probability of progressive osteoarthritis.

References

Slocum B, Slocum TD: Pelvic osteotomy for axial rotation of the acetabular segment in dogs with hip dysplasia. Vet Clin North Am Small Anim Pract 22(3):645–682, 1992.

Smith GK, Beiry DN, Gregor TP, et al: New concepts of coxofemoral joint instability and the development of a clinical stress-radiographic method of quantitating hip joint laxity in the dog. J Am Vet Med Assoc 196:59, 1993.

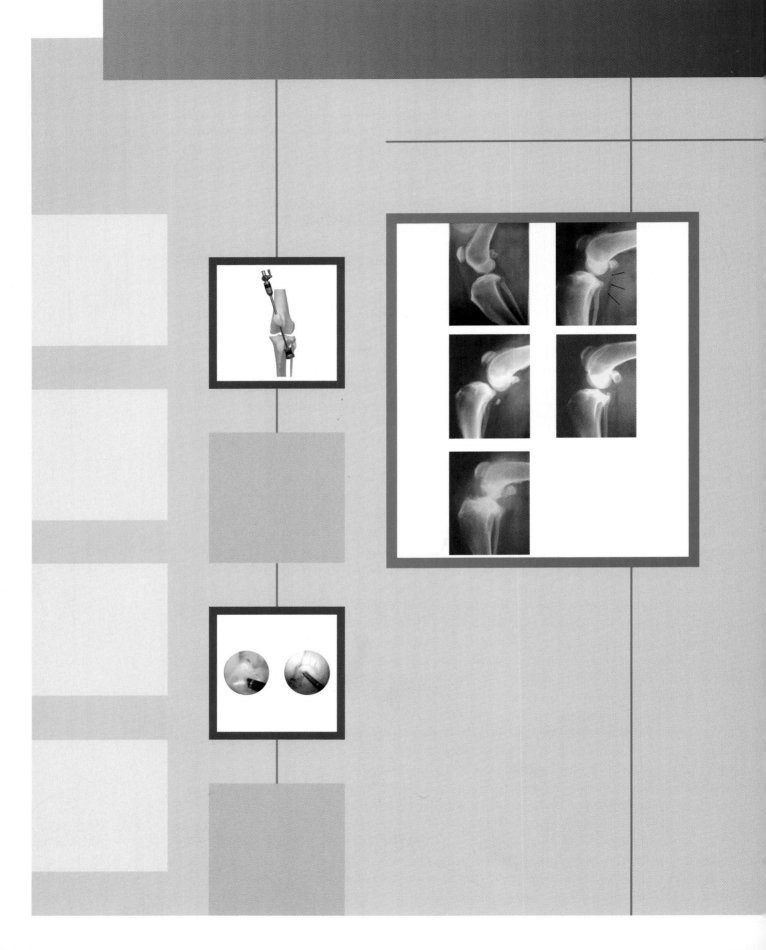

Arthroscopically Assisted Surgery of the Stifle Joint

Wayne O. Whitney

Introduction

Before they attempt to treat clinical cases, surgeons must master basic triangulation skills and become familiar with arthroscopic equipment, instrumentation, and viewing angles. A quality instructional course is well worth the investment. Surgeons who master the basic skills can practice the techniques on bell peppers, sawbones, and cadavers.

Unlike the shoulder and elbow, adequate stifle visualization requires the use of a motorized shaver and electrocautery as well as flow management. Each of these components has an associated learning curve. Another difference between these joints is that the stifle readily bleeds during arthroscopic examination as a result of hyperemia of the synovium and patellar fat pad in response to inflammation. Quick, effective, and precise intraoperative hemostasis is necessary. The formation of periarticular osteophytes is rapid and intense. In addition, periarticular fibrosis and thickening may be pronounced in chronic cases and may make arthroscopy more difficult, especially when the surgeon attempts to access the medial and lateral compartments. If the surgeon has little experience with stifle arthroscopy or if arthroscopic treatment does not resolve the problem, the surgeon should be prepared to convert the procedure to an open arthrotomy. In addition, the surgeon should expect initial cases to proceed slowly and therefore should schedule plenty of time. Once the techniques are mastered, arthroscopic examination and treatment procedures often are much quicker and more accurate than conventional arthrotomy, and the need to convert to an open procedure is rare.

High-quality support staff and precision teamwork are essential. Patient positioning and setup may be laborious and can greatly lengthen anesthesia times if the team is not well trained. The surgeon is highly dependent on a trained assistant because it is not practical for the surgeon to reach for instruments. The assistant plays a vital role in intraoperative limb positioning for proper visualization. Providing arthroscopic fluid support, offering external technical support, and monitoring the patient are demanding tasks for the circulating nurse. Without appropriate teamwork, the length of the procedure, the number of complications, and the level of frustration are all increased. However, after the team masters the necessary skills, arthroscopy typically provides accurate joint examination and treatment with minimal invasion, scarring, and patient discomfort, and rapid return to function.

Arthroscopic Surgery of the Stifle Joint

Equipment and Instrumentation. Appropriate high-quality equipment is essential. Necessary components include a high-resolution monitor, light source (at least a 300-W halogen lamp; xenon is better), high-quality light cable, motorized shaver, sharp shaver blades (disposable), and tissue ablation unit.

A 2.7-mm, 30-degree fore-oblique arthroscope is ideal for most stifles. Both long and short scopes are acceptable. Longer scopes offer better depth of field and require less focusing, but both types have adequate length for large dogs. Short scoops are preferred by some surgeons because they can be easier to manipulate. Arthroscopes that screw directly into the camera are preferred (Fig. 7–1A). Scopes with long eyepieces also work well, are less expensive, and are preferred by some surgeons (see Fig. 7–1B); however, they require a coupler that increases the distance between the camera and the light post. This increased distance makes it difficult to rotate the light post (to change viewing direction) with the same hand that holds the camera. The inability to rotate the light post with one hand becomes a problem when the opposite hand is holding a treatment instrument. Also, couplers occasionally pose fogging problems that are not encountered with C-mount scopes. Extremely long scopes tend to flex considerably and make it more

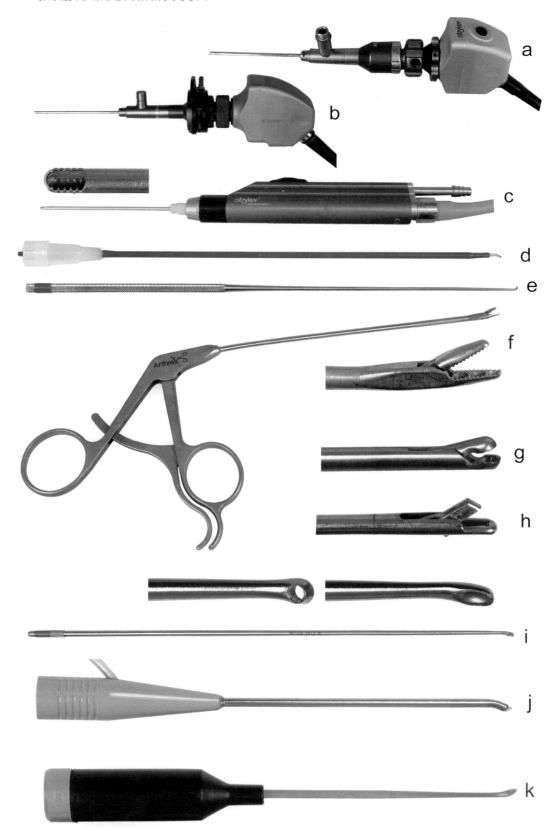

FIGURE 7-1 Instrumentation for stifle arthroscopy. *a,* A C-mount arthroscope with a camera attached. The scope screws directly into the camera. *b,* A 2.7-mm, 30-degree short arthroscope with a coupler and camera attached. *c,* A motorized shaver shown with an aggressive shaver blade. *d,* Arthroscopic electrocautery tip. *e,* Right-angle probe. *f,* Locking small-joint graspers. *g,* Clamshell biopsy forceps. *h,* Straight basket punch. *i,* Ring curette (*left*) and 5–0 curette (*right*). *j,* Bipolar radiofrequency probe. *k,* Monopolar radiofrequency probe.

difficult to cross the trochlear ridges to enter the lateral and medial compartments from the trochlear groove.

Blades of many types, names, and sizes are available for specialized use; however, a 3.5- or 4.0-mm full-radius blade works for most problems encountered in most stifle joints. Shaver blades can be resterilized and reused two or three times, but this practice is not ideal. Small motorized shaver handpieces commonly used in the elbow and shoulder can be used, but larger motorized shaver handpieces are quicker and more durable and are preferred for use in the stifle. After the surgeon becomes comfortable with this blade, more aggressive "toothed" shaver blades (see Fig. 7–1C) can be used to shorten débridement time, but these teeth can more easily cause iatrogenic damage to the articular cartilage. More aggressive (quicker) shaving of tissue is possible with a large handpiece and a larger (4.0-mm) aggressive blade. In giant breeds 5.0-mm blades can be used. Soft tissue is removed in oscillatory mode, and bone and firm cartilage are removed in forward mode. For aggressive bone removal, such as notchplasty, a hooded burr can be used in high-speed forward mode. Alternatively, a blade can be used in high-speed forward mode.

Although it is not mandatory for other joints, some form of specialized intra-articular electrocautery is necessary to control intraoperative hemorrhage in the stifle (see Fig. 7–1D, J, and K). Many instruments are available as disposable handpieces that fit electrocautery consoles that are available in most operating rooms (see Fig. 7–1D). Although these units work well for hemostasis, they are inadequate for most tissue ablation needs (e.g., partial meniscectomy).

Useful hand instruments include a small-joint probe, a small locking grasping forceps, a small-joint curette, a small clamshell forceps to obtain biopsy specimens, and small straight or 15-degree up-biter forceps (basket punch) (see Fig. 7–1E through I). However, even the smallest instruments usually are too large to perform atraumatic partial meniscectomy in dogs. Basket punches and scissors often are too large to open without causing iatrogenic damage to the articular cartilage. Tissue ablation wands are both ideal and necessary for this purpose but require the use of a separate console (see Fig. 7–1J and K). Many have fine tips that can be used for both intra-articular electrocautery and tissue ablation, eliminating the need to use an electrocautery unit for hemostasis alone. The same console accepts slightly larger tips for wider ablation needs. The most important attribute of the tissue ablation wand is its size because it is used primarily for partial meniscectomy within a tight joint space. A probe that is malleable is also important, especially for partial meniscectomy. Very fine tips are used to incise the separate "handles" of bucket handle tears, and slightly larger (approximately 2-mm) rounded-tip probes are ideal for ablation. Both bipolar (ArthroCare) (see Fig. 7–1J) and monopolar (Vulcan EAS by Oratec-Smith and Nephew) versions are available (see Fig. 7–1K). Tissue ablation wands can be used to ablate the fat pad and the cruciate ligament remnants, but this procedure often is faster with a motorized shaver and blade.

A large-diameter fenestrated cannula (Fig. 7–2A) is needed for outflow because hyperplastic synovium often obstructs a single opening. A conical-tipped switching stick (see Fig. 7–2B) is used to place the outflow cannula.

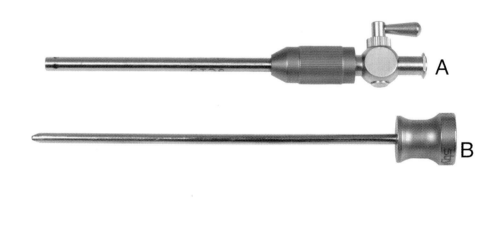

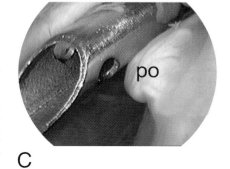
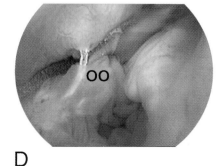

FIGURE 7–2 Outflow instrumentation for stifle arthroscopy. A, A 4.0-mm–diameter multifenestrated cannula. B, Conical-tipped obturator (switching stick) for an outflow cannula. C, Outflow cannula in the medial compartment of the stifle joint, adjacent to periarticular osteophytes (po). D, Cannula that is partially obstructed by the synovium (oo), showing the need for multiple fenestrations.

A fluid ingress pump is helpful but not mandatory. The additional cost of specialized large-diameter intravenous tubing usually is recovered with saved time for both the surgeon and the support staff. A large-volume collection bottle is helpful for the same reason. If gravity ingress is used, large-diameter tubing is necessary to distend the joints adequately.

Anesthetic Considerations and Perioperative Pain Management. Preoperative laboratory evaluation is based on the patient's physical status and surgical risk. Older dogs should undergo a complete blood screen, urinalysis, chest radiographs, and an electrocardiogram. Table 3–1 shows a standard anesthetic protocol, including preemptive pain medication. Long-acting epidural analgesia is routinely used when more severe postoperative pain is anticipated [e.g., tibial plateau leveling osteotomy (TPLO)], but is not necessary for less involved procedures [e.g., osteochondritis dissecans (OCD), diagnostic or second-look arthroscopy]. If an epidural is not performed, local anesthetic (bupivacaine) is instilled into the joint at the conclusion of the procedure. Postoperative pain is controlled with cold therapy, opioids, and nonsteroidal anti-inflammatory drugs (NSAIDs). If arthroscopy is completed early in the day, the patient may be dismissed from the hospital that same afternoon; if arthroscopy is completed later in the afternoon, the patient is discharged the next day. In all cases, cold therapy is recommended as often as possible for 48 hours by alternating 15 minutes on and 10 minutes off for two applications. Commercial cold packs or crushed ice in Ziploc bags can be used. To increase comfort, a thin towel is placed between the cold pack and the skin. The cold pack is applied, followed by layers of towels to insulate the area from the surrounding room temperature. The cold therapy is continued at home when possible for the first 2 days after surgery, especially after walking.

All patients receive preemptive analgesic drugs as part of the premedication protocol. Buprenorphine is preferred because of its effectiveness in patients that have mild to moderate postoperative pain and its relatively long mode of action (6 to 8 hours). When the dog is dismissed from the hospital, NSAIDs and oral butorphanol (Table 3–1) are dispensed for administration at home. NSAIDs are continued for 5 days, and butorphanol is discontinued after 48 hours. If the dog remains in the hospital overnight, a second dose of buprenorphine is administered in the evening. NSAIDs and butorphanol are prescribed for home administration. Alternate methods of pain management, such as transdermal fentanyl patches, can be applied the day before surgery.

Patient Preparation and Positioning. Figure 7–3 shows the arrangement of the operating room for right stifle arthroscopy. The leg is prepared as for open arthrotomy, and the patient is positioned in dorsal recumbency on a vacuum beanbag so that both legs can hang from the end of the table. The table is tilted head-up approximately 30 degrees. The beanbag is positioned to allow the leg to hang straight without deviating to one side (Fig. 7–4A and B). The opposite leg is secured laterally, and the front legs and beanbag are stabilized to prevent the patient from sliding off the table (see Fig. 7–4A and B). Alternately, a metal leg-holding device

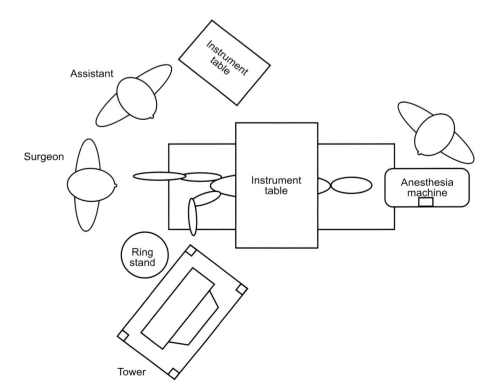

FIGURE 7–3 Arrangement of the operating room for right stifle arthroscopy. The ring stand is used to hold the arthroscope and shaver when they are not in use.

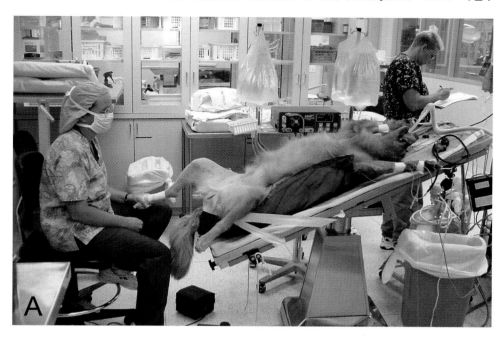

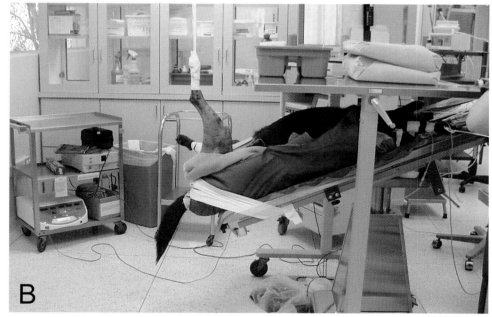

FIGURE 7–4 Positioning of the dog for stifle arthroscopy before draping. *A*, The table is tilted head-up approximately 30 degrees, and a vacuum beanbag is placed under the treated leg to allow it to hang freely. The contralateral leg is placed in an out-of-the-way position. The table and chair are adjusted to a comfortable height for the surgeon and assistant, who are seated. *B*, The instrument table is positioned over the patient, and the leg is hung for aseptic preparation.

affixed to the table can be used. These devices are not readily available commercially and must be constructed. The leg is aseptically prepared, and 10 to 15 mL bupivacaine and epinephrine can be instilled (optional) intra-articularly before the setup procedure is completed (15 to 20 minutes before surgery). The patient is draped as for open surgery because in many cases an additional open procedure is performed (Fig. 7–5). A sterile fluid collection bag may be placed below the stifle (see Fig. 7–5) to aid in keeping the operating area dry. When bilateral stifle arthroscopy is indicated, both legs are prepared in a similar fashion.

Portal Sites. To treat stifle pathology (especially meniscal pathology), portals are placed more distally than what was originally described for diagnostic arthroscopy. Once the technique is mastered, portals can be established in less than 1 minute. The disadvantage of more distal placement of the cranial medial and cranial lateral portals is that the fat pad interferes with visualization. As a result, a motorized shaver, intra-articular electrocautery, and proper flow management are essential for adequate visualization. More distal placement of the portals allows better diagnostic probing and treatment angles for meniscal pathology. Figure 7–6

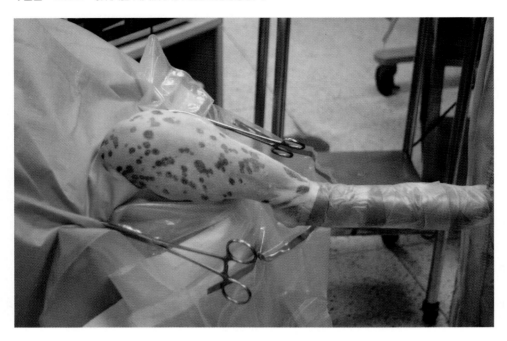

FIGURE 7–5 Sterile preparation of a patient for stifle arthroscopy. The leg is draped with water-impermeable drapes, and a fluid collection bag attached to suction is positioned below the stifle.

shows the landmarks, order and location of portal placement, and important neurovascular anatomy.

The craniolateral portal is established first. Just lateral to the patellar tendon, an eminence of the tibial plateau (known as Gerdy's tubercle in man, unnamed in the dog) is appreciated with deep palpation. This landmark is important because it corresponds to the level of the

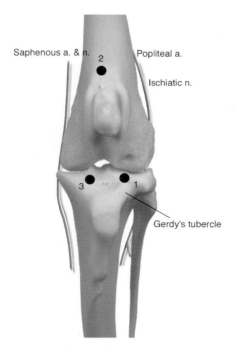

FIGURE 7–6 Cranial view of a bone model showing the portal locations, order of portal establishment, and pertinent anatomy for canine stifle arthroscopy. *1,* Primary arthroscopy portal; *2,* outflow portal; *3,* primary instrument portal.

menisci. A portal that is too proximal will cause difficulty in visualizing and treating the menisci. A portal that is too far lateral may make it difficult to enter the medial compartment and can be interfered with by the long digital extensor tendon. A single (no. 11 blade) stab incision is made into the joint capsule at the level of Gerdy's tubercle, just lateral (1 to 2 mm) to the straight patella tendon (see Fig. 7–6). It is not necessary to first place a needle into the joint because the palpable landmarks are reliable and further distending the joint with fluid may make Gerdy's tubercle difficult to appreciate. Before the arthroscope is introduced, a conical-tipped switching stick is inserted to establish the proximal medial outflow portal. The leg is placed in extension, and the switching stick is gently directed into the cranial lateral portal and through the femoropatellar joint directly beneath the patella until it exits the skin just medial to the quadriceps tendon. The tip of the switching stick is forced bluntly through the joint capsule and skin (Figs. 7–7A and 7–8A). If the tip of the switching stick is blunt instead of conical, it may be necessary to incise the skin. Failure to position the leg in full extension to relieve tension on the quadriceps and patella will make insertion more difficult as well as increase the likelihood of iatrogenic trauma to the articular cartilage. To prevent entrapment of the skin, the proximal outflow cannula must be sized appropriately to fit tightly over the exposed tip of the switching stick. The cannula is slid over the switching stick and into the joint until the cannula tip rests directly beneath the patella (see Figs. 7–7B and 7–8B). The switching stick is removed, and the outflow cannula is repositioned deep into the medial joint compartment adjacent to the medial trochlear ridge of the femur (see Fig. 7–7C and 7–8C). The cannula tip usually must be placed slightly cranially to help it slide over the medial trochlear ridge of the femur, again with the leg in full extension.

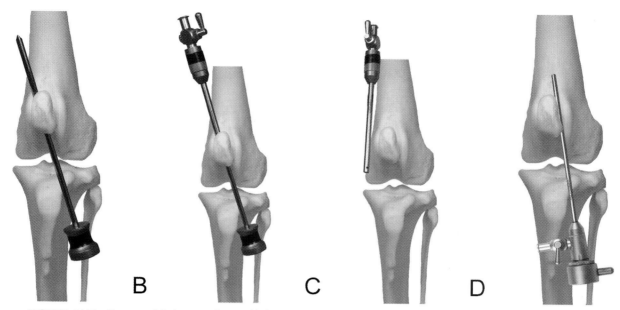

FIGURE 7–7 Bone model showing the establishment of a proximal outflow cannula and insertion of an arthroscope cannula. *A,* With the stifle in full extension, the conical-tipped switching stick is inserted through the craniolateral portal and beneath the patella. Then it is forced through the joint capsule and skin just medial to the quadriceps tendon. *B,* The outflow cannula is slid over the switching stick and advanced into the joint until its tip rests directly beneath the patella. *C,* The switching stick is removed, and the cannula tip is repositioned deep within the medial joint compartment. *D,* The arthroscope cannula with a blunt obturator is inserted in a similar fashion through the same lateral portal but directly toward the midline. When the instrument reaches the proximate joint capsule, the surgeon usually recognizes that a "dead end" has been reached.

Again with the leg in full extension, the scope cannula is introduced with a conical or blunt obturator into the same craniolateral portal and slowly advanced beneath the patella until the tip rests on the midline in the proximal aspect of the proximal pouch (see Figs. 7–7D and 7–8D). A "dead end" usually can be appreciated. The obturator is removed, and inflow is established through the scope cannula with lactated Ringer's solution. Standard suction tubing is used to attach the outflow cannula to a high-volume suction bottle or another collection mechanism. The joint is lavaged with lactated Ringer's solution for 15 to 20 seconds to clear the joint of synovial fluid and blood before the arthroscope and light source are attached. Figures 7–9, 7–10, and 7–11 show correct arthroscopic positioning, proper orientation of the light post, and normal findings in the proximal joint as well as routine findings in the same anatomic locations in stifles with acute compared to chronic changes.

Surgical Anatomy. The most significant difference between open arthrotomy and arthroscopy is the increased ability to see synovial changes, abnormalities of the articular cartilage, and more subtle meniscal and ligamentous tears with arthroscopy. This increased visibility occurs primarily because the anatomy, particularly the synovium and articular cartilage, is greatly magnified, intensely illuminated, and seen floating within a fluid environment. The arthroscopic appearance of normal synovium is dependent on the area of the joint that is being inspected. It is predominantly pale pink, smooth,

and somewhat translucent, with few short villi. The exception is in the most distal aspects of the medial and lateral pouches, where villi are more prominent (both in length and number) but are still thin, wispy, and filamentous in the normal joint. Tiny blood vessels usually can be seen within the villi. With pathology, especially pathology involving the cranial cruciate ligament, the synovium quickly undergoes hyperplastic change and becomes more reddened, vascular, and less translucent. The villi become much longer and thicker but are still filamentous. With more chronic change, the villi become more club-shaped, appear thicker, and sometimes appear shorter. In chronic cases, the villi may appear slightly grayish.

It is not uncommon to see a mixed population of these changes in the villi. These changes are not unique to the stifle and may be similar, but less intense, in the shoulder and elbow. A horizontal plica may be seen as a variation of normal in the superior pouch, just proximal to the proximal pole of the patella and just caudal to the quadriceps tendon (see Fig. 7–9B). Synovial changes also are seen adjacent to large periarticular osteophytes. Occasionally, the synovium has a fibrotic, cobblestone appearance, with few villi where it chronically rubs against the osteophytes. The intensity of the synovial reaction may vary, but the locations of the changes are consistent. Early synovial changes may be reversible if the underlying condition is detected and resolved promptly.

Intra-articular fat is normally yellowish, light and frothy, and similar to a Nerf ball in appearance (Fig. 7–12A). Similar fat often is seen in the normal suprapatellar (or

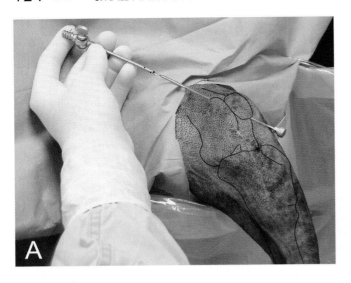 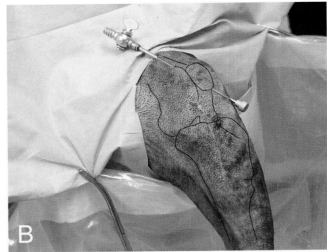

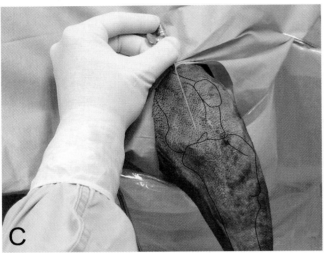 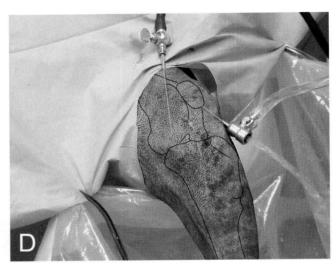

FIGURE 7-8 Establishment of a proximal outflow cannula and insertion of an arthroscope cannula with a blunt obturator in a live dog. *A,* A switching stick obturator is inserted through the lateral portal, under the patella, and through the joint capsule and skin. It exits just medial to the quadriceps tendon. *B,* An outflow cannula is placed over the switching stick obturator until the tip of the cannula is directly beneath the patella. *C,* The outflow cannula is repositioned into the medial joint compartment. *D,* The arthroscope cannula is shown in the lateral portal after the blunt obturator is removed and ingress is established through the scope cannula. The joint is lavaged and the outflow cannula is attached to a high-volume suction collection bottle.

supratrochlear) joint pouch, proximal to the trochlear groove (see Fig. 7–9A). If pathology is present in the stifle, the hypertrophic synovitis quickly becomes intense throughout the knee, especially just caudal to the fat pad (see Fig. 7–12B). The fat pad may become much more dense and vascular as a result of chronic inflammation (steatitis). If chronic disease is present, the fat pad may become fibrotic and thickened but usually is still vascular.

In dogs with cranial cruciate ligament injury, periarticular osteophytes form rapidly and are apparent arthroscopically within 3 to 4 weeks. These changes are not specific to cranial cruciate ligament injury but are less intense when seen with other stifle pathology. They occur in three predicable locations: the proximal trochlear groove, the medial trochlear ridge of the femur, and the lateral trochlear ridge of the femur (see Figs. 7–9D,

7–10C, and 7–11C). The size and number of changes are directly related to chronicity. In some joints, they occur within the trochlear notch. If examination is performed before osteophytes develop, neovascularization of the articular cartilage may occur in the location of future osteophyte sites. Neovascularization is seen as small spider web–like networks of vessels that appear on the surface and penetrate the periphery of the articular cartilage on the medial and lateral femoral condyles and at the proximal extent of the trochlea (see Figs. 7–9C, 7–10B, and 7–11B).

Because of this intense inflammatory reaction in pathologic joints, only the proximal joint is examined before the anterior medial instrument portal is established. Examination of the intra-articular ligaments, menisci, and weightbearing surfaces requires arthroscopic débridement and hemostasis.

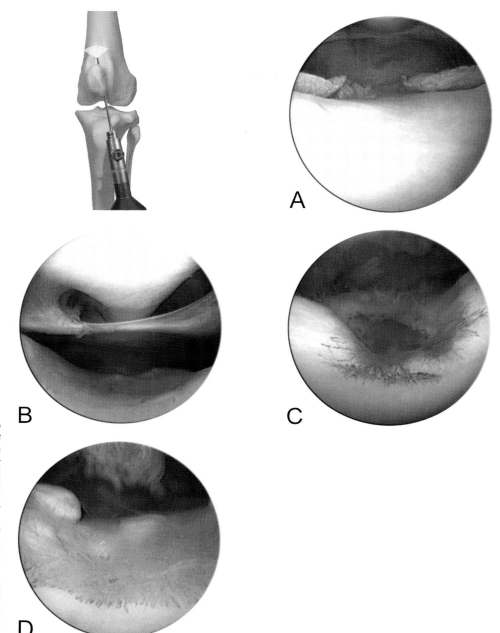

FIGURE 7-9 Positioning of the arthroscope, orientation of the light post, and superior (suprapatellar) pouch views of typical findings during exploration of the proximal stifle in a normal dog, a dog with an acute (<3 weeks) cranial cruciate ligament injury, and a dog with a chronic cranial cruciate ligament (months) injury. *A*, Normal findings. *B*, A horizontal plica, which is a variation of normal. The quadriceps tendon is seen directly above the horizontal plica. *C*, Acute changes. Neovascularization of the articular cartilage is seen before osteophytes develop. *D*, Chronic changes. Periarticular osteophytes and hyperplastic synovitis are seen. Note the penetration of blood vessels into the articular cartilage.

Arthroscopic Exploration of the Proximal Stifle. The proximal stifle (supratrochlear pouch, lateral and medial pouches) is explored before the craniomedial instrument portal is established. The cruciate ligaments and menisci usually cannot be examined at this time because they are obscured by hyperplastic synovium and the fat pad. A 2.7-mm short or long, 30-degree oblique arthroscope is introduced, and the proximal joint is systematically explored in the following order: superior (supratrochlear) pouch and proximal trochlear groove (see Fig. 7–9), lateral pouch and lateral trochlear ridge (see Fig. 7–10), and medial pouch and medial trochlear ridge (see Fig. 7–11). The trochlear ridges of the femur are closely inspected because periarticular

osteophytes commonly form in these areas. The synovium is inspected in all pouches, and the articular cartilage is examined for evidence of neovascular invasion, chondromalacia, and fibrillation. Figures 7–9 to 7–11 show the proper scope positioning and light post orientation to provide ideal viewing angles (scope direction). The light post is rotated 180 degrees to visualize the quadriceps tendon, the proximal and distal poles of the patella, and the articular surface of the patella and its articulation with the trochlear groove. Photographs of the proximal stifle should be taken for the medical record and should include the proximal trochlear groove, patella, and the proximal and distal aspects of the medial and lateral trochlear ridges. Attempts to inspect

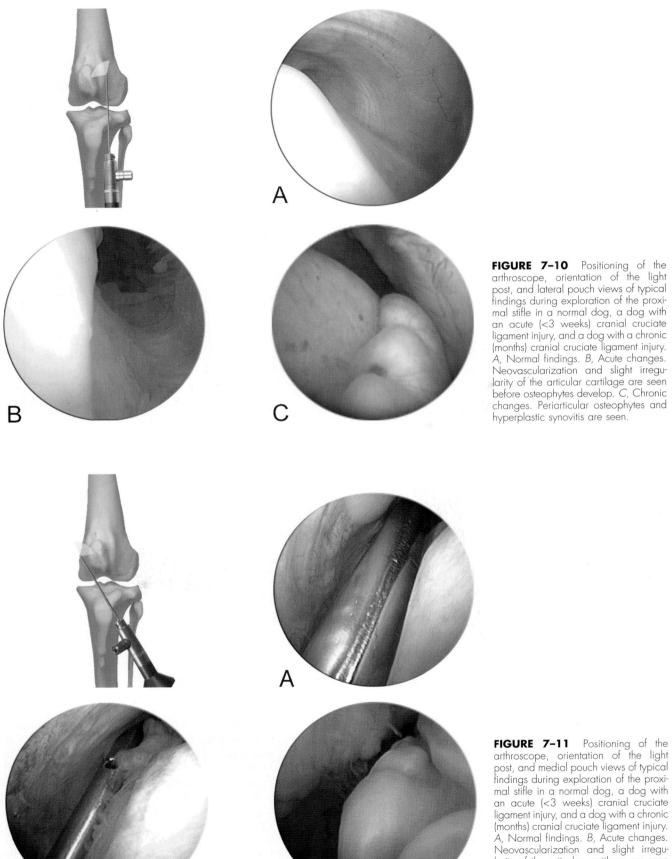

FIGURE 7-10 Positioning of the arthroscope, orientation of the light post, and lateral pouch views of typical findings during exploration of the proximal stifle in a normal dog, a dog with an acute (<3 weeks) cranial cruciate ligament injury, and a dog with a chronic (months) cranial cruciate ligament injury. *A,* Normal findings. *B,* Acute changes. Neovascularization and slight irregularity of the articular cartilage are seen before osteophytes develop. *C,* Chronic changes. Periarticular osteophytes and hyperplastic synovitis are seen.

FIGURE 7-11 Positioning of the arthroscope, orientation of the light post, and medial pouch views of typical findings during exploration of the proximal stifle in a normal dog, a dog with an acute (<3 weeks) cranial cruciate ligament injury, and a dog with a chronic (months) cranial cruciate ligament injury. *A,* Normal findings. *B,* Acute changes. Neovascularization and slight irregularity of the articular cartilage are seen before osteophytes develop. *C,* Chronic changes. Periarticular osteophytes and hyperplastic synovitis are seen.

pathologic joints further without débridement with a motorized shaver are time-consuming and frustrating. Figures 7–9 to 7–11 show the typical appearance of a normal proximal stifle as well as acute (<3 weeks) and chronic (months) cranial cruciate ligament injuries.

Cranial Medial Portal Establishment. The cranial medial portal is the primary instrument portal; however, sometimes it is beneficial to interchange the scope and instrument portals. The tip of the arthroscope is positioned just cranial to the intercondylar notch, with the notch in the field of view (Fig. 7–12). To minimize obstruction by the inflamed synovium and fat pad, the tip of the arthroscope is placed close to the midline of the trochlear articular cartilage and the knee is slowly flexed to bring the notch into view. Often, the notch cannot be visualized if marked synovitis is present. Occasionally, the notch is visible only as a tiny slit as a result of the formation of osteophytes within the trochlear notch.

Without moving the scope or the limb, the craniomedial portal is established with a similar stab incision just medial to the straight patellar tendon and at the same level as the cranial lateral portal. A blunt obturator is inserted as a "trailblazer," and its tip is visualized just cranial to the intercondylar notch. Visualization at this point may be almost completely obliterated by inflamed synovium and a frothy or steatotic fat pad (see Fig. 7–12). Often, it is helpful to "feel" the shaft of the scope

with the obturator tip and then to slide the obturator toward the scope tip to bring it into view. After the tip of the obturator is in view (Fig. 7–13), the surgeon should steady the leg and the scope, remove the obturator, and introduce a motorized shaver (3.5- to 4.0-mm full-radius blade) at the same angle and direction (see Fig. 7–13). The orifice of the shaver is visualized (positioned up) (Fig. 7–14A), suction is attached, and the fat pad is carefully débrided to create a "viewing window" just cranial to the intercondylar notch. The shaver should be set at 1800 to 2700 RPM in the oscillatory mode (see Fig. 7–14B). Initially, the shaver is held steady while suction pulls adjacent tissue into the orifice for débridement. As débridement proceeds, the shaver is slowly rotated and moved to enlarge the viewing window. Once the femoral articular cartilage is in view, débridement can proceed more aggressively, although the surgeon must take care not to débride the remnants of the cranial cruciate ligament before they are inspected and photographed. Adequate flow is imperative because hemorrhage is likely. Before attempting to cauterize bleeders, the surgeon should attempt to obtain a viewing window that is at least three times the diameter of the shaver. With a smaller window, the source of bleeding is much more difficult to locate. Small bleeders are managed by increasing the flow rate while the viewing window is created. Large bleeding vessels are controlled with electrocautery or a radiofrequency unit through the same craniomedial portal. Inflow may be temporarily

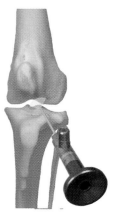

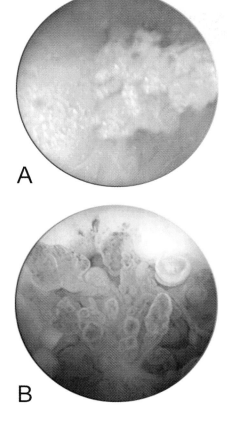

FIGURE 7–12 Positioning of the arthroscope and orientation of the light post immediately before the medial instrument portal is established. The intertrochanteric notch is often obliterated by a frothy fat pad in the normal joint (A) and by hyperplastic synovium in dogs with cranial cruciate ligament injury (B).

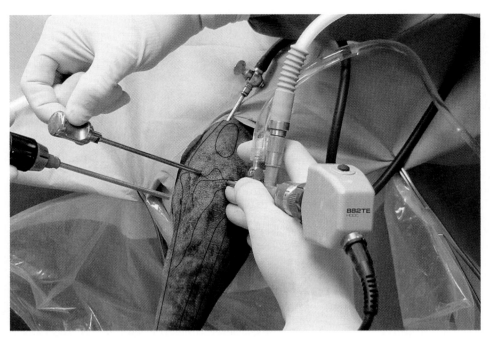

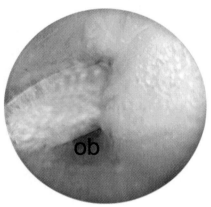

FIGURE 7-13 Establishment of a medial instrument portal and insertion of a motorized shaver. A blunt obturator (*ob*) is inserted into the medial portal, and its tip is visualized within the fat pad. The shaver is positioned adjacent to the obturator at the same angle and direction, and the obturator is removed.

increased to dilute hemorrhage and to slow the rate of bleeding by increasing intra-articular pressure until hemostasis is obtained with electrocautery. To prevent subcutaneous extravasation of fluid, lower flow rates are restored after hemostasis is obtained. The viewing window must be developed distally enough to allow proper visualization and treatment of the menisci. This treatment includes removal of the tough, leading caudal edge of the fat pad just proximal to the intermeniscal ligament. It is often helpful to partially remove or transect this tissue with a punch or an ablation wand to give the shaver an "edge" to facilitate shaving. Alternately, this tissue can be caramelized with a tissue ablation wand.

Arthroscopic Exploration of the Intra-articular Structures. After the viewing window reaches the level of the intermeniscal ligament and hemostasis is achieved, the cranial cruciate ligament and caudal cruciate ligament are inspected. Each structure is palpated with a small-joint probe. Figure 7–14C shows the typical appearance

of the normal cruciate ligaments. The two distinct bands of the cranial cruciate ligament are readily apparent. Articular cartilage is carefully inspected and probed for areas of chondromalacia, fibrillation, or eburnation. These lesions are described in the section on osteoarthritis. Correct portal placement is critical to allow for adequate visualization and treatment of menisci.

Inspection of the Medial Meniscus. Visualization of the caudal aspect of the medial meniscus often is best obtained with the joint in approximately 30 degrees of flexion, external rotation, and valgus stress. The light post is positioned medially (3 o'clock for a right leg and 9 o'clock for a left leg). The arthroscope must be maneuvered laterally and just cranial to the insertion of the cranial cruciate ligament to obtain the desired view (Fig. 7–15). Visualization is much easier if the torn cranial cruciate ligament is débrided (see the discussion of cranial cruciate ligament injuries). With the caudal aspect of the medial meniscus visualized, the cranial tibial thrust maneuver is performed several times to aid

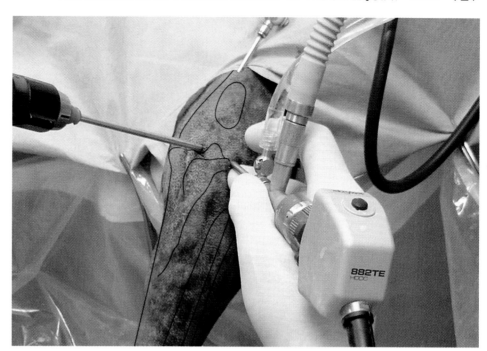

FIGURE 7-14 Establishment of a medial instrument portal, insertion of a motorized shaver, and débridement of the fat pad. The obturator is removed, and the shaver is inserted at the same angle and direction. *A,* After the orifice of the shaver is visualized, the shaver is attached to suction and shaving is begun with minimal movement. *B,* After enough tissue is removed to improve visualization, the shaver is moved and rotated until a viewing window (*vw*) is established to reveal the femoral condyle (*fc*). The surgeon should note the appearance of the femoral articular cartilage. *C,* Normal appearance of the caudal cruciate ligament (*cdcl*) and cranial cruciate ligament (*crcl*), showing the two distinct bands of the cranial cruciate ligament.

in the detection of nondisplaced bucket handle tears. The menisci are probed carefully to detect tears. The oyster curl, or flounce, of the meniscal edge is normal (see Fig. 7–15) but is not always seen and can be influenced by stressing the joint. Inspection is often aided by hooking the anterior horn of the meniscus with a probe and retracting it cranially. If the tissue is normal,

photographs are taken at this point. If pathology is detected, photographs are taken both before and after treatment. The anterior horn of the medial meniscus usually is best seen with the light post at the 10 o'clock position for a right leg and at the 2 o'clock position for a left leg. Various types of meniscal tears and the principles of treatment are discussed later.

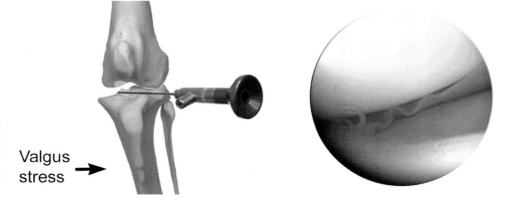

FIGURE 7-15 Positioning of the arthroscope and orientation of the light post for visualization of the caudal aspect of the medial meniscus. Valgus stress is placed on the distal limb. The medial meniscus, including the oyster curl, or flounce, is normal.

Inspection of the Lateral Meniscus. Figure 7–16 shows the proper arthroscope position and light post orientation for inspection of the lateral meniscus. Varus stress is applied with the knee in approximately 30 degrees of flexion, although the angle can vary. If the cranial cruciate ligament has been débrided, the large, easily identified meniscofemoral ligament (see Fig. 7–16B) is inspected first. For a left leg, the light post is positioned in the 9 o'clock position. The 3 o'clock position is used for a right leg. The meniscal edge is followed antero-laterally by slowly withdrawing the arthroscope to visualize its termination at the meniscotibial attachment cranially. Common arthroscopic appearance and treatment recommendations are discussed later.

Indications for Arthroscopic Surgery of the Stifle Joint

In humans, the knee is the most common site for arthroscopic procedures. The most common procedures are reconstruction of the anterior cruciate ligament and treatment of meniscal injury. Although isolated meniscal injury is not common in dogs as it is in humans, the incidence of cranial cruciate ligament rupture in dogs is high. Cranial cruciate ligament rupture represents both the greatest need and the greatest challenge in canine arthroscopy. Lameness caused by complete or partial tear of the cranial cruciate ligament is common, but the diagnosis is often delayed. Unlike in humans, osteo-arthritis advances rapidly (within weeks) in large-breed dogs that have complete rupture of the cranial cruciate ligament. Osteoarthritis also advances rapidly in pal-pably stable stifles that have only partially torn cranial cruciate ligaments, emphasizing the need for early diagnosis and treatment. Many veterinarians are reluctant to perform exploratory arthrotomy in the absence of palpable instability. Arthroscopy provides a minimally invasive means of obtaining an early diagnosis of partial tears before these changes occur; moreover, it is readily accepted by pet owners. Arthroscopic examination of a normal joint causes minimal postoperative lameness or morbidity that typically resolves within a day. Compared with arthrotomy, arthroscopy allows for more accurate assessment of partial tears of the cranial cruciate liga-ment, synovial pathology, articular cartilage pathology, and meniscal injuries. Meniscal tears can be treated more precisely, and partial or complete cranial cruciate ligament remnants can be more thoroughly débrided than with an open technique. When used in conjunction with various intra-articular and extra-articular tech-niques, arthroscopy reduces morbidity. Regardless of the surgeon's preference of stabilization technique, arthroscopy allows for more precise assessment, intra-articular débridement, and meniscal treatment without the pain associated with cutting the highly innervated joint capsule as performed with traditional arthrotomy.

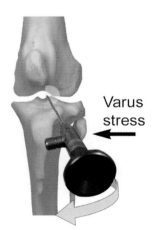

Varus stress

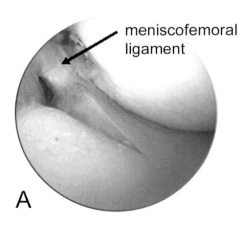

meniscofemoral ligament

A

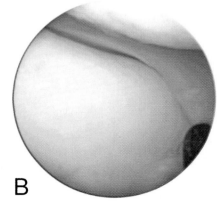

B

FIGURE 7-16 Positioning of the arthroscope and orientation of the light post for visualization of the lateral meniscus. Varus stress is placed on the distal limb, and the cranial cruciate ligament remnants have been removed. *A,* The meniscofemoral ligament (*arrow*) at the caudal horn. This structure must be visualized and preserved during débride-ment of the remnants of the cranial cruciate liga-ment. *B,* The midbody of the lateral meniscus is normal. The arthroscope is maneuvered medially to follow the edge of the meniscus cranially to visualize the anterior horn, the area where radial tears are commonly seen. The curved arrow represents the path of the arthroscope.

Other successful applications of arthroscopy in the stifle include the diagnosis and treatment of OCD lesions of both the lateral and medial femoral condyle, repair and débridement of avulsion fractures of the cranial cruciate ligament and caudal cruciate ligament, débridement of septic osteomyelitis, removal of implants, and percutaneous placement of temporary transarticular pins. The benefits of arthroscopic synovectomy as an adjunct to the medical management of chronic osteoarthritis are just beginning to be realized. Poststabilization late-onset meniscal injury in dogs previously treated for cranial cruciate ligament rupture can be readily diagnosed and treated without arthrotomy. Finally, the research implications for arthroscopically transected cranial cruciate ligament and caudal cruciate ligament studies, meniscal studies, drug efficacy studies, and serial reevaluations to evaluate the response to various osteoarthritis treatments and stabilization procedures are tremendous. However, the greatest benefits of arthroscopy are more accurate patient assessment, more precise intra-articular treatment, decreased postoperative pain, earlier return to function, preservation of range of motion, and minimal scarring.

Injuries of the Cranial Cruciate Ligament

Many clinicians are concerned about the increasing incidence of cranial cruciate ligament injuries in healthy athletic dogs, especially retrievers, and the growing incidence of this injury in younger adult dogs. The etiology of these injuries is unknown. Several authors speculate that increased tibial slope predisposes dogs to rupture of the cranial cruciate ligament, although the role of tibial slope in this injury is not known. Neutralization of active cranial tibial thrust likely plays an important role in the efficacy of stabilization techniques, especially in light of patient compliance, which is typically poor.

The cranial cruciate ligament loses strength with age, and this degenerative process likely plays a significant role in its clinical pathophysiology. Most cranial cruciate ligament injuries likely begin as partial tears that eventually become complete tears. Most clinicians believe that partial tears seldom heal with conservative treatment and almost invariably become complete tears. This tendency may explain why many dogs have a history of low-grade intermittent lameness before they become dysfunctional and require treatment. Clinicians must recognize the signs of partial cranial cruciate ligament ruptures to aid in early diagnosis. Arthroscopic examinations of dogs with chronic lameness as a result of partial cranial cruciate ligament ruptures show severe synovial hyperplastic changes, the formation of periarticular osteophytes, and advanced osteoarthritis, even though these dogs have palpably stable knees under general anesthesia. However, radiographic findings are rarely normal in dogs with partial tears, although the abnormal findings may be subtle. Early intervention with arthroscopic examination is recommended to confirm partial tears prior to the rapid onset of osteoarthritis. Arthroscopic examination has negligible morbidity (if negative), and most stabilization techniques can be arthroscopically assisted during the same examination when a partial tear is confirmed. This approach decreases both surgical morbidity and the advancement of osteoarthritis due to delayed intervention. It is a common misconception that a "wait-and-see" approach with symptomatic treatment is appropriate if the knee lacks cranial drawer.

The primary advantage of arthroscopically assisted treatment is more accurate assessment and more precise treatment of intra-articular pathology, especially if the menisci and articular surfaces are affected. Also, torn ligament remnants can be more thoroughly débrided. Additionally, scarring is minimal, and postoperative lameness and pain are greatly reduced because disruption of the highly innervated joint capsule is minimized.

History and Signalment. All breeds are affected, spayed females are overrepresented, and dogs can be affected at any age over 1 year of age. The incidence of avulsion fractures is higher in juvenile dogs. Most dogs have lameness of varying degree. Many cases are precipitated by adrenalin-associated everyday activities, such as a quick start or torsional movement, but in some cases, no precipitating event is associated with the onset of lameness. In competitive athletes, such as field trial participants, lameness may become apparent during or after work.

Most dogs with partial tears present with a history of weightbearing lameness that may be intermittent and that usually can be overridden with excitement. Lameness often resolves with rest and NSAIDs and is exacerbated by exercise. Occasionally, dogs are sound for several days or weeks before they have a recurrence. Dogs may sit with the affected leg slightly extended laterally because they are reluctant to fully flex the stifle. Dogs that have partial tears usually present with low-grade to moderate lameness, but some may have a short history of inability to bear weight. In many cases, the excitement associated with the hospital visit masks the lameness. Bilateral partial tears are occasionally seen, and dogs may have a history of shifting leg lameness, difficulty rising, and reluctance to get up or walk. In addition, many dogs have a history of low-grade unilateral rear leg lameness. As noted earlier, most partial tears eventually progress to complete tears.

Dogs that have complete tears may have acute or chronic weightbearing or non-weightbearing lameness. In some reportedly acute cases, careful review of the history shows previous intermittent low-grade lameness prior to becoming more severely lame. Some cases truly are acute or appear acute because a partial tear becomes a complete tear or sudden meniscal damage occurs. With time, most non-weightbearing cases become partially weightbearing, but lameness persists. Most dogs sit with the hock and affected stifle extended away from the body, and some owners report an audible popping that usually is related to displacement of a bucket handle tear of the medial meniscus. Bilateral complete tears are common and are often misdiagnosed as spinal cases because the dog may appear ataxic or paretic as a result of the effort to bear as much weight on the front legs as possible. These patients often have a history of unilateral rear leg lameness, and many are unable or unwilling to rise.

Physical Examination Findings. Weightbearing lameness is the most common finding, but some dogs have non-weightbearing lameness. Most patients have palpable joint effusion, which may be subtle. In chronic cases, a palpable medial buttress routinely can be appreciated by simultaneously palpating each stifle for medial thickening. Thickening is most apparent in dogs with chronic complete rupture but occurs to a lesser extent in those with chronic partial rupture.

Classically, dogs with complete tears have a palpable anterior drawer and a positive finding on the cranial tibial compression test (cranial tibial thrust). This result may be difficult to appreciate in large dogs unless they are under anesthesia or heavy sedation, or in chronic cases due to fibrosis of the joint capsule or other secondary restraint mechanisms. In dogs with a bucket handle tear of the medial meniscus, a dull pop may be palpated during the cranial tibial compression test or cranial drawer testing. Most cases have palpable stifle joint effusion, but this finding may be subtle. Most are uncomfortable when the stifle is manipulated, especially in hyperextension, but this discomfort may be difficult to elicit.

Partial tears are difficult to diagnose. A high index of suspicion is warranted because many large dogs with occult rear leg lameness have partial cruciate tears. Joint effusion may be appreciated with palpation. Asymmetrical stifle discomfort on hyperextension is a reliable sign and usually exacerbates lameness. This test can be performed in sedated dogs that are difficult to examine. Flexion may cause a painful response, and flexion testing for 20 to 30 seconds may exacerbate lameness. Most dogs sit with the affected leg extended, with the hock positioned away from the body. Patients with partial tears may have no cranial drawer or only subtle cranial drawer. Because of this, patients should be carefully examined under general anesthesia. Testing should be performed in both flexion and extension and compared to the contralateral stifle. If the anterior medial band is markedly torn, examination shows subtle anterior drawer in flexion only with an ill-defined endpoint. It is important to realize that partial tears frequently have stable knees in both flexion and extension.

Differential Diagnosis. The differential diagnosis includes medial patellar luxation, osteochondrosis, hip dysplasia, panosteitis (in young dogs), lumbosacral disease, intervertebral disk disease (in bilateral cranial cruciate ligament rupture), septic discospondylitis, calcaneal tendon disease, and septic arthritis.

Radiographic Findings. Most partial and complete ruptures can be preliminarily diagnosed radiographically. Radiographs typically show nonspecific changes that suggest cranial cruciate ligament rupture. Radiographic diagnosis is based on the finding of swelling of the joint capsule, formation of periarticular osteophytes, and occasionally, cranial and proximal translation of the tibia.

The first and most subtle radiographic finding in acute cases is soft tissue swelling in the caudal joint. Lateral radiographs show increased soft tissue density in the caudal joint causing obliteration or caudal deviation of the fat line of the gastrocnemius muscle planes in the popliteal fossa. Similar soft tissue swelling causes loss of the triangular detail of the infrapatellar fat pad in the cranial joint (Fig. 7–17B). The soft tissue changes are the same for partial and complete tears. In some cases of complete rupture, cranial and proximal translation of the tibia in relation to the femur is seen as mild to severe subluxation (see Fig. 7–17C). In subacute cases (3 to 6 weeks), early formation of osteophytes may be noted, especially on the proximal and distal poles of the patella and the medial and lateral trochlear ridges of the femur (see Fig. 7–17D). In chronic cases (months), these osteophytes may be large and may be accompanied by similar changes along the medial, lateral, and caudal aspects of the tibia (see Fig. 7–17E). Subchondral sclerosis may be present.

Diagnosis. Diagnosis is based on history, physical findings, radiographic findings, and if necessary, confirmation during arthroscopic examination.

Treatment. Conservative treatment consists of NSAID therapy, chondroprotective agents, weight control, and regular low-impact exercise. Without surgical intervention, most patients have persistent lameness and rapid progression of osteoarthritis. Large dogs appear to progress more rapidly than smaller dogs but studies documenting this are lacking. Some small patients eventually become sound without treatment, but recovery is greatly hastened by surgical intervention. If advanced osteoarthritis is present, surgery may not alleviate the need for concurrent conservative treatment.

Anesthetic Considerations and Perioperative Pain Management. Aspirin is discontinued at least 1 week before surgery. Ideally, Cox II inhibitor NSAIDs are discontinued 1 to 2 days before surgery, but discontinuation is not mandatory. Healthy, young patients require minimal preoperative laboratory evaluation. Older patients should be adequately screened to exclude underlying metabolic disorders. Preferred pain management includes preoperative long-acting epidural opioid therapy, cold therapy for 48 hours (20 minutes on and 20 minutes off as often as possible), use of a fentanyl transdermal patch for 4 days, and administration of NSAIDs for 15 to 30 days. Alternately, parenteral and oral opioids can be used, with or without NSAID therapy, especially in patients that are sensitive to NSAIDs. Surgical pain is reduced considerably when the intra-articular component of the procedure is performed arthroscopically because disruption of the highly innervated joint capsule is minimized. Additionally, intra-articular injection of 10 to 15 mL bupivacaine with epinephrine 15 to 20 minutes before and immediately after surgery provides analgesia to help reduce the concentration of inhalant anesthetics and improve recovery in patients not treated with epidural opioids. Intra-articular opioids such as morphine may also be given and may be superior to other routes of administration.

Surgical Intervention. Most small dogs (<15 kg) undergo repair with various open lateral imbrication

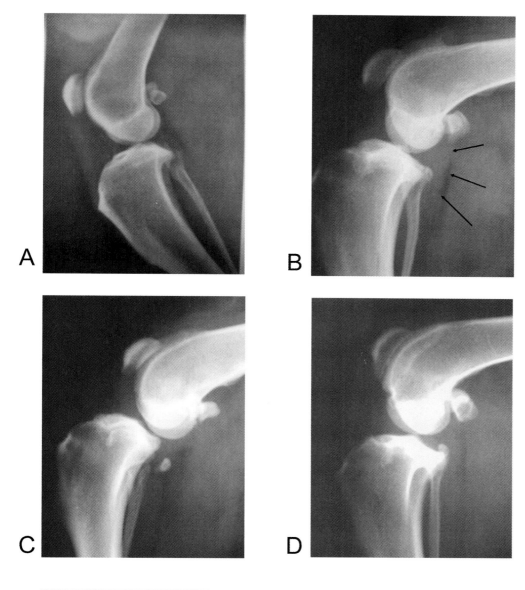

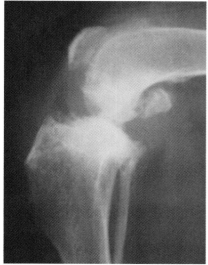

FIGURE 7-17 Lateral stifle radiographs showing a normal stifle and the progression of change in dogs with injury of the cranial cruciate ligament. *A,* A normal stifle showing the smooth poles of the patella, the triangular infrapatellar fat pad (patellar tendon to weightbearing articular surfaces), and the close, distinct approximation of the lucent fat line to the caudal joint surfaces. *B,* Typical radiograph of a dog with joint effusion, but without osteophyte formation, showing joint swelling, caudal deviation, and partial obliteration of the fat line in the caudal joint (*arrows*). Obliteration of the fat line may be the most reliable indicator of early joint effusion. In the cranial joint, the triangular detail of the infrapatellar fat is lost as a result of radiodense effusion located just cranial to the weightbearing articular surfaces. These changes are compatible with acute partial or complete tears. *C,* Lateral radiograph of a stifle showing marked cranial and distal translation that often is associated with complete acute rupture of the cranial cruciate ligament. The lack of periarticular osteophyte formation supports the diagnosis of acute injury. *D,* Radiographic changes typical of chronic osteoarthritis, showing pointed osteophytes off the proximal and distal poles of the patella and a row of osteophytes along the trochlear ridges of the femur. Effusion is evident. These changes are compatible with chronic partial or complete tears. *E,* End-stage osteoarthritis in a Labrador retriever with long-term untreated instability of the cranial cruciate ligament.

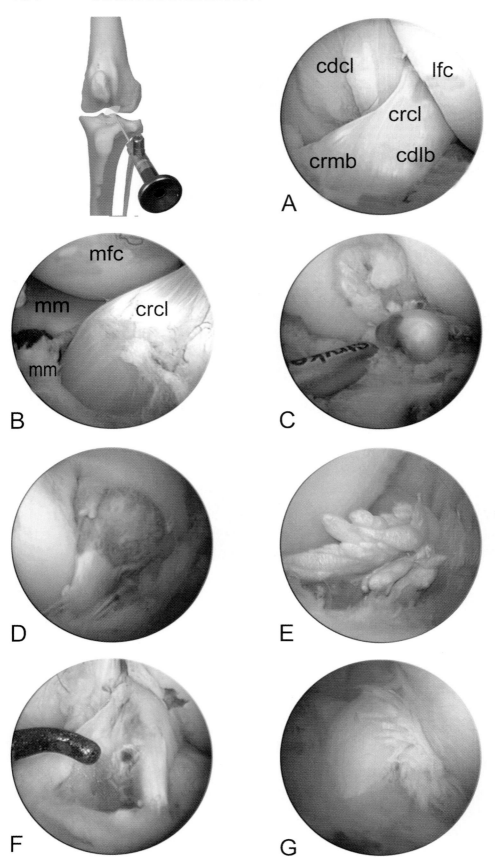

FIGURE 7-18 Positioning of the arthroscope, orientation of the light post, and normal and abnormal findings in dogs with injuries of the cranial cruciate ligament. *A,* Normal arthroscopic appearance of the caudal cruciate ligament (*cdcl*) and cranial cruciate ligament (*crcl*). The two distinct bands of the cranial cruciate ligament [craniomedial band (*crmb*), caudolateral band (*cdlb*)], the broad origin of the caudal cruciate ligament, and the lateral femoral condyle (*lfc*) are seen. *B,* Normal insertion of the cranial cruciate ligament (*crcl*). The cranial cruciate ligament passes directly beneath the edge of the cranial horn of the medial meniscus (*mm*) before it inserts. The medial femoral condyle (*mfc*) also is shown. *C,* Complete chronic tear of the cranial cruciate ligament with a nodular formation (Cyclopes lesion) on the end of the torn ligament. *D,* Acute complete tear with swelling and hemorrhage at the end of the ligament. *E,* Complete tear without associated hemorrhage. *F,* Iatrogenic lesion caused by preoperative arthrocentesis. *G,* Partial tear of the posterior lateral band. Note the bowed, stretched-out appearance of the remaining nonfunctional ligament.

techniques or with open TPLO that is performed with small instruments and implants. If the tibial slope is severe, TPLO is preferred, especially for revision. Arthroscopic examination and treatment can be performed in small dogs and cats if desired. In medium (>15 kg) and larger dogs, stabilization techniques are combined with arthroscopic examination and treatment of the intra-articular structures. In dogs >15 kg, arthroscopic intra-articular therapy is preferred to reduce surgery-related lameness, reduce scarring, improve visualization, and more accurately treat intra-articular pathology. This therapy includes examination of the joint, débridement of the remnants of the cranial cruciate ligament, and treatment of the meniscus. Osteotomy to level the tibial plateau is the treatment of choice, although other techniques also may provide satisfactory results. When TPLO is performed on dogs with complete rupture and intact medial menisci, the meniscus can be released arthroscopically if the surgeon elects to do so. As in humans, intra-articular allografts, autografts, and synthetic grafts are placed arthroscopically within bone tunnels with mixed results. Fibular head transposition and extracapsular prosthetic ligament techniques (imbrication techniques) can also be used to stabilize the stifle after the intra-articular procedure is performed endoscopically to reduce surgical morbidity.

Arthroscopic Technique. Positioning, portal placement, and systematic arthroscopic examination and photographic documentation of the joint were described earlier.

With few exceptions, dogs with complete or partial tearing of the cranial cruciate ligament also have pathologic changes in the proximal compartments. Figures 7–18 and 7–19 show the typical appearance of common partial and complete tears of the cranial cruciate ligament. Occasionally, some fraying of the caudal cruciate ligament is noted in dogs with cranial cruciate ligament rupture.

In cases of complete rupture, the cranial cruciate ligament should be removed completely, although the value of removing the ligament remnants in decreasing joint inflammation is not known. Débridement of the cranial cruciate ligament is most quickly accomplished with the motorized shaver (2000 to 2700 RPM, oscillatory mode) and should be performed before the menisci are inspected to facilitate their examination. When stable knees are examined for partial tears, the surgeon should carefully probe the origin and insertion of both bands of the cranial cruciate ligament to locate tears and ensure the stability of intact ligament. When a tear is identified in a palpably stable knee, the surgeon should débride only the torn portion with tissue ablation probes, leave the remaining portion intact, and perform TPLO. TPLO alters the mechanics of the stifle joint and improves stability of the joint under weightbearing load. Because stress on the remaining fibers of the cranial cruciate ligament is reduced, the ligament remains intact in most cases. Some report that saving the partially torn cranial cruciate ligament maintains enough joint stability that it is unnecessary to compromise the function of the meniscus by releasing it.

In some cases, arthroscopy shows a normal-appearing cranial cruciate ligament, despite knee instability. The cranial cruciate ligament must be carefully palpated for stretching and attenuation. These ligaments likely have significant interstitial tears, are nonfunctional, and should be treated as complete tears when palpable instability is present (Fig. 7–20).

The articular surfaces of the joint are carefully examined and palpated to detect areas of chondromalacia, fibrillation, or eburnation, and these lesions are documented. The arthroscopic appearance, grading, and management of these lesions are discussed in Chapter 4 and later in this chapter.

Meniscal Examination and Treatment. Proper inspection of the menisci is one of the most difficult arthroscopic procedures performed on the canine stifle. The surgeon must have thorough knowledge of the arthroscopic anatomy as well as excellent assistance to provide proper limb positioning. Both valgus and varus stress are required to allow visualization and probing of both menisci. Proper visualization requires careful attention to the placement of the arthroscope, the orientation of the light post, and the position of the limb. Placement of the portal in an overly proximal location and failure to débride the hyperplastic synovium and fat

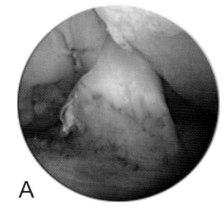
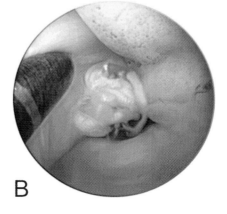

FIGURE 7–19 Partial cranial cruciate ligament tears. *A*, Partial tear at insertion with hemorrhage and active inflammation at cranial cruciate ligament insertion. *B*, Small partial tear of the anterior medial band by probing beneath the postlateral band. Sometimes it is difficult to differentiate which band is torn.

A   B

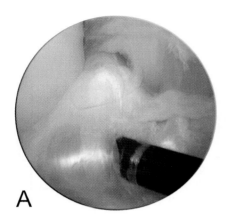

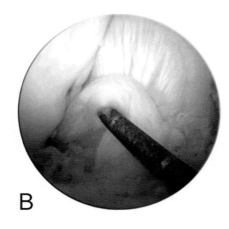

FIGURE 7-20 *A and B,* Nonfunctional tears of the cranial cruciate ligament. These tissues may appear intact initially, but careful palpation shows a stretched-out, attenuated ligament, usually associated with visible partial tears. In addition, the knee is palpably unstable.

pad far enough distally may preclude effective visualization and treatment of the menisci. To maintain visualization during treatment and avoid iatrogenic injury to the cartilage, proper instrumentation must be teamed with appropriate operative assistance. Inspection of the menisci is more difficult with intact cranial cruciate ligament tears but still almost always possible.

Inspection of the Medial Meniscus. Visualization of the caudal aspect of the medial meniscus is best obtained in approximately 30-degree flexion with external rotation and valgus stress and with the light post at 3 o'clock for a right leg and 9 o'clock for a left leg. In most cases, the arthroscope must be maneuvered laterally to obtain adequate visualization. When the caudal aspect of the medial meniscus is visualized, the cranial tibial thrust maneuver is used several times to aid in the detection of nondisplaced bucket handle tears. Careful probing of the menisci is critically important. The oyster curl, or flounce, of the meniscal edge is normal (Fig. 7–21A) but is not always seen and can be influenced by stressing the joint. Photographic documentation is performed at this point if the tissue is normal and both before and after débridement if pathology is detected. Figure 7–21 shows proper scope position and the typical arthroscopic appearance of a normal medial meniscus, a typical bucket handle tear, an oblique tear, and a complex degenerative meniscal tear. Meniscectomy may be performed with small-joint hand instruments, but this procedure often causes iatrogenic trauma to the articular surface, especially in caudal tears. A small, malleable tissue ablator is used in conjunction with a small-joint grasper, and even the most caudal tears are accessible in dogs as small as 10 to 15 kg. The anterior horn of the medial meniscus usually is best seen with the light post at the 10 o'clock position for a right leg and at the 2 o'clock position for a left leg, with the arthroscope oriented slightly deeper within the joint.

Inspection of the Lateral Meniscus. Figure 7–22 shows proper arthroscope position and light post orientation for examination of the lateral meniscus. Varus stress is applied with the knee in approximately 30 degrees of flexion, although the angle can vary. If the cranial cruciate ligament has been débrided, then inspection begins posteriorly with the large, easily identified meniscofemoral ligament (see Fig. 7–22B). The arthroscope is maneuvered medially to follow the edge of this ligament anterolaterally to the lateral meniscal edge and continued to its termination at the meniscotibial attachment cranially. In a series of 100 consecutive cases of naturally occurring tears of the cranial cruciate ligament (79 complete, 21 partial), 77 had some degree of lateral meniscal tearing (most small) compared with 58 medial meniscal tears in the same population. Most of these are short, radial tears of the cranial horn and may not be clinically significant (see Fig. 7–22D). However, several were long tears that had a macerated component and likely were painful (see Fig. 7–22F). The significance and etiology of these radial tears are not thoroughly understood. Many small tears may be clinically insignificant, but some may propagate with time. For this reason, and because débridement is performed quickly and easily with a tissue ablation wand, débridement is recommended. These lesions may be caused by the combination of pivot shift and rotational instability and cranial tibial thrust that causes the anterior horn of the lateral meniscus to slide repeatedly up the lateral tibial spine. This sliding has been visualized arthroscopically during a cranial tibial compression test (Fig. 7–23A and B). The same edge of the anterior horn of the lateral meniscus is sometimes visualized being pinched between the lateral tibial spine and lateral femoral condyle during full extension with cranial tibial thrust. In humans, meniscal edges caught between articular surfaces are painful. Deep areas of chondromalacia and fibrillation often are seen on the lateral tibial spine and lateral femoral condyle in conjunction with these tears (see Fig. 7–23C). These lesions may be caused by abrasive wear from the lateral meniscus, direct impact from the articular cartilage surfaces, or abrasive wear from the lateral band of the cranial cruciate ligament on the lateral femoral condyle during rotation, which has also been visualized arthroscopically. It is not known whether these chondral lesions cause symptoms in dogs.

Lateral meniscal tears have been seen in conjunction with OCD lesions of the lateral femoral condyle, but rarely. Bucket handle tears and horizontal cleavage tears

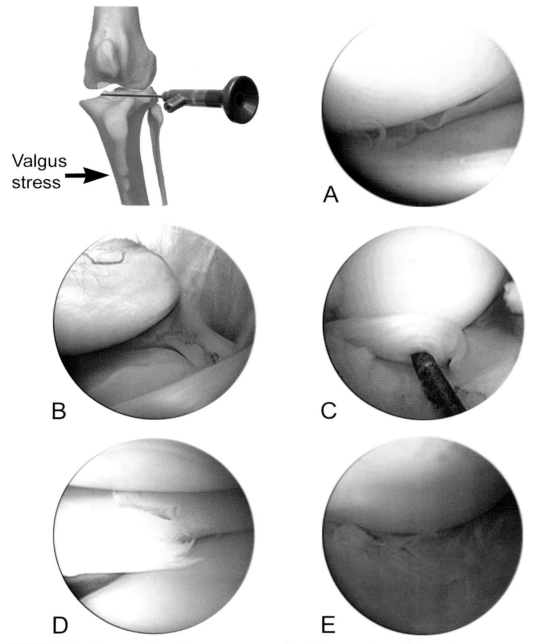

Valgus stress

FIGURE 7–21 Positioning of the arthroscope, orientation of the light post, and typical findings during inspection of the medial meniscus in a valgus-stressed stifle. *A,* Normal medial meniscus. The oyster curl, or flounce, of the meniscal edge is normal and is affected by stressing the knee. *B,* Normal caudal meniscofemoral ligament. *C,* Typical bucket handle tear that is displaced cranially with a probe. *D,* Oblique flap tear, or parrot beak tear, of the midbody. *E,* Macerated complex degenerative tear.

(see Fig. 7–22*C*) sometimes are seen in the lateral meniscus in conjunction with rupture of the cranial cruciate ligament.

Classification of Meniscal Tears. Although variations and combinations occur, there are four basic types of meniscal tears (Fig. 7–24). The fifth type is typically a complex combination of the four, resulting in a macerated meniscus. These may also be termed degenerative tears.

1. Vertical longitudinal tears include the common bucket handle tear (see Figs. 7–21*C* and 7–24*A*) and many variations, including short vertical tears that have not yet become displaced bucket handle tears and incomplete vertical tears. Incomplete vertical tears usually can be seen or palpated only by carefully probing a well-stressed joint and, as a result, are easily missed. Vertical tears may progress to become oblique or

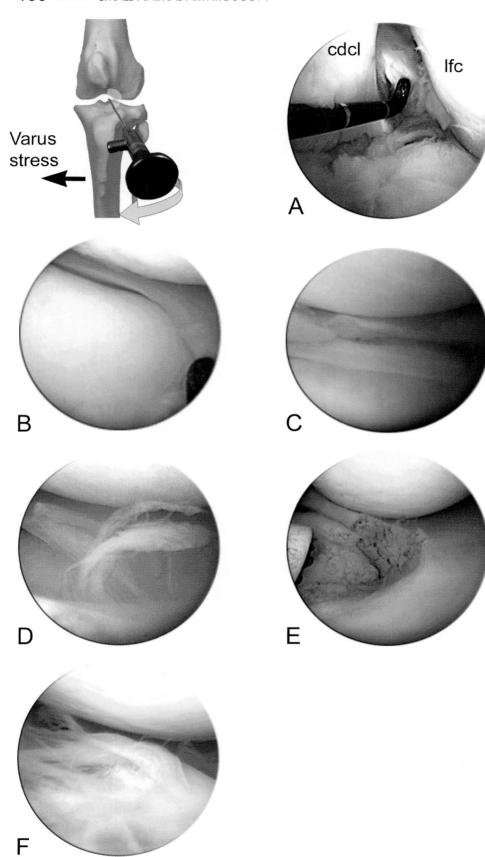

Varus stress

cdcl   lfc

A

B

C

D

E

F

FIGURE 7–22 Positioning of the arthroscope, orientation of the light post, and typical findings during inspection of the lateral meniscus in a varus-stressed stifle. *A,* Normal meniscofemoral ligament (*probe*) in caudal aspect of joint in relation to the caudal cruciate ligament (*cdcl*) and lateral femoral condyle (*lfc*). The cranial cruciate ligament remnants have been débrided with a motorized shaver. *B,* Normal lateral meniscus. *C,* Horizontal cleavage tear of the mid-body. The arthroscope is moved medially and withdrawn slightly to follow the meniscal edge to the cranial horn. *D,* Radial tear of the cranial horn. *E,* The radial tear shown in *D* after radiofrequency ablation. *F,* Long radial tears of the anterior horn with a degenerative and macerated component.

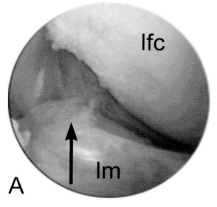

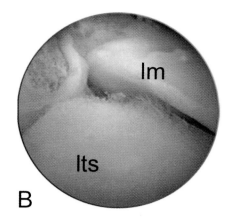

FIGURE 7-23 Chondral lesions commonly seen on the lateral femoral condyle and lateral tibial spine in cranial cruciate ligament–deficient stifles. *A* and *B*, Fibrillation and chondromalacia of the lateral tibial spine. The cranial horn of the lateral meniscus (*lm*) slides up the tibial spine (*lts, arrow*). The associated chondromalacia of the adjacent lateral femoral condyle (*lfc*) is shown. *C*, Chondromalacia and fibrillation of the lateral femoral condyle. The close approximation of the lateral band of the cranial cruciate ligament is seen contacting the lesion with external rotation of the distal limb.

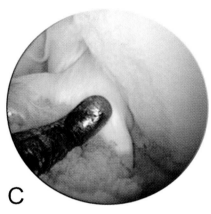

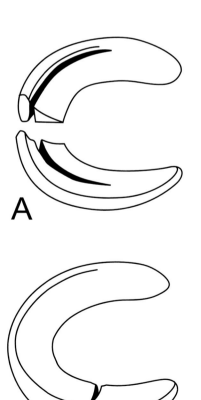

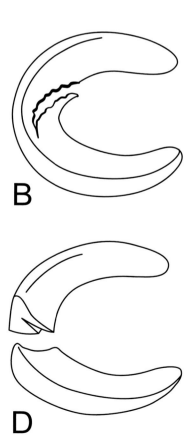

FIGURE 7-24 Classification of meniscal tears. *A*, Longitudinal vertical tear, commonly called a bucket handle tear. *B*, Oblique, or flap, tear. Short oblique tears often are called "parrot beak tears." *C*, Radial tear. In dogs, these tears commonly occur in series on the cranial horn of the lateral meniscus associated with tears of the cranial cruciate ligament. *D*, Horizontal, or horizontal cleavage, tear.

flap tears, or when chronic, degenerative or macerated tears. Approximately half of medial meniscal tears are bucket handle tears. In some cases, two bucket handle tears are seen on the same meniscus.

2. Oblique, or flap, tears may be single or double, and include parrot beak tears (see Figs. 7–21*D* and 7–24*B*). Many flap tears probably start as vertical tears, become bucket handle tears, and then break off at either handle end to become a flap or break off midway to become a double flap. As the dog continues to walk on the injured area, many of these tears have a macerated component as well.
3. Radial, or transverse, tears most commonly occur as a series of tears in the anterior horn of the lateral meniscus (see Figs. 7–22*D* and F and 7–24*C*). These tears may propagate if left untreated. It is not known how long they must become to cause lameness.
4. Horizontal, or horizontal cleavage, tears (see Figs. 7–22*C* and 7–24*D*) are less common and often occur in conjunction with other tears, especially after they become macerated or degenerative. Incomplete horizontal tears are probably present in many cases but go undiagnosed. This may play a role in late-onset meniscal tears that occur after surgical stabilization. These tears can be visualized with magnetic resonance imaging in humans and likely in dogs as well. To diagnose these tears arthroscopically, the surgeon must probe the edge of the meniscus and view it end-on rather than from above.
5. Degenerative, or macerated, tears (see Figs. 7–21*E* and 7–22*F*) can be seen with any type of tear and often result from delayed treatment and chronic trauma when dogs continue to walk on injured menisci. These tears have numerous filamentous strands and often occur in conjunction with adjacent articular cartilage chondromalacia, fibrillation, and occasionally, eburnation.

The source of meniscal pain in dogs is not well understood. Humans who have meniscal tears and undergo arthroscopy under local anesthesia feel no pain when the flaps are moved, although traction on the flap causes sensations similar to the clinical symptoms. Therefore, most authors believe that pain from meniscal tears is caused by repeated traction on the capsule and synovial border when the flap is caught in the joint. The situation is likely the same in dogs. It is interesting to speculate on the intensity of meniscal pain during cranial tibial thrust in dogs with cranial cruciate ligament–deficient stifles. In humans, meniscal tears usually are repaired if the patient is young and the tear is neither too complex nor macerated. Postoperative patient compliance, which ranges from the use of crutches to the need for reduced activity for as long as 6 weeks, is also required. Most canine tears do not fit these criteria, similar postoperative

control of activity is not possible in dogs, and limited visualization makes repair demanding in the few tears that are suitable for treatment. In humans, meniscectomy leads to significant long-term osteoarthritis; the same is likely true in the canine stifle.

Principles of Arthroscopic Meniscectomy. The principles of arthroscopic meniscectomy are as follows:

1. Mobile fragments that displace beyond the normal rim of the meniscal edge are removed because they may become caught between joint surfaces and cause pain and propagation of the tear.
2. Sudden changes in the rim contour must be corrected. It is not necessary to leave the meniscus the same width throughout, but a long, slow, gentle curve should be reestablished.
3. A perfectly smooth rim is not necessary. Follow-up arthroscopy in humans shows that the rim will become smooth in 6 to 9 months, although similar studies are lacking in the dog.
4. Probing should be performed frequently to evaluate the area for mobility and texture. When possible, the surgeon should probe and inspect the area or blindly probe the underside of the meniscus and apply cranial traction to test for an unstable but nondisplaced tear.
5. The texture of the meniscus should guide evaluation and treatment. Soft, mushy tissue should be excised, whereas firm areas should be left undisturbed. This guideline primarily applies to procedures that are performed with hand instruments. Texture is more difficult to appreciate when an ablation wand is used. However, with some effort, texture can be appreciated with the probe. Close inspection of the meniscal surface often shows roughness associated with an underlying incomplete tear. Horizontal probing of this area often shows a soft spot that tears easily with continued probing.
6. The meniscocapsular junction must be protected. If the surgeon is uncertain, then more, rather than less, meniscal rim should be left. This principle is violated when meniscal release is performed, which can also be done arthroscopically. Studies of the long-term effects of meniscal release are needed as well as studies documenting the efficacy of meniscal release in preventing future tears.
7. Iatrogenic damage to the articular cartilage can be avoided if care is taken to use small tissue ablation wands, to avoid placing the camera tip too close to the articular cartilage, and to avoid the use of jawed instruments in the joint space when their opening is traumatic to adjacent articular cartilage. Further, the surgical assistant should manipulate the joint slowly and carefully, and only when the surgeon is prepared.

Partial Medial Meniscectomy of Bucket Handle Tears. Bucket handle tears of the medial meniscus often are seen during canine stifle arthroscopy, and their treatment can be technically demanding. The use of proper instrumentation and sequential technique aids in visualization and instrumentation, facilitates removal, and significantly reduces iatrogenic damage to cartilage. Cutting the bucket handles out of order may cause obstruction of the view by the meniscal fragment. Adequate synovial débridement, especially distally and laterally, must be performed before the meniscus is grasped.

The step-by-step procedure for removal of a typical bucket handle tear is listed below.

1. A probe is used to displace the tear forward. Cranial traction on the probe is maintained while the grasper is inserted through the same portal.
2. A locking small-joint grasper is inserted through the same portal. The midportion of the tear is grasped, and the probe is removed. Ideally, the surgeon will obtain a strong bite on the first attempt. Smaller bites invariably give way, and iatrogenically damaged tissue may be difficult to grasp again. The assistant should maintain traction on the grasper.
3. While the assistant applies cranial traction with the graspers, the joint is stressed slightly valgus and the abaxial handle is visualized at its attachment to the body of the meniscus, which usually is near the medial collateral ligament. Occasionally, additional hyperplastic synovium must be débrided for adequate visualization. The abaxial handle is incised with the tip of the smallest tissue ablation wand, cutting from cranial to caudal. Larger wands may obstruct the surgeon's view. The wand is inserted through the shared craniomedial portal, proximal to the grasper. Occasionally, the probe must be bent to make a precise cut. In rare cases, a small-joint punch can be used, but care must be taken to avoid causing iatrogenic damage to the articular cartilage.
4. Finally, the axial bucket handle is incised, usually near its tibial attachment caudally. Gentle traction is directed proximally on the grasper to allow visualization of the attachment between the handle and the caudal horn of the meniscus. Then the ablation wand is introduced distal to the grasper, within the shared anterior medial portal. After transection is performed, the ablation probe is removed, followed by the grasper holding the fragment. The joint is opened again, with valgus stress, and reexamined and reprobed to reveal additional tears. The remaining meniscal edge is sculpted according to the principles of meniscectomy.

Release of the Medial Meniscus. To prevent future tearing of the medial meniscus, meniscal release is often performed at the same time as osteotomy to level the tibial plateau. This procedure is considered when the knee is unstable and the medial meniscus is intact. The efficacy of this procedure and the long-term effect on the articular cartilage are unknown, and the technique is controversial. Some argue that meniscal release renders the meniscus nonfunctional and predisposes the patient to osteoarthritis, whereas others argue that the incidence of meniscal tears after TPLO is unacceptably high without release. When partial meniscectomy is required for significant naturally occurring tears, release is not indicated. Instead of meniscal release, some surgeons elect to perform prophylactic partial meniscectomy on uninjured menisci. In dogs that have partial tears, but palpably stable knees, TPLO usually saves the ligament, and some consider meniscal release unnecessary. Clinically some dogs that undergo meniscal release later tear the meniscus, whereas tears do not always occur in other dogs that do not undergo the procedure. Controlled studies are needed to determine the need, efficacy, and induced morbidity associated with this procedure. Release of the medial meniscus can be performed arthroscopically by transecting the caudal meniscotibial ligament or by transversely incising the meniscus caudal to the attachment of the medial collateral ligament. It is not known whether either location of release is superior or whether meniscal release is superior or inferior to prophylactic partial ablation.

Medial meniscal release is most quickly and easily performed at the caudal meniscotibial ligament.

To release the caudal meniscotibial ligament, a palpation probe is placed directly beneath the ligament at its origin on the meniscus, and its caudal border is hooked with the probe. While craniodistal traction is applied on the probe handle, a fine-tipped radiofrequency ablation wand is inserted through the same portal (craniomedial portal) and an incision is made directly over the probe (Fig. 7–25A and B). A distinct pop can be felt when the meniscus is released and the tension on the palpation probe is suddenly relaxed. The caudal horn of the medial meniscus should displace caudally and medially when the meniscotibial ligament is completely transected, and the meniscus can be seen actively moving during direct arthroscopic visualization while the cranial tibial compression test is applied.

For midbody release, a radiofrequency probe is used to make a transverse incision of the medial meniscus, caudal to its attachment to the medial collateral ligament. This procedure can be performed arthroscopically, although this technique may be difficult to visualize peripherally. Alternatively, the meniscus can be incised with a no. 11 scalpel blade that is introduced through the skin into the joint from the caudomedial aspect of the stifle. The meniscus is visualized arthroscopically while a 22-gauge spinal needle guide is inserted just caudal to the medial collateral ligament, over the intended site of meniscal transection. The no. 11 blade is introduced alongside the guide needle into the joint. The meniscus is transected as pressure is applied to the blade (see Fig. 7–25C and D). When the meniscal incision is complete, the caudal horn of the meniscus

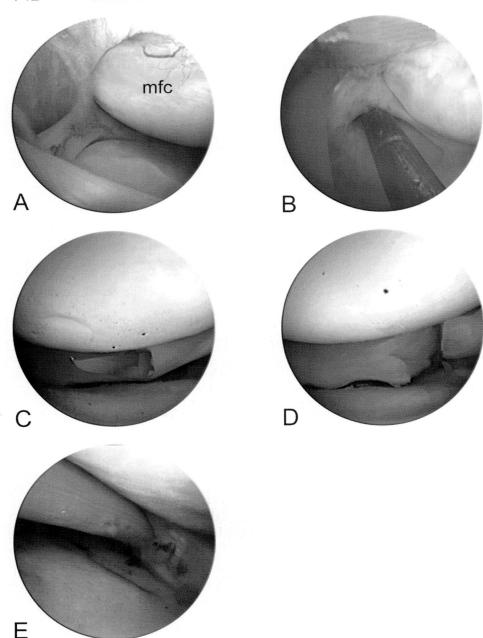

FIGURE 7-25 Two techniques of meniscal release for prophylactic treatment of the medial meniscus after tibial plateau leveling osteotomy. *A,* Site of release of the medial meniscus at the caudal meniscofemoral ligament. *B,* Caudal medial meniscal release. A probe is placed beneath the meniscotibial ligament, and transection is performed with a fine-tipped radiofrequency probe. *C,* Midbody medial meniscal release. Guided by an arthroscopically visualized needle that is inserted percutaneously just caudal to the medial collateral ligament, a no. 11 blade is inserted percutaneously to transect the meniscus. *D,* After the midbody is released, complete transection creates a visual gap. *E,* Prophylactic partial meniscectomy. A radiofrequency probe is used to ablate the caudal aspect of the outer third of the meniscus.

displaces caudally and a gap is seen in the body of the meniscus (see Fig. 7–25D).

Partial meniscal ablation can be performed in lieu of meniscal release. Meniscal ablation may better preserve meniscal function by maintaining the hoop-stress mechanism that is lost when transverse tearing of the meniscus occurs. This procedure is performed with a radiofrequency probe (see Fig. 7–25E). The inner third of the caudal horn of the medial meniscus is ablated to remove the region of the meniscus that is most susceptible to tearing. Meniscal ablation is used to discourage meniscal tears after osteotomy to level the tibial plateau, but future tears may occur despite the use of this technique.

Surgical stabilization is performed after joint débridement and meniscal treatment, according to the surgeon's preferred technique. TPLO is currently the treatment of choice, but other techniques provide satisfactory results in many cases.

Postoperative Care. Intra-articular bupivacaine with or without morphine is injected at the conclusion of surgery if an epidural was not performed. The application of a Robert Jones bandage for the first 12 to 24 hours is optional, but bandaging helps alleviate discomfort from postsurgical swelling. Preferred pain management includes preoperative long-acting epidural opioid therapy, cold therapy (20 minutes on and 20 minutes off as often as possible) for the first 48 hours, the use of a fentanyl transdermal patch for 4 days, and administration of NSAIDs for 15 to 30 days. Alternately, parenteral and oral opioids can be used in patients that are sensitive to NSAIDs or in conjunction with NSAID therapy when additional analgesia is needed. Bandages usually are not necessary in isolated meniscal treatment or simple diagnostic or second-look arthroscopy. These cases are routinely treated on an outpatient basis with NSAIDs alone. Most cranial cruciate ligament repair patients are released the morning after surgery.

Complications. Complications associated with arthroscopy are minimal and uncommon. The most common complication is swelling as a result of subcutaneous fluid extravasation. Edema is uncomfortable, and these cases benefit from the application of a Robert Jones bandage for 24 hours. If the patient is released from the hospital with a bandage the owners should be cautioned that slippage is likely as the swelling subsides and if it occurs the bandage should be removed. Some hock swelling often develops within the first 1 to 2 postoperative days as a result of gravitation of subcutaneous fluids. Iatrogenic damage to the articular cartilage usually occurs when the stifle is not fully extended while instruments or arthroscopes are manipulated beneath the patella, when the tip of the scope is allowed to get too close to the articular cartilage during attempts to view the menisci, and as a result of instrument manipulation during partial meniscectomy. Most hand instruments are too large for use in atraumatic partial meniscectomy in dogs. The use of small tissue ablation wands has almost eliminated this problem. Extreme caution must be exercised to avoid thermal injury to the articular cartilage. Electrocautery burns may occur if patients are not properly grounded when necessary. Infections are rare. Meniscal injuries can be overlooked if the meniscus is not thoroughly probed and carefully inspected. The reader is referred elsewhere for complications associated with various stabilization techniques.

Prognosis. The prognosis depends on many factors, including the timing of intervention, the degree of osteoarthritis present at the time of surgery, the size of the patient, and the severity of meniscal injury. Other factors that affect outcome include whether the disease is unilateral or bilateral, whether the patient has undergone previous stifle surgery, whether concurrent stifle pathology is present, and whether additional orthopedic problems are present. In addition, the experience of the surgeon, the activity level of the dog, and the stabilization technique used may affect the prognosis. Excessive tibial slope may play a role in the prognosis of non-TPLO procedures. Finally, the individual willpower, drive, and pain tolerance of the patient likely affect the outcome, but these factors are difficult to measure or predict. It is not known whether meniscal release affects prognosis. Many experienced clinicians believe that it reduces the incidence of late-onset meniscal tears, whereas others argue that it may predispose the patient to osteoarthritis by rendering the meniscus nonfunctional because the hoop-stress mechanism is disrupted. Despite these

variables, treatment results for uncomplicated rupture of the cranial cruciate ligament rupture are good if osteoarthritis is absent or minimal, and many dogs do well despite having advanced osteoarthritis at the time of intervention.

Avulsion Fractures of the Cruciate Ligament

Avulsion fractures of the cruciate ligament can be repaired successfully with traditional open arthrotomy, an arthroscopic procedure, or a combination of techniques. If the knee is stable and the avulsion fragment is small, treatment may involve only removal of the arthroscopic fragment and rest. If all or much of the ligament is avulsed, treatment options include open repair augmented with extracapsular techniques or external coaptation, complete removal and stabilization, and arthroscopic repair. Ideally, for repair, the entire ligament is intact and the bony avulsion is large and in one piece. Unfortunately, this situation does not always occur, and the ligament should be closely examined for structural damage. The avulsions may be seen from both the proximal and distal ends of both the cranial cruciate ligament and caudal cruciate ligament. Involvement of the caudal cruciate ligament must be excluded before osteotomy to level the tibial plateau is considered for stabilization. These patients often have open growth plates that may contraindicate some techniques. Finally, if repair of the avulsion fragment is too tenuous or if the ligament is severely damaged, removal and traditional repairs for ligament-deficient stifles are warranted unless growth plate issues prevail. The age and growth potential of the dog should be considered when these decisions are made.

History and Signalment. Avulsion fractures are seen almost exclusively in dogs younger than 1 year old because juvenile bones are softer than adult bones. They sometimes occur in older dogs and may be related to violent trauma, such as vehicular accidents. Otherwise, the history and signalment are the same as for other cruciate ligament injuries.

Physical Examination Findings. Lameness ranges from partial to non-weightbearing. Avulsions are often associated with effusion or hemarthrosis, and the joint is often painful on manipulation. Instability is usually pronounced and dependent on which ligament (cranial cruciate ligament or caudal cruciate ligament) is avulsed. Isolated tears of the caudal cruciate ligament are stable in extension, but have marked drawer in flexion, with a sharp endpoint created by the intact cranial cruciate ligament. Cranial cruciate ligament instabilities have drawer in both flexion and extension and usually have a positive result on cranial tibial compression test. Findings should always be compared to the contralateral limb as many puppy stifles have considerable laxity.

Differential Diagnosis. The differential diagnosis includes medial patellar luxation, septic arthritis, hip

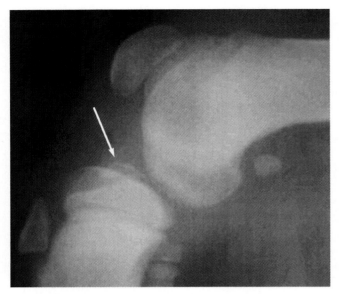

FIGURE 7–26 Lateral radiograph of a 3-month-old Labrador retriever with a distal avulsion fracture of the cranial cruciate ligament. The fracture fragment is visible within the joint (*arrow*). Note the marked subluxation.

dysplasia, panosteitis (in young dogs), lumbosacral disease, and tibial tuberosity avulsion.

Radiographic Findings. Bony avulsion is usually apparent on quality films with standard projections (Fig. 7–26). Other radiographic signs include swelling of the posterior joint capsule, loss of triangular detail of the infrapatellar fat pad, and formation of periarticular osteophytes if chronic. Cranial and proximal translation of the tibia in relation to the femur is appreciated as mild to severe subluxation. In some chronic cases, early osteophyte formation is noted off either or both poles of the patella and along the medial and lateral trochlear ridges of the femur. In more chronic cases, these osteophytes may be large and may be accompanied by similar changes along the medial, lateral, and caudal aspects of the tibia. However, unlike most cases of cranial cruciate ligament rupture, these cases present acutely.

Diagnosis. The diagnosis is based on the history, physical findings, radiographic findings (see Fig. 7–26), and if necessary, confirmation during arthroscopic examination. When trauma is involved, the full extent of injury must be determined to exclude stifle derangement of multiple ligaments, especially if both the cranial cruciate ligament and caudal cruciate ligament or the collateral ligaments are involved.

Treatment. If marked swelling is present, a Robert Jones bandage may be applied for 24 to 48 hours to reduce swelling. NSAIDs, with or without opioids, are used to control pain. Conservative treatment consists of NSAID therapy, chondroprotective agents, weight control, and regular low-impact exercise. Without surgical intervention, most dogs have persistent lameness. In dogs that have advanced osteoarthritis at the time of surgery, surgery does not alleviate the need for concurrent conservative treatment.

Anesthetic Considerations and Perioperative Pain Management. Cox II NSAIDs are discontinued 1 to 2 days before surgery, although discontinuation is not mandatory. Healthy, young patients require minimal preoperative laboratory evaluation. Older patients are adequately screened to exclude underlying metabolic disorders. Routine chest radiographs are recommended if vehicular trauma is the cause of injury. Preferred pain management is preoperative administration of long-acting epidural opioids, cold therapy for 48 hours, application of a fentanyl transdermal patch for 4 days, and NSAID administration for 15 days. Alternately, parenteral and oral opioids can be used, with or without NSAID therapy. Surgical pain is reduced considerably when the intra-articular component of the procedure is performed endoscopically because joint capsule disruption is minimized.

Surgical Intervention. The avulsion fragment is either removed or incorporated into the repair. Small dogs (<15 kg) are usually treated with open arthrotomy for fragment removal and extracapsular stabilization. In larger dogs, options include open primary repair with adjunctive lateral imbrication or external coaptation, fragment removal and stabilization, arthroscopic débridement and extracapsular stabilization, and arthroscopic primary repair with temporary external coaptation, which is considered ideal if the avulsion fragment is large. Dogs usually do well with caudal cruciate ligament–deficient stifles if the bony avulsion fragment is removed, although when feasible, it is preferable to repair the avulsion and save the ligament. In addressing avulsion fracture injuries, it is important to confirm that the ligament has not been torn in conjunction with avulsion. In these cases, the avulsion fragment is débrided and stabilization is performed when indicated.

Positioning, portal placement, and systematic arthroscopic examination and photographic documentation are performed. Most avulsion cases are acute, and the patient may have minimal proximal compartment changes. The joint is aggressively lavaged before the arthroscope is introduced because these patients often have marked hemarthrosis. The avulsion fragment is identified, and the associated ligament is probed to verify that it is intact (Fig. 7–27A). The avulsion bed and avulsion fragment are débrided of hematoma and fibrous tissue. Care must be taken to avoid removing soft underlying cancellous bone (see Fig. 7–27B). A probe is used to inspect the area of avulsion to identify its boundaries and exclude comminution. With the probe, the fragment is maneuvered over the avulsion bed to confirm its fit and anatomic orientation (see Fig. 7–27C). For distal avulsions of the cranial cruciate ligament, the switching stick is used to establish an additional instrument portal immediately lateral to the patella. A small metal instrument cannula is slid over the switching stick, and the switching stick is removed. The cannula tip is used to hold reduction of the fragment under direct visualization.

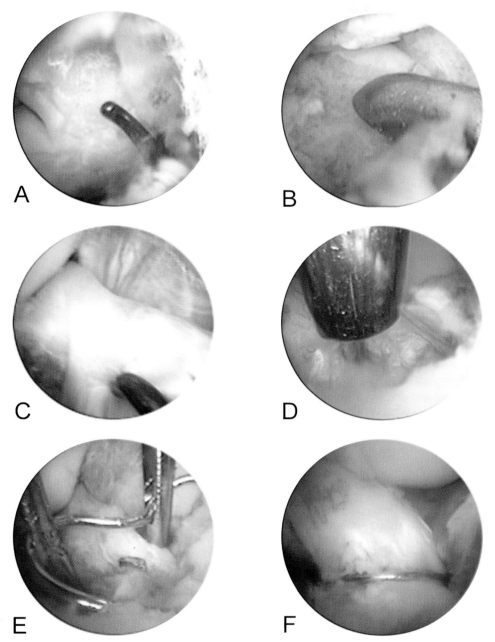

FIGURE 7–27 Arthroscopic repair of a distal avulsion fracture of the cranial cruciate ligament. *A,* The fracture fragment is identified with a palpation probe. *B,* The fracture bed is gently débrided with a small curette. *C,* A probe is used to perform reduction. *D,* An instrument cannula is placed through an additional proximal portal. A small K-wire is centered through the fragment, driven until it exits the tibial cortex and skin, and withdrawn distally until only 1 mm protrudes from the bony fragment. *E,* An eyed K-wire is driven in similar fashion, both medial and lateral to the fragment, and threaded with cerclage wire. *F,* The eyed pins are withdrawn distally and the wires twisted to complete the modified tension band.

The lumen of the cannula is centered over the bulk of the fragment. While reduction is held with the cannula, an appropriately sized small K-wire (usually 0.045 to 0.0625 inches) is inserted through the cannula and drilled with power until it exits the medial cortex proximal to the tibia and skin (see Fig. 7-27D). The exposed proximal tip of the pin is clipped with pin cutters. The proximal instrument portal is maintained, and the drill is placed on the distally protruding pin. Under direct arthroscopic visualization, the pin is slowly advanced distally until only 2 mm of the pin protrudes from the fragment. With a similar technique and the additional instrument portal, a small eyed K-wire is drilled on each side of the fragment (medial and lateral) until the eyed portion of the K-wire protrudes slightly above the fragment (see Fig. 7-27E). A grasper is used to insert the tip of a cerclage wire (0.8 to 1.0 mm) through the anterior medial portal and through the tip of one of the eyed K-wires. The involved pin is removed with a Jacobs hand chuck, without twisting, until the cerclage wire exits the skin. The cerclage wire is tagged with a hemostat. These steps are repeated for the other end of the cerclage wire and the other eyed pin (see Fig. 7-27E). To employ a modified tension band principle, the cerclage wire must pass caudal to the tip of the K-wire exposed within the joint. The skin is incised between the ends of the cerclage wire. The wire is hand twisted until the loop appears tight around the avulsion fragment (see Fig. 7-27F). The opposite (distal) ends of the K-wires are bent onto the tibial cortex to prevent migration into the joint (Fig. 7-28).

If the animal has significant growth potential, the pin and tension band device are removed after acceptable radiographic union is achieved. For avulsion fractures of the proximal cranial cruciate ligament, the knee must be flexed for adequate visualization. Because of the very caudal location of the origin of the cranial cruciate ligament, adequate visualization is difficult if the instrument cannula is used for reduction. A notchplasty is performed to aid visualization. If the fragment is large enough, it is helpful to pull the avulsion fragment through the anterior medial portal, drill a small transverse hole, and place a no. 0 or no. 2 nylon suture through the hole. An eyed K-wire is drilled through the avulsion bed, the suture is threaded onto the eye, and the pin is pulled with a Jacobs chuck until it exits proximally. The suture is pulled to aid in reduction of the fragment. When reduction is accomplished, it is held with the instrument cannula. The previously described technique is used to stabilize the fragment with a modified tension band. If necessary, the suture is removed immediately before the K-wire is drilled. For avulsion fractures of the proximal caudal cruciate ligament, pins are run proximally to exit the medial distal femur. The routine portals are used, but the camera is switched to the instrument portal and vice versa to facilitate drilling. Most dogs do well with caudal cruciate ligament–deficient stifles, and excision of the ligament and avulsion is another option. For avulsion fracture of the distal caudal cruciate ligament, this method is preferred because of the inaccessibility of the injury for repair.

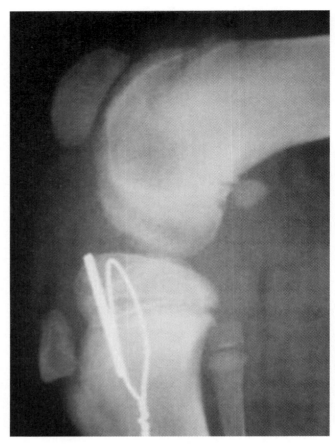

FIGURE 7-28 Postoperative radiograph after arthroscopic repair of a distal avulsion fracture of the cranial cruciate ligament.

Postoperative Care. Lateral fiberglass splintage is maintained for 2 to 4 weeks if the patient's age and skin will allow. Sedatives are prescribed if necessary to prevent overactivity. If necessary for growth, the pins and wires are removed after healing is confirmed radiographically.

Complications. The primary complication is pull-out of the avulsion fragment, which is most likely to occur when pin fixation is used without the addition of cerclage wire and a tension band. Overactivity in young animals also may contribute to this complication and must be avoided. This problem should be taken into consideration when deciding when to attempt repair.

Prognosis. The prognosis is good to excellent for full return to function.

Tear of the Caudal Cruciate Ligament

Isolated caudal cruciate ligament tears are rare. Most are caused by violent trauma to the cranial tibia while the knee is in flexion and are seen in conjunction with other, more serious ligamentous injuries. Dogs do well clinically without a caudal cruciate ligament. During physical examination, caudal cruciate ligament injury is easily misdiagnosed as cranial cruciate ligament injury.

Osteotomy to level the tibial plateau is contraindicated in the caudal cruciate ligament–deficient stifle.

History and Signalment. Any age, sex, or breed may be affected. Vehicular trauma is often involved.

Physical Examination Findings. The stifle is carefully palpated for concurrent injuries, especially instability of the collateral ligaments. Most caudal cruciate ligament tears occur in conjunction with other ligamentous injuries. True isolated caudal cruciate ligament tears have a marked drawer motion in flexion that is easily confused with cranial drawer. To differentiate between these two conditions, careful palpation is performed in both flexion and extension. Complete caudal cruciate ligament tears have marked drawer in flexion that has a sharp endpoint created by the intact cranial cruciate ligament. The knee is stable in extension. Cranial cruciate ligament tears have drawer in both flexion and extension and usually have a positive result on the cranial tibial compression test, whereas caudal cruciate ligament injuries do not. Partial cranial cruciate ligament tears involving the anterior medial band are stable in extension and have drawer in flexion with an ill-defined endpoint. Careful palpation is always performed under general anesthesia, and the findings are compared with the contralateral limb.

Differential Diagnosis. The differential diagnosis includes cranial cruciate ligament injury, multiple ligamentous instability, and concurrent meniscal injury.

Radiographic Findings. Findings are usually unremarkable but may include mild joint swelling. Chronic cases do not have the advanced periarticular osteophytes typically seen in cases of cranial cruciate ligament rupture.

Diagnosis. The diagnosis is based on the history, physical examination findings, and results of direct arthroscopic examination (Fig. 7–29).

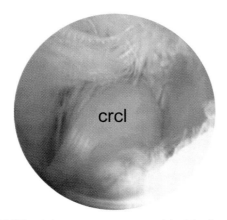

FIGURE 7–29 Arthroscopic appearance of the left stifle of a 2-year-old bulldog with spontaneous rupture of the caudal cruciate ligament (cdcl). The contralateral limb had a similar lesion. The case was treated with débridement alone.

Treatment. If concurrent ligamentous injury or meniscal injury is not overlooked, most dogs do well without surgical stabilization. Arthroscopic examination is preferred to confirm the diagnosis, débride the remnants of the caudal cruciate ligament, and treat or exclude meniscal injury.

Anesthetic Considerations and Perioperative Pain Management. Cox II NSAIDs are discontinued 1 to 2 days before surgery, although this practice is not mandatory. Young, healthy patients require minimal preoperative laboratory evaluation. Older patients should be adequately screened to exclude underlying metabolic disorders. Surgical pain is minimal, and NSAID administration for 15 days in conjunction with cold therapy for 48 hours usually provides adequate pain relief. Alternatively, parenteral or oral opioids or a fentanyl transdermal patch can be used, with or without NSAID therapy. Surgical pain is reduced considerably when the procedure is performed endoscopically because it minimizes disruption of the highly innervated joint capsule.

Surgical Intervention. Positioning, portal placement, systematic arthroscopic examination, and photographic documentation of the joint are performed. In patients with isolated caudal cruciate ligament injury, the ligament remnants are débrided arthroscopically with a motorized shaver. At the same time, meniscal injuries are inspected and treated. If avulsion of the proximal origin is present and the fragment is large, repair is preferred if the ligament is intact (see section on avulsion fractures). Stabilization techniques may be used if the response to treatment is inadequate.

Postoperative Care. Cold therapy is provided for 48 hours, and Cox II NSAIDs are administered for 15 days. Immediate weightbearing is allowed. The dog is restricted to controlled leash walking for 2 weeks, and normal activity is gradually resumed as tolerated. If the avulsion fragment is repaired, lateral splintage and exercise control are used. Unless significant growth is anticipated, removal of the implant is not necessary.

Complications. One potentially serious complication is misdiagnosing a caudal cruciate ligament injury as a cranial cruciate ligament injury and treating it with tibial plateau leveling osteotomy. Collateral ligament tears can be easily overlooked.

Prognosis. The prognosis is good for full return to function. Radiographic follow-up does not show the aggressive osteoarthritis that is commonly seen with cranial cruciate ligament tears.

Osteochondritis Dissecans of the Stifle

OCD lesions are the result of a failure of endochondral ossification in the epiphyseal complex of developing bones. The unmineralized endochondral cartilage and its overlying articular cartilage become too thick to receive adequate nutrition from the synovial fluid and subchondral bone. The result is chondrocyte death, lack of structural support, cleft formation, cartilage collapse, and flap development. The etiology of OCD is unknown, and most cases are likely multifactorial. Contributing factors include genetic predisposition, rapid growth, over-nutrition, and activity. Everyday trauma likely precipitates the condition clinically. As the cartilage becomes more unstable and the fissures and clefts communicate with the joint, the products of cartilage degradation reach the joint and mediate inflammation. Mechanical incongruency develops and results in a corresponding increase in cartilage wear. Clinical signs can be seen even when only partial flap detachment occurs. Localized synovitis is seen arthroscopically adjacent to the lesion during partial detachment and may become generalized if the condition becomes chronic. Left untreated, flaps may detach or collapse and may become mineralized.

OCD is much less common in the stifle than in the shoulder. Although it usually involves the medial aspect of the lateral femoral condyle, it is seen in the medial femoral condyle as well. Because the condition is often bilateral, the contralateral limb must be evaluated carefully.

History and Signalment. Large and giant purebred dogs are most commonly affected, both males and females. Common breeds include the rottweiler, Labrador retriever, golden retriever, and Great Dane. Most dogs have onset of weightbearing lameness as puppies (age 5 to 7 months) but may not present for treatment until much later. Common complaints include early morning stiffness that may "warm out" partially but is exacerbated by exercise. The lameness is usually helped by NSAIDs and rest, but it returns when activity is resumed.

Physical Examination Findings. Most dogs show weightbearing lameness of various degrees that may be exacerbated by hyperflexion of the stifle. Effusion is often present and is more prominent in chronic cases. The knee is palpably stable, although joint laxity is common in immature dogs and may be present. The patella tracks normally, and the dog is afebrile.

Differential Diagnosis. The differential diagnosis includes medial patellar luxation, panosteitis, hip dysplasia, septic arthritis, and partial tearing of the cranial cruciate ligament.

Radiographic Findings. The condition is often bilateral. Quality radiographs in the two standard projections are usually adequate for the diagnosis. The lateral view typically shows a radiolucent concavity or flattened area of the lateral or medial femoral condyle (Fig. 7–30A). Radiographic evidence of joint effusion is often present. In chronic cases, other degenerative changes, such as periarticular osteophyte formation and subchondral sclerosis, may be present. Only rarely are mineralized joint mice seen.

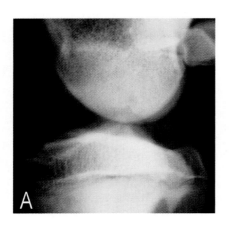

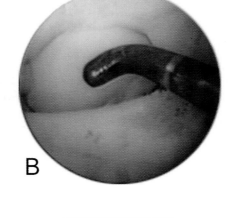

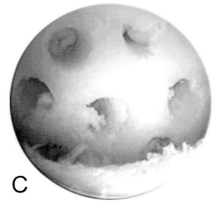

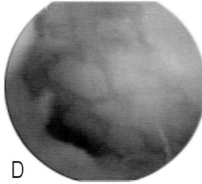

FIGURE 7–30 Radiographic and arthroscopic images of a dog with osteochondritis dissecans of the stifle. *A*, Lateral radiograph showing a radiolucent region of the medial femoral condyle. *B*, Arthroscopic view of an osteochondritis dissecans lesion of the medial femoral condyle with the unstable flap in place. *C*, Medial femoral condyle after removal of the flap, curettage, and forage. *D*, Second-look arthroscopy of the lesion 3.5 months later, showing islands of fibrocartilage stimulated by forage.

Diagnosis. The diagnosis is based on radiographic findings in dogs with appropriate history, physical findings, and signalment. A complete orthopedic examination is performed to exclude other juvenile orthopedic conditions. The contralateral stifle is examined as well. If the condition is bilateral, both stifles are routinely treated during the same anesthetic procedure. Occasionally, asymptomatic radiographic lesions are seen on the contralateral limb. If articular cartilage "blisters" are seen, these lesions are carefully palpated arthroscopically and treated during the same procedure. If no lesion is detected arthroscopically, morbidity as a result of diagnostic arthroscopy during the same anesthetic episode is negligible.

Treatment. Conservative treatment includes NSAID therapy, chondroprotective agents, weight control, and regular low-impact exercise. Most dogs have persistent lameness and more rapid progression of osteoarthritis without surgical intervention, but in most cases, surgery does not alleviate the need for concurrent conservative treatment.

Anesthetic Considerations and Perioperative Pain Management. Cox II NSAIDs are discontinued 1 to 2 days before surgery. Aspirin therapy is discontinued at least 1 week before surgery. Healthy young patients require minimal preoperative laboratory evaluation. Surgical pain is minor and is easily controlled with pre-emptive opioid pain medication, NSAIDs, intra-articular long-acting local anesthetics, and optional cold therapy.

Surgical Intervention. These lesions can be treated by open arthrotomy, but surgical morbidity is considerably higher. Osteochondral autografting techniques and open arthrotomy have been used to treat a limited number of larger, more severe weightbearing defects, with promising results. Portal placement, complete examination, and documentation of the proximal joint were discussed earlier.

Depending on chronicity, varying degrees of hyperplastic synovial changes are routinely seen, but they usually are not as intense as with cranial cruciate ligament rupture. The fat pad is partially débrided, and the cruciate ligaments and menisci are inspected. OCD affects both the medial (see Fig. 7–30A and B) and lateral femoral condyles. The lateral site is more common. These lesions are readily visualized and treated arthroscopically, but a considerable amount of flexion, often more than 90 degrees, is needed to see the entire lesion in some cases. Varus and valgus stress are applied as needed. Free fragments are easily removed with loose body forceps and small grasping forceps. Nondetached cartilage is removed in small bites with a grasper or a motorized shaver. The underlying bed is débrided with the shaver or a small hand curette until bleeding subchondral bone is seen. To avoid overaggressive débridement, inflow is periodically discontinued to check for bleeding. Care is taken to avoid freeing fragments before they are grasped. Smoothing of the bed is best accomplished with the shaver in reverse mode. A

chondral pick can be used for microfracture technique, or a small Kirschner wire can be used for forage to stimulate fibrocartilage response (see Fig. 7–30C and D). Follow-up arthroscopic examination in dogs shows earlier development of fibrocartilage in areas treated with these techniques compared with areas treated with abrasion chondroplasty alone (see Fig. 7–30D). The posterior pouch occasionally contains fragments of cartilage. These fragments can be accessed by inserting the arthroscope between the cruciate ligaments and into the caudal pouch of the knee. In some cases, a smaller (1.9-mm) scope must be used to gain access into the caudal pouch. If fragments are seen, it may be necessary to establish a caudal portal for instrument retrieval, taking care to avoid the popliteal artery.

Postoperative Care. Soft, padded bandages are applied for the first 24 hours. Cold therapy (20 minutes on, 20 minutes off) is applied as often as possible for the first 48 hours. Controlled leash walking is allowed as necessary for elimination. NSAID therapy with Cox II inhibitors is recommended for 2 to 4 weeks but may be needed for a longer period.

Long-term management often includes chondroprotective agents, weight control, and regular low-impact exercise. In most cases, surgery does not alleviate the need for concurrent conservative treatment.

Complications. Complications are rare, but swelling and soreness as a result of hemarthrosis may occur if the patient is not confined for the first 2 weeks postoperatively. Seromas are seen in dogs treated with osteochondral autografting techniques, but this complication is less common when the donor site is packed with generous amounts of Gelfoam after the graft is harvested.

Prognosis. The prognosis for OCD of the stifle is not as favorable as it is in the shoulder. Without treatment, most dogs have persistent lameness and advancement of osteoarthritis. With surgical treatment, some dogs become asymptomatic or minimally symptomatic, despite the inevitable advancement of osteoarthritis. Most dogs are helped, but not cured, and eventually experience recurrent stiffness and lameness. Although patients no doubt have earlier return to function and less short-term morbidity and pain, no studies have compared long-term results for cases treated with arthroscopic versus open procedures.

Osteoarthritis of the Stifle

With few exceptions, osteoarthritis of the stifle is a secondary condition. It develops rapidly in the dog and is most common in those with cranial cruciate ligament injury. Although it appears to develop most severely and rapidly in the cranial cruciate ligament deficient stifle, the changes are similar with other conditions. It is rarely primary in young patients and is usually present to some degree in older patients. Although this condition

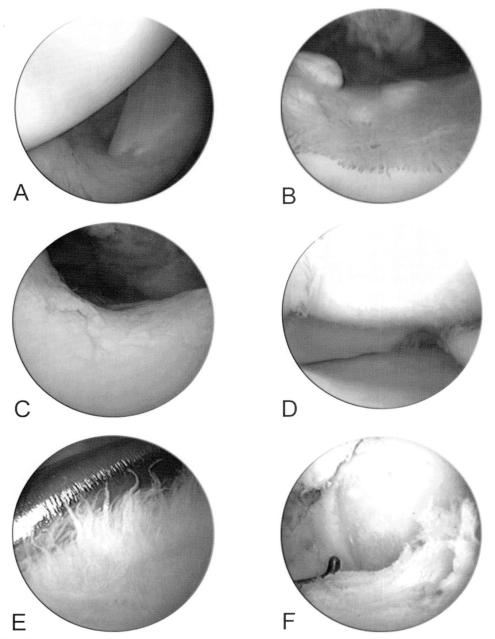

FIGURE 7–31   Arthroscopic images of articular cartilage changes associated with osteoarthritis of the canine stifle. *A,* Normal articular cartilage of the femoral condyle. *B,* Marked neovascularization and pannus of the proximal trochlear groove. *C,* Chondromalacia with fissures of the proximal trochlear groove. *D,* Fine fibrillation and chondromalacia of the medial femoral condyle and tibial plateau during second-look arthroscopy 1 year after tibial plateau leveling osteotomy. Note the unhealed midbody medial meniscal release site. *E,* Deep fibrillation of the medial trochlear ridge of the femur associated with medial patellar luxation. *F,* Full-thickness eburnation of the lateral femoral condyle of a 2-year-old Blue Healer that had a partial cranial cruciate ligament tear and a palpably stable stifle.

is most common in association with cranial cruciate ligament instability, the arthroscopic appearance of osteoarthritis is similar, regardless of etiology.

The anatomy and pathology of the articular cartilage is underappreciated with open arthrotomy. The articular cartilage is smooth and white and indents only slightly when palpated with a probe (Fig. 7–31A). The articular cartilage changes rapidly in dogs with stifle pathology, especially cranial cruciate ligament pathology. Early in stifle osteoarthritis, the articular surface may show neovascularization or pannus formation (see Fig. 7–31B) at three primary sites: the medial trochlear ridge of the femur, the lateral trochlear ridge of the femur, and the trochlear notch. In most cases, this change is seen as a small network of vessels on the surface and penetrating the periphery of the articular cartilage, on the medial and lateral femoral condyles, and at the proximal extent of the trochlea. These sites represent the location of future osteophytes as the condition becomes more chronic. Occasionally, this network of vessels is superficial and only loosely adhered to the articular surface, especially when it arises from a synovial tag in the area of the trochlear notch. Closer inspection of the adjacent articular cartilage usually shows chondromalacia (see Fig. 7–31C). Arthroscopically, the articular cartilage is less smooth and has a slight cobblestone appearance, is slightly gray, and may contain small fissures (see Fig. 7–31C). Classically, it appears soft when probed and marks easily. Lesions of the articular cartilage are graded on a scale of I to V, using a modified Outerbridge system. According to this system, chondromalacia is a grade I lesion (Table 4–1). A grade II lesion has superficial fissures (see Fig. 7–31C) that may be obvious but more often are discrete and easily overlooked. For proper examination and grading, the cartilage must be inspected closely and at a tangent angle. Grade III lesions have full-thickness fissures down to the subchondral bone as well as more obvious fibrillation. Often, it is helpful to stop inflow temporarily to allow close inspection of the articular cartilage for fibrillation. High fluid flow causes invisible movement of the fine fibrillation (see Fig. 7–31D). In the dog, it is difficult to differentiate grade II lesions from grade III lesions because the articular cartilage is so thin. For most practical purposes, if fibrillation is easy to see, the lesion is classified as grade III, and if it is difficult to see, the lesion is classified as grade II. Grade IV lesions are full-thickness regions of deep fibrillation (see Fig. 7–31E). They are identified arthroscopically by the ability to see pinkish-yellow areas of exposed bone. Grade V lesions are areas of full-thickness articular cartilage loss. They have a polished appearance (eburnation) and often have corresponding kissing lesions (see Fig. 7–31F).

When describing articular cartilage lesions, grade refers only to depth. The size and location of the lesions also must be noted. Also, some lesions contain mixed grades of cartilage injury. For this reason, the use of descriptive terms, such as "chondromalacia," "fissuring," "fibrillation," and "eburnation," in conjunction with the size and location of the lesion is often less confusing than attempting to refer to a lesion as a specific grade or

a mixture of grades. Also, some authors prefer to grade the lesion after treatment rather than before, further confusing the issue.

Periarticular osteophytes form rapidly and become large in the canine stifle. Osteophytes occur at four primary sites: the proximal trochlear groove, the medial and lateral trochlear ridges of the femur, and within the intercondylar notch. In addition to their location, osteophytes are classified as follows:

Early: osteophytes are barely visible (Fig. 7–32B)
Advanced: a few isolated osteophytes are seen; they are clearly visible and mostly smooth (see Figs. 7–31B and 7–32C)
Severe and coalescing: a continuous series of medium to large osteophytes is seen; they have a knobbly appearance (see Fig. 7–32D).

Documenting changes in articular cartilage, including osteophytes, helps to determine the efficacy of treatment when second-look arthroscopy is performed and allows the actual findings to be compared with the preoperative radiographic assessment. Osteophytes may be visible arthroscopically before they are readily apparent radiographically.

History and Signalment. In most cases, osteoarthritis of the stifle joint is caused by cranial cruciate ligament insufficiency, but it may occur in any dog as a result of traumatic, infectious, immune-mediated, or developmental causes. Some dogs have subtle to severe lameness; others have difficulty rising without lameness. Patients may "warm out" of the lameness with light exercise and sit with the affected leg away from the body. In mild cases, lameness may be apparent only after aggressive exercise. Dogs commonly "override" their lameness (completely or partially) with excitement.

Physical Examination. Physical examination findings are dependent on the etiology and chronicity of the condition. Manipulation of the stifle may show pain during hyperextension or hyperflexion or decreased range of motion, primarily in flexion. Palpation of the stifle joint may show mild to severe effusion. As the disease progresses, palpable thickening as a result of fibrosis and bony proliferation may become apparent, especially medially. Muscle atrophy is common. In mild cases, minimal abnormal findings may be noted on orthopedic examination.

Differential Diagnosis. The differential diagnosis includes osteochondrosis, rupture of the cranial cruciate ligament, neoplasia, immune-mediated arthritis, medial patellar laxation, panosteitis, septic arthritis, lumbosacral disease, hip dysplasia, and neurologic disease.

Diagnostic Findings. Diagnostic tests include radiography and arthrocentesis. Radiographic findings vary dramatically with the severity of disease. As the osteoarthritis progresses, osteophytosis and sclerosis increase. Arthrocentesis usually shows cell counts of 2000 to

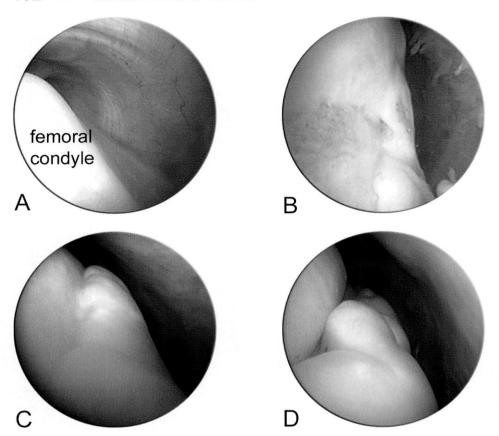

FIGURE 7–32 Arthroscopic images of osteophytes of the lateral trochlear ridge of the femoral condyle. *A*, Normal; *B*, early; *C*, advanced; *D*, severe and coalescing.

5000/μL, with a predominance of mature mononuclear cells.

Treatment. Medical treatment consists of anti-inflammatory medication and control of activity and body weight. Surgical treatment is directed toward the underlying cause of the osteoarthritis in conjunction with arthroscopic treatment of identified articular cartilage and synovial pathology.

Anesthetic Considerations and Perioperative Pain Management. A standard anesthetic protocol, including preemptive pain medication, is used (see Table 3–1). Postoperative pain is controlled with cold therapy, opioids, and NSAIDs.

Surgical Intervention. Portal sites and surgical anatomy were discussed earlier. With the advent of arthroscopy, in bilateral cases, both stifles may be treated simultaneously. In more severe cases, the joints may be staged to limit weightbearing on the operated limb postoperatively. Standard portal placement and complete stifle examination and documentation of the joint were discussed earlier.

In humans, pain is significantly reduced by aggressive removal of hyperplastic synovium in affected joints. Although total synovectomy is not possible, aggressive subtotal synovectomy has been used successfully in dogs with mixed but generally favorable results. Additional maximal portals may be necessary for effective removal of hyperplastic synovium in the proximal compartments. A motorized shaver is used in oscillatory mode to remove as much hyperplastic synovium as possible. Arthroscopic synovectomy should be recommended as an adjunct to medical management, weight control, and physical therapy. The procedure may be repeated periodically if results are rewarding and clinical signs return. After the joint is thoroughly explored and the extent of the lesion is defined, an instrument portal is created. The surgeon should visually evaluate and palpate the areas of cartilage damage and note the size and severity of the lesion based on the scale shown in Table 4–1.

Areas of chondomolacia and mild fibrillation (grades I to II) are generally left undisturbed. Grade III lesions are areas of full-thickness fibrillation and may be treated, although the efficacy of treatments is controversial. A curette or burr is used to remove the diseased cartilage, taking care to avoid damaging the surrounding, more normal cartilage. The resulting subchondral bone bed is treated by abrasion or light curettage to expose bleeding subchondral bone. Microfracture technique or forage may be added for larger lesions. Grade IV cartilage damage is full-thickness loss of cartilage and exposure, and, in some cases, eburnation of the subchondral bone. These lesions are treated in similar fashion.

To perform abrasion arthroplasty, a hand burr, or preferentially, a power shaver used in forward mode with a blade or hooded burr, is inserted through the instrument portal. Because both methods produce significant bone debris that can clog the egress portal and impede visualization, it is important to monitor and maintain the flow of fluid through the joint. The burr or blade is spun to remove subchondral bone over the area of the lesion. Inflow of fluid is stopped periodically to allow the surgeon to check for resulting bleeding. In addition, adequate outflow must be ensured to decrease the pressure in the joint. When bleeding is observed diffusely from the lesion bed, the joint is lavaged to remove the remaining bone debris and routine closure is performed.

To perform microfracture, an appropriately angled micropick is inserted into the joint and the tip is pressed against the subchondral surface of the bone. An assistant should lightly tap the pick handle with a mallet once or twice. The pick must be held securely to avoid gouging the surface and adjacent healthy cartilage. The micropick is applied diffusely across the diseased area. The surgeon should check for resulting bleeding often by stopping the inflow of fluid and ensuring adequate outflow. When bleeding is observed diffusely from the lesion bed, the joint is lavaged to remove the remaining bone debris and routine closure is performed.

In some joints, it is relatively easy to produce diffuse, effective bleeding, whereas in others, it is much more difficult. Combining abrasion and microfracture may increase subchondral bleeding. If eburnation is present, the surgeon may have difficulty achieving significant bleeding with these techniques. The forage technique can be used in lieu of microfracture to allow deeper penetration of subchondral bone. After abrasion chondroplasty is performed, a small K-wire (0.045- to 0.0624-inch) is used to drill small, equally spaced holes in the lesion (see Fig. 7–30C and D and Fig. 7-33B).

Postoperative Management and Complications. Postoperative management and complications are identical to those associated with routine stifle arthroscopy. Typically, osteoarthritis requires lifelong medical management. Treatment includes exercise, physical therapy, and control of body weight in combination with NSAIDs and chondroprotective medications.

Prognosis. The efficacy of arthroscopic treatment in the management of osteoarthritis of the stifle is unknown. The efficacy is likely to be much greater when combined with medical management, physical therapy, and weight control. Severe cases may be unresponsive, and some cases may require additional arthroscopic débridement or surgical intervention, including corrective osteotomy, arthrodesis, or joint replacement.

Septic Osteomyelitis

In cases of septic arthritis, arthroscopic evaluation allows precise assessment of the articular surface and improves prognostic accuracy. Large-diameter catheters and high flow volumes are effective in joint lavage after specimens are collected for culture and sensitivity tests.

Idiopathic septic arthritis of the stifle occasionally is seen in young dogs and sometimes is related to hematogenous osteomyelitis of the metaphysis. Unfortunately, in most cases, there is no good alternative to treating the aftermath of septic arthritis in the stifle. Placement of implants to provide arthrodesis in a previously infected area must be recommended cautiously and only after months of successful antibiotic therapy. Successful stifle arthrodesis eliminates pain, but causes considerable gait abnormality. Amputation is an alternative that satisfactorily relieves pain and should be considered, especially in cases of life-threatening sepsis. Another alternative for salvage is aggressive arthroscopic débridement of infected cartilage and diseased tissues combined with medical management and physical therapy. Although this procedure does not result in a normal joint, many dogs have a surprising amount of function, even after aggressive removal of large amounts of articular cartilage. The owner must understand that this procedure is a salvage attempt and should realize that amputation or arthrodesis may be the final outcome.

History and Signalment. Any age, sex, or breed can be affected. Most cases present with lameness and may have a history of a puncture wound, bite wound, or draining tract. Most spontaneous cases occur in immature dogs, although the majority of cases are associated with previous stifle surgery. Lethargy, depression, and anorexia also may be present. Affected dogs may have responded well to previous antibiotic therapy.

Physical Examination. Most patients are nonweightbearing. Manipulation of the joint elicits pain, and effusion is evident. Popliteal lymphadenopathy may be evident as well. In long-standing disease, pitting edema of the distal extremity may be present and the limb may be warm to the touch. Pyrexia is common.

Differential Diagnosis. The differential diagnosis includes immune-mediated joint disease, fractures of the stifle, OCD, avulsion fractures of the cruciate ligaments, panosteitis, injury of the collateral ligaments, patellar tendon injury, partial cruciate tears, and neoplasia.

Radiographic Findings. Radiographs are usually unremarkable but may show soft tissue swelling. Most cases present acutely. Bony lysis may be evident if hematogenous metaphyseal osteomyelitis is present or is the source of disease or if osteomyelitis is associated with an implant. Lytic changes in the area of the intercondylar notch or implants may be the result of previous intraarticular repair of a cranial cruciate ligament injury.

Diagnosis. Diagnosis is based on the history, physical examination findings, and arthrocentesis results. Joint fluid is typically yellow or brown and cloudy, has poor viscosity, and is increased in volume. Fluid analysis is usually diagnostic. Cytology shows large numbers of polymorphonuclear leukocytes (usually >100,000 cells/μL), many of which are usually toxic. Cases that were treated and responded to long-term antibiotic therapy may be

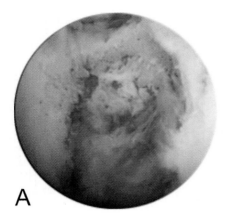

A

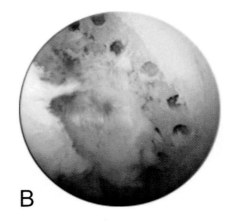

B

FIGURE 7–33 *A,* Septic osteomyelitis of the intertrochanteric notch before treatment. *B,* The same lesion after biopsy, culture, aggressive shaver débridement, and forage. The caudal cruciate ligament is intact.

less obvious. Figure 7–33*A* shows the typical appearance of an area of septic osteomyelitis.

Treatment. These cases are treated as surgical emergencies. The joint is aggressively lavaged as quickly as possible to minimize damage to the articular cartilage. Culture and sensitivity testing should be performed before antibiotic therapy is initiated. Treatment with broad-spectrum intravenous antibiotics that provide good aerobic and anaerobic coverage is initiated immediately. When osteomyelitis is involved, long-term antibiotic therapy is necessary, and antibiotic selection is based on the results of aerobic and anaerobic culture and sensitivity testing.

Anesthetic Considerations and Perioperative Pain Management. A complete blood count and chemistry panel should be obtained, but processing of laboratory tests should not delay intervention. If the source of infection is unknown, urinalysis, blood cultures, abdominal ultrasound, and thoracic radiographs may be necessary. Cox II NSAIDs, in conjunction with opioids, are used to control pain. Alternately, parenteral or oral opioids or a fentanyl transdermal patch can be used, with or without NSAID therapy. Most cases are painful acutely, but treatment relieves pain and improves attitude dramatically.

Surgical Intervention. Positioning, portal placement, and systematic arthroscopic examination and photographic documentation of the joint were discussed earlier. Before the arthroscope is introduced, the joint is aggressively lavaged with large volumes of lactated Ringer's solution. If the patient has sepsis and is systemically ill or has severe periarticular swelling, treatment is staged. A large-diameter cannula system is used to lavage the joint and arthroscopic examination is delayed until the patient is more stable and the swelling subsides. If swelling is severe, prearthroscopic intravenous antibiotic therapy with a bandage and drainage (grenade) for 24 to 48 hours may facilitate arthroscopic examination, which can be performed later. The joint is examined arthroscopically, diseased tissue is débrided, the articular cartilage is evaluated, and implants are removed if

necessary. The surgeon may find it helpful to periodically change ingress from one portal to the other and even to provide ingress through the superior portal to help dislodge fibrinopurulent material from the joint pouches. In severe cases, superior portals are established both medially and laterally. High inflow rates are used, and a motorized shaver or an instrument cannula are used to remove and suction fibrinopurulent material. In addition, the caudal pouch is inspected as described earlier, and an additional caudal instrument portal is established for removal of fibrinopurulent material if indicated.

The goal of arthroscopic treatment is to identify the nidus of infection and débride it and the infected tissue. If the infection is diagnosed early, no nidus may be identifiable, especially in spontaneously occurring septic arthritis. In previously operated cases, pieces of suture or areas of necrotic bone may be found. If intra-articular grafts have been implanted, osteomyelitis of the intracondylar notch may be identified. This tissue is usually readily identifiable as abnormal and may have a covering of inflamed granulation tissue, with or without synovial adhesions (see Fig. 7–29*A*). The tissue should be débrided aggressively with a motorized shaver until healthy, bleeding subchondral bone is seen. To avoid excessive débridement, the surgeon should periodically discontinue the ingress and check for bone bleeding. Involved articular cartilage is débrided similarly. To stimulate the response of fibrocartilage, a small K-wire is used to drill several closely spaced holes (forage) in the denuded subchondral bone to stimulate fibrocartilage response (see Fig. 7–33*B*). Alternately, a chondral pick is used to perform microfracture. The joint pouches are checked for fibrinopurulent material and it is removed when found. At the conclusion of the procedure, the joint is lavaged aggressively.

Postoperative Care. Aggressive intravenous antibiotic therapy with good aerobic and anaerobic coverage is initiated pending culture and sensitivity results. Antibiotic treatment is adjusted based on culture and sensitivity results. Bandage and drainage (grenade) are optional but may not be necessary if aggressive débridement and lavage were performed. The recommended approach is to leave the portals open, perform aggressive hydrotherapy and massage postoperatively, and allow walking as tolerated. Aggressive postoperative physical therapy is ideal. Intravenous antibiotics should be maintained for several days prior to switching to longer term oral antibiotics.

Complications. Complications include residual infection, recurrent infection, persistent lameness, osteoarthritis, and osteomyelitis. Residual lameness may be caused by previous or secondary cranial cruciate ligament rupture; however, septic joints usually undergo considerable periarticular fibrosis that leads to stabilization. Definitive stabilization procedures such as TPLO may be required after the infection is resolved.

Prognosis. The prognosis is good to excellent if treatment is provided before significant articular cartilage damage occurs and if the intra-articular ligaments are intact. It is guarded in patients that have significant articular loss. The prognosis also depends on the integrity of the intra-articular and collateral ligaments. The prognosis may be refined after the articular surfaces are examined arthroscopically.

Medial Patellar Luxation

Most cases of medial patellar luxation are too severe to be treated arthroscopically. The exception may be acute traumatic patellar luxations and grade I and II luxations in dogs that have good conformation. These cases may be treated arthroscopically, but case selection is critical and results are mixed in a small number of cases. Additional work is needed to determine the ideal case selection and efficacy. Procedures have been performed with complete informed consent by the owners and with the understanding that this technique is new and unproven and that more invasive open procedures may be necessary if reluxation occurs. Although scarring is minimal, the benefit of decreased pain is not as remarkable with this procedure as with most stifle arthroscopic procedures because the highly innervated joint capsule is incised.

History and Signalment. Any age, sex, or breed may be affected. If the cause of injury is traumatic, lameness may be severe and is often intermittent. Grade I and II congenital patellar luxations may cause low-grade lameness that may be chronic or intermittent and associated with exercise.

Physical Examination Findings. Physical examination shows grade I to II medial patellar luxation and weightbearing lameness. Swelling and discomfort are often present in traumatic cases. Some cases are not obviously lame until the patella is manipulated during examination.

Differential Diagnosis. The differential diagnosis includes partial rupture of the cranial cruciate ligament,

fracture, contusion, and injury to the quadriceps tendon or patellar tendon.

Radiographic Findings. Radiographs are performed to exclude fracture. Usually, they are normal or show mild effusion. Skyline views may be beneficial.

Diagnosis. Diagnosis is based on the history, physical findings, and exclusion of other causes of lameness.

Treatment. Conservative treatment with Cox II NSAIDs should be attempted before surgical intervention is performed, especially in patients with grade I luxation.

Anesthetic Considerations and Perioperative Pain Management. NSAIDs are discontinued 1 to 2 days before surgery, although discontinuation is not mandatory if Cox II NSAIDs are used. Young, healthy patients require minimal preoperative laboratory evaluation. Older patients should be adequately screened to exclude underlying metabolic disorders. Administration of NSAIDs for 15 days in conjunction with cold therapy for 48 hours is usually adequate. Alternately, parenteral or oral opioids or a fentanyl transdermal patch can be used, with or without NSAID therapy.

Surgical Intervention. Positioning, portal placement, systematic arthroscopic examination, and photographic documentation of the joint were described earlier. However, the technique is modified slightly to place the superior portal lateral to the quadriceps tendon instead of medial. The articular cartilage of the medial trochlear ridge of the femur and the lateral articular cartilage of the patella are inspected carefully. In chronic cases, fibrillation or eburnation may be present in both areas (Fig. 7–34A). The joint should be maximally distended and the light post positioned in the 6 o'clock position for adequate visualization. Under direct arthroscopic visualization, a hook-tipped electrocautery or radiofrequency probe is inserted through the instrument portal and placed just medial to the cranial pole of the patella. The joint capsule and medial retinacular tissue are incised, including the medial fibrocartilage wing of the patella and the medial femoropatellar ligament from inside to out (see Fig. 7–34B and D). Care is taken not to include the skin. The incision is continued distally, in a straight line adjacent to the patellar tendon, to the instrument portal. If the incision is adequate, extravasation of fluid into the subcutaneous tissue should be evident.

Arthroscopically, an obvious dark subcutaneous cavity is seen as fluid fills the subcutaneous space. The goal of the procedure is to release the tissues medially to allow dynamic realignment of the patella.

Postoperative Care. A Robert Jones bandage is applied for the first 24 hours to reduce swelling. The bandage is changed and maintained for an additional 5 days. The patella may reluxate during the first 1 to 2 postoperative weeks. As discomfort resolves and muscle function improves, realignment usually ensues.

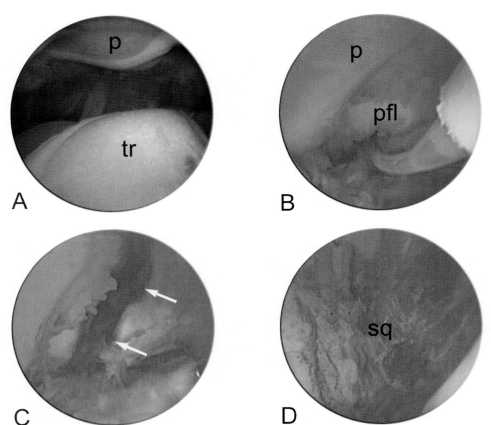

FIGURE 7–34 Arthroscopic images of pathology associated with medial patellar luxation and arthroscopic release of the medial retinaculum. *A,* Eburnation of the medial trochlear ridge (*tr*) of the femur and corresponding eburnation of the lateral aspect of the patella (*p*). *B,* Intraoperative view of arthroscopic release of the medial retinaculum with a hook-tipped radiofrequency probe immediately before transection of the patello-femoral ligament (*pfl*). *C,* The same view immediately after treatment, showing the transected ligament (*arrows*). *D,* Completed procedure after the remaining retinacular tissue is released, showing the dark cavity formed by extravasation of fluid into the subcutaneous space (*sq*).

Complications. Overaggressive electrosurgical incision can result in cutting through the skin. The most common complication is reluxation, which is directly related to incorrect case selection. These cases often require more invasive surgical procedures (e.g., tibial tuberosity transposition, wedge recession trochleoplasty). This procedure is more painful than routine arthroscopic examination because the highly innervated joint capsule is incised. Physical therapy should be provided for at least 1 month before the result is considered a failure because this dynamic realignment requires adequate reestablishment of muscle function.

Prognosis. The prognosis is excellent if reluxation does not occur. Patients that have significant articular cartilage show significant improvement, likely because direct bone-on-bone contact is reduced and the force is redistributed to healthier articular cartilage.

Suggested Readings

Beale BS: Arthroscopic-assisted stabilization of the cruciate-deficient stifle in dogs using a percutaneous prosthetic ligament-suture anchor technique. Vet Surg 29(5):457, 2000.

Chandler JC, Whitney WO, Beale BS: Management of partial cranial cruciate ruptures with arthroscopic assisted tibial plateau leveling osteotomy. Proceedings of the 29th Annual Conference of the Veterinary Orthopedic Society, The Canyons, Utah, 2002.

Hulse DA, Beale BS: Arthroscopically assisted "under and over" reconstruction of the cranial cruciate ligament in the dog. Proceedings of the 27th Annual Conference of the Veterinary Orthopedic Society, Val d'Isere, France, March 2000, p. 22.

Kivumbi CW, Bennett D: Arthroscopy of the canine stifle joint. Vet Rec 109:241–249, 1981.

Lewis DD, Goring RL, Parker RB, et al: A comparison of diagnostic methods used in the evaluation of early degenerative joint disease in the dog. J Am Anim Hosp Assoc 23:305–315, 1987.

McGinty, John B. M.D.: In Operative Arthroscopy, Preface to Second Edition, Philadelphia, Lippincott-Raven, 1996.

McLaughlin RM, Hurtig RM, Fries CL: Operative arthroscopy in the treatment of bilat stifle osteochondritis dissecans in a dog. Vet Compar Orthop Traum 4:158–161, 1989.

Miller CW, Presnell KR: Examination of the canine stifle: arthroscopy versus arthrotomy. J Am Anim Hosp Assoc 21:623–629, 1985.

Person MW: A procedure for arthroscopic examination of the canine stifle joint. J Am Anim Hosp Assoc 21:179–186, 1985.

Ralphs SC, Whitney WO: Arthroscopic evaluation of meniscal tears in dogs with cranial cruciate ligament injuries: 100 consecutive cases. Accepted for publication, J Am Vet Med Assoc, 2002.

Siemering GB: Arthroscopy of dogs. J Am Vet Med Assoc 172:575–577, 1978.

Siemering GB, Eilert RE: Arthroscopic study of cranial cruciate ligament and medial meniscal lesions in the dog. Vet Surg 15:265–269, 1986.

Van Gestel, MA: Arthroscopy of the canine stifle joint. Vet Q 7:237–239, 1985.

Van Gestel, MA: Diagnostic accuracy of stifle arthroscopy in the dog. J Am Anim Hosp Assoc 21:757–763, 1985.

Whitney WO: Arthroscopic reconstruction of the cranial cruciate ligament in the dog. Proceedings of the Eighth Annual ACVS Symposium, Chicago, 1998.

Whitney WO: Arthroscopy of the canine stifle. Proceedings of the Third Annual International Arthroscopy Workshop, Ghent, Belgium, 1998.

Whitney WO: Basic arthroscopy of the canine stifle. In Slatter Textbook of Small Animal Surgery, Philadelphia, WB Saunders, in press.

Whitney WO: Basic arthroscopy of the canine stifle. Arthroscopy Proceedings of the Nineth Annual ACVS Symposium, San Francisco, 1999.

Whitney WO: Arthroscopic observation in dogs with cranial cruciate ligament deficient stifles. Proceedings of the Tenth Annual ACVS Symposium, Arlington, Virginia, 2000.

Whitney WO: Principles of arthroscopic meniscal treatment and stifle débridement. Proceedings of the 2001 Advanced International Arthroscopy Workshop, Ghent, Belgium, 2001.

Whitney WO, Chandler JC, Beale BS: Proceedings of the First World Orthopaedic Veterinary Congress, Munich, Germany, September 2002.

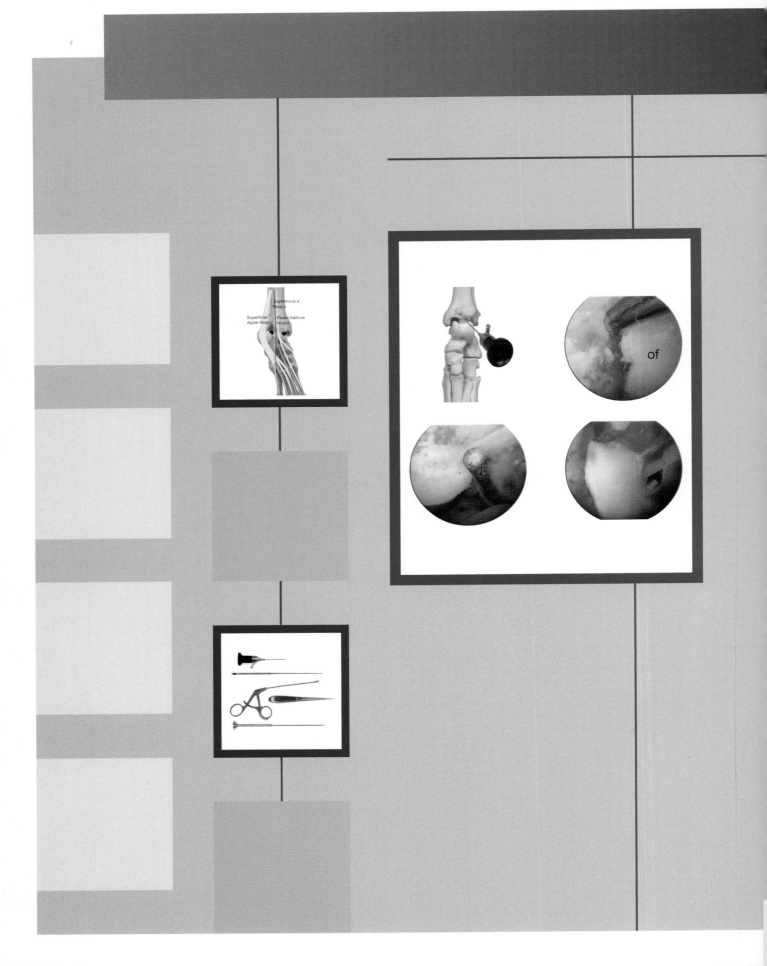

Arthroscopically Assisted Surgery of the Tarsal Joint

Introduction

The canine tarsal joint is challenging to examine arthroscopically. An experienced surgeon can use arthroscopy to evaluate the articular surfaces of the tibiotarsal joint, remove osteochondral flaps associated with osteochondritis dissecans (OCD), and remove or assist in the reduction of fracture fragments. Early intervention is recommended because arthroscopy becomes more difficult as joint capsule fibrosis and osteoarthritis progress. Arthroscopy of the tarsus is only in its infancy; future applications will grow as expertise and experience are gained.

Arthroscopy of the Tarsal Joint

Equipment and Instrumentation. For tarsal arthroscopy, the surgery table is adjusted to a position that allows the surgeon and assistants to hold the arms as close to the body as possible (Fig. 8–1). The surgeon's shoulders should be held in neutral position with the elbows close to 90 degrees. This position prevents fatigue and improves the efficiency of the operating team. The imaging tower is positioned at the head of the patient or opposite the surgeon. Fluid ingress is achieved with a pressurized gravity bag or an infusion fluid pump administered through the arthroscope cannula. Fluid can be evacuated by allowing it to flow freely through the egress needle (or cannula) or through a working cannula. Evacuation of fluid can be assisted with suction attached to the egress needle (or cannula). If suction is used, it must be set at a low level or bubbles will be produced that obscure the surgeon's view.

A 30-degree fore-oblique arthroscope is commonly used. Because the tibiotarsal joint space is small, in most dogs, a 1.9-mm arthroscope is the best choice. In large breeds, a 2.4- to 2.7-mm arthroscope may be used

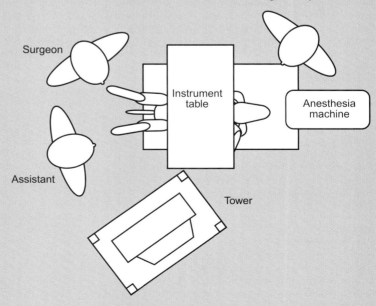

Surgeon

Instrument table

Anesthesia machine

Assistant

Tower

FIGURE 8–1 Arrangement of the operating room for tarsal arthroscopy.

successfully if the joint capsule can be distended. Even in large dogs, a smaller scope is suggested to prevent iatrogenic damage to the cartilage. Whichever size arthroscope is chosen, the surgeon must consider the outside diameter of the arthroscope cannula because it too must enter the joint. Each arthroscope cannula is fitted with a blunt, canonical obturator and a sharp trocar. In most cases, the sharp trocar is not needed to enter the joint. When it is used, caution must be exercised to prevent iatrogenic damage to the cartilage. A blunt, conical obturator is recommended for entering the joint.

Tarsal arthroscopy requires an assortment of hand instruments (Fig. 8–2). Recommended are instruments to assist in the inspection of intra-articular structures (probes), grasping forceps to remove free bodies, biopsy forceps, and instruments to perform surface abrasion and synovectomy. Instruments can be inserted into the joint through an open instrument port, instrument cannulas, or a combination of the two. If the surgeon works through an instrument cannula, different-sized cannulas and switching sticks are helpful.

Anesthetic Considerations and Perioperative Pain Management. Preoperative laboratory workup is based on the patient's physical status and surgical risk. Young, healthy patients with no underlying systemic problems require minimal laboratory evaluation. Older dogs should undergo a complete blood screen, urinalysis, chest radiographs, and an electrocardiogram. Table 3–1 shows a standard anesthetic protocol, including preemptive pain medication. Postoperative pain is minimal, but pain management with epidural analgesia, opioids, and nonsteroidal anti-inflammatory drugs (NSAIDs) can be used if necessary. If arthroscopy is completed early in the day, the patient may be dismissed from the hospital the same afternoon unless an associated surgical procedure requires hospitalization. If arthroscopy is completed later in the afternoon, the patient is discharged the next day.

All patients receive preemptive analgesic drugs as part of the premedication protocol. Buprenorphine is the preferred agent because of its effectiveness in dogs that have mild to moderate postoperative pain and its relatively long mode of action (6 to 8 hours). When the dog is dismissed from the hospital, NSAIDs and oral butorphanol (see Table 3–1) are dispensed for administration at home. NSAIDs are continued for 5 days, and butorphanol is discontinued after 48 hours. If the dog remains in the hospital overnight, a second dose of buprenorphine is administered in the evening, and NSAIDs and butorphanol are prescribed for home administration. Fentanyl transdermal patches also may be used to manage postoperative pain.

Patient Preparation and Positioning. The patient is clipped and prepared for open arthrotomy in case the arthroscopy procedure must be aborted for technical reasons and an open arthrotomy performed. This situation is more common when the surgeon is beginning to learn arthroscopy. The damaged region of the articular surface is identified by thoroughly assessing the joint radiographically before surgery. The tarsus is divided into the following four quadrants for evaluation: dorsomedial, plantaromedial, dorsolateral, and plantarolateral. Once a lesion is classified to a specific region of the tarsus, a surgical approach or an arthroscopic portal can be selected that gives access to the area of interest. A hanging limb preparation is recommended. If the dorsal aspect of the joint is to be approached, the patient is positioned in dorsal recumbency with the hind legs extended (Fig. 8–3). If the plantar aspect of the joint is to be approached, the patient is best assessed in ventral recumbency with the hind legs extended (Fig. 8–4). Ventral or dorsal recumbency allows for bilateral tarsal arthroscopy and may allow easier manipulation of working instruments. An experienced arthroscopist may be able to access all four portals from either a dorsal or a ventral recumbency position by flexing or extending the joints of the hindlimb as needed to gain access to the underside of the joint. Although this approach may be awkward for the beginning arthroscopist, it avoids the need to reposition the dog and allows access to all regions of both hocks. Lateral recumbency with the affected leg placed uppermost can be used if only one tarsus needs to be evaluated. It is often helpful to allow the tarsus and foot to protrude past the end of the table. By preventing the surgical table from interfering with the scope, this position allows adjustment of the tarsus position and greater manipulation of the scope. The leg is surgically draped with four quadrant towels and a sterile cloth, paper, or adhesive drape. A clear adhesive sterile drape repels water, keeps the patient dry, and reduces the opportunity for contamination from wet towels and drapes (Figs. 8–5 and 8–6).

Portal Sites. Depending on the purpose of arthroscopic intervention, two or three portal sites are used. Visual exploration requires an egress portal and an

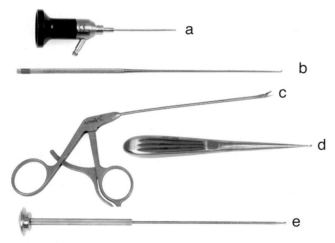

FIGURE 8–2 Instrumentation for tarsal arthroscopy. A 1.9-mm arthroscope (a) is ideal for most patients. A blunt probe (b) is useful for evaluation of the articular cartilage and ligaments. Grasping forceps (c) are used to remove small osteochondral fragments or synovium. A curette (d) is used for débridement of damaged cartilage and curettage of eburnated bone. A hand burr (e) is used for débridement of damaged cartilage and eburnated bone.

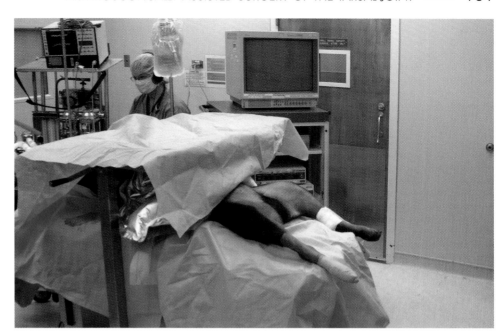

FIGURE 8–3 Positioning of the dog before draping for bilateral arthroscopy of the dorsal portion of the tibiotarsal joint.

arthroscope portal. However, if tissue biopsy or treatment of joint pathology is undertaken, then an additional instrument portal is required. Alternatively, the egress portal may be converted to an instrument portal.

The egress portal usually is established first, followed by the scope portal. The four commonly used scope portals are the dorsomedial, dorsolateral, plantaromedial, and plantarolateral portals (Figs. 8–7 and 8–8). The scope portal usually is located medially if the lateral aspect of the joint is to be viewed and laterally if the medial aspect of the joint is to be viewed. For example, a dorsomedial scope portal is used to view the dorso-

lateral aspect of the tibiotarsal joint. When this technique is used to examine the joint, a longer length of the scope is located inside the joint and inadvertent dislodgement is less likely. The necessary regions of the joint also can be examined with an arthroscopic portal that is made directly over the affected quadrant of the joint. For example, a plantaromedial scope portal can be used to view an osteochondrosis flap that is located on the plantar aspect of the medial trochlear ridge. With this technique, a shorter length of the scope sits in the joint, increasing the likelihood of accidental dislodgement. A dorsolateral or dorsomedial scope portal can be used to

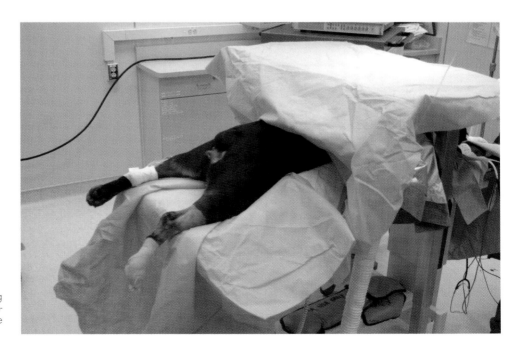

FIGURE 8–4 Positioning of the dog before draping for bilateral arthroscopy of the plantar portion of the tibiotarsal joint.

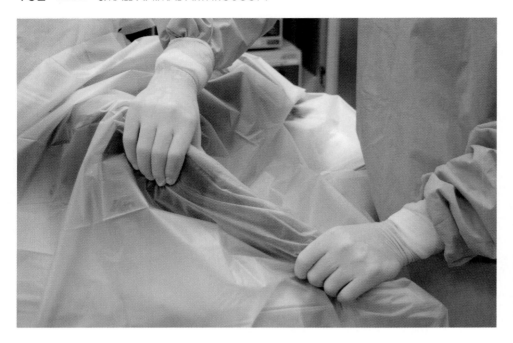

FIGURE 8–5 A patient prepared for tarsal arthroscopy of the dorsal aspect of the joint with four quadrant towels and a clear adhesive sterile drape. The drape repels water, keeping the patient dry and reducing the opportunity for contamination from wet towels and drapes. This method of preparation permits good manipulation of the limb during arthroscopy and allows the surgeon to convert to an open arthrotomy if needed. The tarsus is extended for dorsal arthroscopy.

examine the dorsal aspect of the joint. Examination of the plantar aspect of the joint requires a plantarolateral or plantaromedial portal. The surgeon should be familiar with all of the arthroscopic portals of the tarsus because complete visualization and access to the joint may require the use of multiple portals. If visualization is inadequate or if the scope is difficult to maintain in an intra-articular position, the surgeon should not hesitate to change to a new portal. Often, different portals allow access to similar regions of the tarsus. With time and experience, the surgeon will learn which portals to use for specific applications. For conditions that affect the

tarsus, such as OCD, arthroscopic treatment is a viable alternative to arthrotomy. Arthroscopy is flexible and effective and has a low morbidity rate.

General Surgical Procedure. An 18- to 20-gauge (1.5-inch) spinal needle is used to distend the joint with saline. This needle functions as an egress cannula and is positioned on the side of the joint opposite the intended location of the scope portal. For example, if the scope portal is dorsomedial, the egress portal is dorsolateral. If an instrument portal is needed, the egress cannula can be placed in a different location to allow three func-

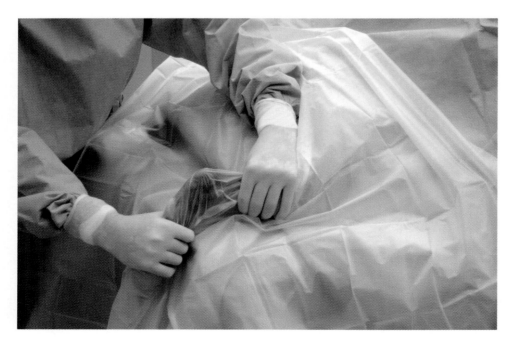

FIGURE 8–6 A patient prepared for tarsal arthroscopy of the plantar aspect of the joint with four quadrant towels and a clear adhesive sterile drape. The drape repels water, keeping the patient dry and reducing the opportunity for contamination from wet towels and drapes. This method of preparation permits good manipulation of the limb during arthroscopy and allows the surgeon to convert to an open arthrotomy if needed. The tarsus is flexed for plantar arthroscopy.

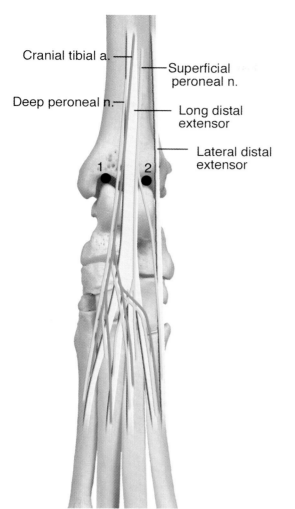

FIGURE 8-7 Portal locations and pertinent anatomy for canine tarsal arthroscopy. *1*, Dorsomedial arthroscope portal location; *2*, dorsolateral arthroscope portal location.

tional portals. For example, to treat an OCD lesion that involves the plantaromedial aspect of the trochlea, the following portals are established: a plantarolateral scope portal, a plantaromedial instrument portal, and a dorsolateral egress portal.

The tibiotarsal joint and the trochlear ridge of the talus are palpated. These structures may be easier to identify if palpation is performed while the joint is flexed and extended. The needle is inserted perpendicular to and just over the palpable ridge of the trochlear ridge into the joint. The surgeon often feels a popping sensation when the joint is entered. To ensure placement within the joint, a syringe is attached to the needle and synovial fluid is aspirated. In most cases, when the needle is properly placed, synovial fluid is easily aspirated. If synovial fluid is not aspirated and the surgeon believes that the joint has been entered, lactated Ringer's solution is instilled into the joint. If the needle is located in the joint, fluid is easily instilled. Also, as the joint cavity begins to fill with fluid, reverse pressure is felt on the syringe plunger. This sensation ensures proper place-

ment of the needle into the joint. The joint cavity is distended with 3 to 6 mL lactated Ringer's solution, and distension is maintained by leaving the syringe attached to the needle (the assistant maintains pressure on the plunger). The fluid ingress line can be temporarily attached to the egress needle (replacing the syringe) to sustain joint distension while the scope cannula is inserted. The needle is maintained as the egress cannula. Evacuation of fluid maintains fluid flow through the joint, enhancing visualization. Intravenous or suction tubing can be attached to the needle to capture fluid as it leaves the joint. Alternatively, fluid is allowed to spill onto the floor for capture by a floor suction unit, a basin, or towels.

A guide needle (20- to 22-gauge) is inserted at the intended site for the scope portal. If the needle is positioned correctly, fluid leaks from its hub. A no. 11 Bard-Parker blade is used to make a small entry wound through the skin and superficial soft tissues adjacent to the needle. A scalpel blade should not be used to enter the joint because extravasation of fluid outside the joint cavity is more likely. However, in patients that have marked thickening of the joint capsule, a small stab incision made into the joint capsule can greatly aid atraumatic insertion of the arthroscope cannula. Fluid extravasation is not a problem if the incision is small and good egress flow is maintained. The needle is removed, and the arthroscope cannula is inserted with the attached pointed, blunt obturator in the same

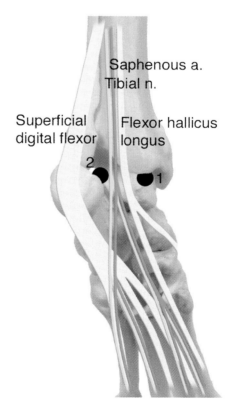

FIGURE 8-8 Portal locations and pertinent anatomy for canine tarsal arthroscopy. *1*, Plantaromedial arthroscope portal location; *2*, plantarolateral arthroscope portal location.

direction as the needle. The tip of the blunt obturator can be walked off the edge of the trochlear ridge to aid localization of the joint space. When a pointed, blunt obturator is used, pressure must be applied to penetrate the joint capsule. With experience, the surgeon will learn to feel when the joint is entered. After the joint is entered, the obturator is removed from the cannula. Fluid flows freely from the cannula, confirming that placement is correct. The fluid ingress line is attached to the cannula, and the arthroscope is inserted.

Manipulation of the arthroscope should be minimized to avoid inadvertent damage to the cartilage surface and reduce the likelihood of accidental dislodgement of the arthroscope. The tip of the scope can be tipped slightly or carefully advanced and withdrawn to increase the viewable area. The light post is rotated to change the orientation of the oblique lens to further increase the field of view. If the cartilage surface is difficult to visualize as a result of synovial proliferation, the joint is distended further by temporarily occluding the egress cannula. If the view remains obstructed, a mini-shaver is inserted through an instrument portal and synovectomy is performed. Fluid ingress flow is increased as needed to control intra-articular hemorrhage. Intra-articular cautery can be used to control bleeding. Systematic exploration of all accessible intra-articular structures is recommended.

The instrument portal is established if biopsy of intra-articular tissue or treatment of joint pathology is required. Like the egress portal, the instrument portal usually is made on the side of the limb opposite the scope portal. To improve access to the necessary structures, the instrument portal can be made directly adjacent to the scope portal. For arthroscopy of the tarsus, the locations of the portals may need to be adjusted because of variations in the locations of pathologic lesions, subtle anatomic differences, thickening of the joint capsule, and the range of motion of the joint. If three portals are used, the position of the scope and instrument portals must be established to permit visualization and treatment of the lesion. The egress needle can be shifted to a convenient location that allows drainage but does not interfere with the other two portals. The egress portal also can function as the instrument portal, especially in small dogs in which the surgeon has difficulty establishing and maintaining three functional portals. The surgeon must learn to triangulate the instrument relative to the position of the arthroscope tip within the joint. A 20-gauge (1.5-inch) hypodermic needle is helpful to use as a guide needle to locate the appropriate site for the instrument portal. The guide needle must penetrate the surface of the skin at a 75- to 90-degree angle and maintain this orientation through the soft tissues. As the needle enters the joint and is seen on the monitor, it appears to be entering at a very oblique angle. This illusion is created by the 30-degree fore-oblique arthroscope and does not represent the actual angle of penetration. The most common reason for failing to locate the appropriate instrument portal site is entering the skin at too oblique an angle. When the angle of entry is too oblique, the triangulation needle (to locate the instrument port) crosses the arthroscope and cannot be visualized on the monitor. If the triangulation needle cannot be visualized, the needle is inserted at a different location at a 75- to 90-degree angle.

Dorsomedial Scope Portal. The egress portal is established first. If an instrument portal is needed, the egress portal is located either plantaromedially or plantarolaterally. If an instrument portal is not needed, the egress portal can be located in a dorsolateral position. The scope portal is placed second, medial to the extensor tendons (Fig. 8–9). The instrument portal is placed last, lateral to the extensor tendons (see Fig. 8–9). The dorsomedial scope portal commonly is used to assess the dorsolateral joint compartment, the dorsal aspect of the lateral trochlear ridge, and the trochlea of the talus. The dorsal aspect of the medial trochlear ridge also can be evaluated, but inadvertent dislodgement of the arthroscope tip is likely. The arthroscope cannula and blunt obturator are introduced medial to the extensor tendons, just over the palpable medial trochlear ridge and cranial to the medial malleolus. The cannula is directed laterally, below the extensor tendons. The tip is directed into the dorsolateral compartment. The obturator is removed and replaced with the scope. The tip of the scope is tipped slightly or carefully advanced and withdrawn to increase the extent of viewable area. When the dorsal aspect of the tarsus is viewed, the tibiotarsal joint is extended to maximize the viewable area of the trochlea. The basic technique for establishment of portals was described earlier.

Dorsolateral Scope Portal. The egress portal is established first. If an instrument portal is needed, the egress portal is located either plantaromedially or plantarolaterally. If an instrument portal is not needed, the egress portal can be located in a dorsomedial position. The scope portal is placed second, lateral to the extensor tendons (Fig. 8–10). The instrument portal is placed last, lateral to the extensor tendons (see Fig. 8–10). The dorsolateral scope portal often is used to assess the dorsomedial joint compartment, the dorsal aspect of the medial trochlear ridge, and the trochlea of the talus. The dorsal aspect of the lateral trochlear ridge also can be evaluated, but inadvertent dislodgement of the arthroscope tip is likely. The arthroscope cannula and blunt obturator are introduced lateral to the extensor tendons, just over the palpable lateral trochlear ridge and cranial to the lateral malleolus. The cannula is directed medially, below the extensor tendons. The tip is directed into the dorsomedial compartment. The obturator is removed and replaced with the scope. The tip of the scope can be tipped slightly or carefully advanced and withdrawn to increase the extent of viewable area. When the planter aspect of the tarsus is viewed, the tibiotarsal joint is a flexed to maximize the viewable area of the trochlea. The basic technique for establishment of portals was described earlier.

Plantaromedial Scope Portal. The egress portal is established first. If an instrument portal is needed, the

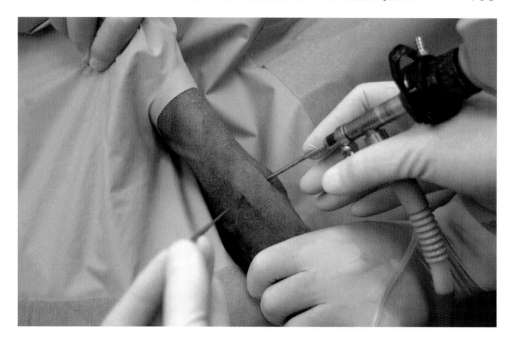

FIGURE 8–9 Dorsomedial arthroscope portal and dorsolateral instrument portal for canine tarsal arthroscopy. The tarsus is evaluated in an extended position. The articular surface of the distal tibia is viewed (with the light post down) while the articular cartilage is probed.

egress portal is located in either a dorsomedial or dorsolateral position. The egress portal can be located in a plantarolateral position if an instrument portal is not needed. The scope portal is placed second, medial to the flexor tendons (Fig. 8–11). The instrument portal is placed last, lateral to the flexor tendons (see Fig. 8–11). The plantaromedial scope portal often is used to assess the plantarolateral joint compartment, the plantar aspect of the lateral trochlear ridge, and the trochlea of the talus. The arthroscope cannula and blunt obturator are introduced medial to the extensor tendons, just over the palpable medial trochlear ridge and caudal to the medial

malleolus. The plantar aspect of the medial trochlear ridge also can be evaluated, but inadvertent dislodgement of the arthroscope tip can occur in this position. This portal is often used to view lesions associated with OCD, especially if a plantarolateral portal provides an inadequate view because of synovial hyperplasia and diminished range of motion. The scope is directed laterally, below the extensor tendons. The tip is directed into the plantaromedial compartment, and the obturator is removed and replaced with the scope. The tip of the scope can be tipped slightly or carefully advanced and withdrawn to increase the extent of viewable area.

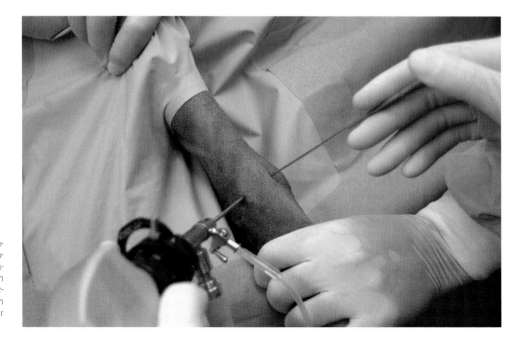

FIGURE 8–10 Dorsolateral arthroscope portal and dorsomedial instrument portal for canine tarsal arthroscopy. The tarsus is evaluated in an extended position. The articular surface of the distal tibia is viewed (with the light post down) while the articular cartilage is probed.

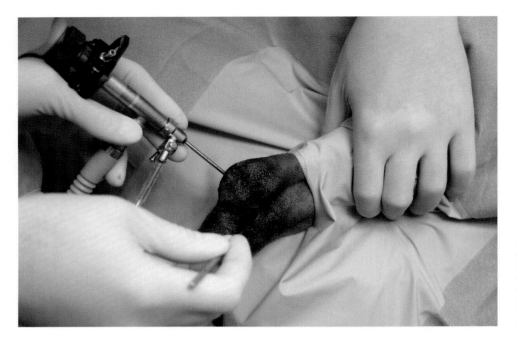

FIGURE 8-11 Plantaromedial arthroscope portal and plantarolateral instrument portal for canine tarsal arthroscopy. The tarsus is evaluated in a flexed position. The articular surface of the distal tibia is viewed (with the light post down) while the articular cartilage is probed.

When the dorsal aspect of the tarsus is viewed, the tibiotarsal joint is extended to maximize the viewable area of the trochlea. The basic technique for establishment of portals was described earlier.

Plantarolateral Scope Portal. The egress portal is established first. If an instrument portal is needed, the egress portal is located in either a dorsomedial or dorsolateral position. The egress portal can be located in a plantaromedial position if an instrument portal is not needed. The scope portal is placed second, lateral to the flexor tendons (Fig. 8–12). The instrument portal is placed last, lateral to the flexor tendons (see Fig. 8–12). The plantarolateral scope portal is commonly used to assess the plantaromedial joint compartment, the plantar aspect of the medial trochlear ridge, and the trochlea of the talus. The plantar aspect of the lateral trochlear ridge also can be evaluated, but inadvertent dislodgement of the arthroscope tip can occur in this position. The arthroscope cannula and blunt obturator are introduced lateral to the flexor tendons, just over the palpable lateral trochlear ridge and caudal to the lateral malleolus. The scope is directed medially, below the flexor tendons, with the tip directed into the

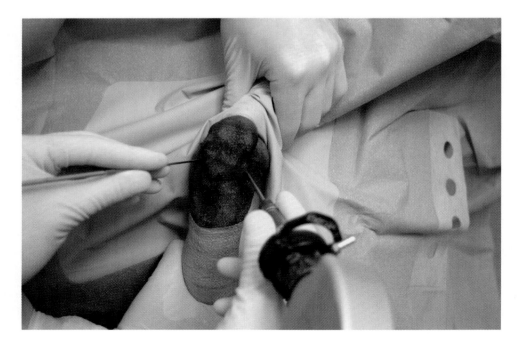

FIGURE 8-12 Plantarolateral arthroscope portal and plantaromedial instrument portal for canine tarsal arthroscopy. The tarsus is evaluated in a flexed position. The articular surface of the distal tibia is viewed (with the light post down) while the articular cartilage is probed.

plantaromedial compartment. The obturator is removed and replaced with the scope. The tip of the scope can be tipped slightly or carefully advanced and withdrawn to increase the viewable area. When the planter aspect of the tarsus is viewed, the tibiotarsal joint is flexed to maximize the viewable area of the trochlea. The basic technique for establishing portals was described earlier.

Surgical Anatomy. The tarsus is a complex hinge joint that is composed of many individual smaller joints. It primarily moves in flexion and extension, and more than 95% of the range of motion occurs at the tibiotarsal joint. Unlike other joints, the tibiotarsal joint usually is amenable to arthroscopy. The mortise character of the joint, the joint capsule, the collateral ligaments, the intertarsal and tarsometatarsal ligaments, and the strong plantar ligaments provide joint stability.

When the tarsus is evaluated arthroscopically, anatomic structures on the side of the joint opposite the scope portal usually are viewed more easily and more completely than structures on the same side as the portal. Multiple scope portals may be needed to permit thorough examination of the joint. When the arthroscope enters the joint, the camera is positioned in a way that provides proper spatial orientation on the monitor. Orientation is correct when right is shown on the right, left is shown on the left, ventral is shown down, and dorsal is shown up on the monitor. The controls on the camera will face upward. Most surgeons initially prefer to view 30 degrees down. The proper spatial orientation and fore-oblique view are obtained when the light post and the controls on the camera head are upright. When the camera and light post are in this position, the articular surface of the distal tibia and the trochlear ridges of the talus are visible. If necessary, the scope is carefully withdrawn slightly to increase the viewing window. To improve visualization of the articular surfaces, the joint may be hyperflexed and hyperextended to separate the joint surfaces and increase the amount of articular surface visible from each portal. When the dorsal (cranial) aspect of the tibiotarsal joint is viewed, the tarsus is extended. The position of the camera head is maintained, and the light post is rotated to the side to view other regions of the trochlear ridges, trochlear sulcus, synovial membrane, and collateral ligaments (Figs. 8–13 and 8–14). The articulation of the tibia, fibula, and talus is visible as well. As the light post is rotated to the ventral position, the articular surface of the distal tibia is seen. When the plantar (caudal) aspect of the tibiotarsal joint is viewed, the tarsus is positioned in flexion. The position of the camera head is maintained, and the light post is rotated to the side to view other regions of the trochlear ridges, trochlear sulcus, flexor hallucis longus tendon, synovial membrane, and collateral ligaments (Figs. 8–15 and 8–16). The articulation of the tibia, fibula, and talus is also visible. As the light post is rotated to the ventral position, the articular surface of the distal tibia is seen. The articular cartilage of the trochlear ridge, the synovial membrane, and the recess of the joint capsule as it attaches to the tibia and talus are seen as well. The medial and lateral collateral ligaments also are visible.

Indications for Arthroscopic Surgery of the Tarsal Joint

Tarsal arthroscopy is a new treatment modality in small animal surgery. As small animal surgeons become more adept at arthroscopy, more conditions will be treated arthroscopically or with arthroscopic assistance. Potential indications include OCD, malleolar and intra-articular fractures, osteoarthritis, joint instability, and diagnostic examination (biopsy or culture of bone, cartilage, or synovial membrane). The arthroscope also can be used to place a drain within the joint capsule to allow ingress and egress flushing in patients with septic arthritis.

Osteochondritis Dissecans

OCD is a manifestation of osteochondrosis in which a flap of cartilage is lifted from the articular surface. The loose flap is often composed of both bone and cartilage. Osteochondrosis is believed to precede OCD and is caused by a disturbance in endochondral ossification. The articular cartilage becomes thickened and is susceptible to fissure and loosening as the deeper chondrocytes undergo necrosis as a result of inadequate nutrition and a suboptimal microenvironment. In the tarsus, osteochondrosis is usually evidenced as a flap of cartilage found on the plantar aspect of the medial trochlear ridge. Osteochondral flaps associated with OCD have been reported to occur in all four quadrants of the trochlea of the talus (plantaromedial, dorsomedial, plantarolateral, and dorsolateral). The abnormal cartilage may fissure and cause a loose flap of cartilage to protrude into the joint, or the cartilage may detach from the underlying bone and float within the joint pouch. The condition may be unilateral or bilateral. The patient is evaluated carefully for evidence of OCD in other joints, including the shoulder, elbow, and stifle.

History and Signalment. Large and giant breed dogs are most commonly affected, and males are affected more often than females. Rottweilers and Labrador retrievers are overrepresented. Any breed of dog may be susceptible to OCD, including smaller breeds, such as the Australian cattle dog, Border collie, chow chow, and American pit bull. Clinical signs often develop between 4 and 8 months of age; however, some dogs may not be presented for veterinary evaluation until they are mature or middle-aged. Dogs usually are presented for examination because of unilateral or bilateral hindlimb lameness. Owners usually report a gradual onset of lameness that improves after rest and worsens after exercise.

Physical Examination Findings. The patient often stands with the tarsus hyperextended. Many dogs have a straight-legged conformation of the hindlimbs. Most dogs have weightbearing or non-weightbearing lameness that is exacerbated by exercise. On physical examination, the tarsus is palpated and moved through a complete range of motion. In most cases, crepitation or palpable swelling of the joint is evident, and pain is elicited when

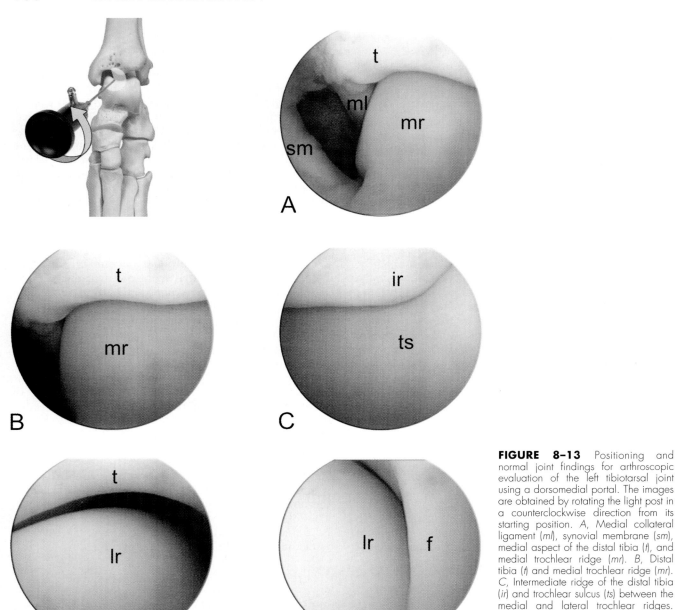

FIGURE 8-13 Positioning and normal joint findings for arthroscopic evaluation of the left tibiotarsal joint using a dorsomedial portal. The images are obtained by rotating the light post in a counterclockwise direction from its starting position. *A*, Medial collateral ligament (*ml*), synovial membrane (*sm*), medial aspect of the distal tibia (*t*), and medial trochlear ridge (*mr*). *B*, Distal tibia (*t*) and medial trochlear ridge (*mr*). *C*, Intermediate ridge of the distal tibia (*ir*) and trochlear sulcus (*ts*) between the medial and lateral trochlear ridges. *D*, Lateral trochlear ridge (*lr*) and distal tibia (*t*). *E*, Lateral trochlear ridge (*lr*) and lateral malleolus of the fibula (*f*).

the tarsus is moved into hyperextension or forced flexion. Loss of range of motion is common, especially loss of flexion. Muscle atrophy of the hindlimb is evidenced by loss of muscle mass, most noticeably in the thigh region.

Differential Diagnosis. The differential diagnosis includes osteoarthritis, joint instability, and septic arthritis.

Radiographic Findings. Although lameness may be apparent in only one limb, both tarsi should be radiographed because this condition is often bilateral. Sedation may be required to obtain quality radiographs, particularly in large or hyperactive dogs. Complete radio-

graphic assessment usually requires standard craniocaudal, mediolateral, oblique, and skyline views. The defect is localized to one of the four quadrants of the talus (dorsolateral, dorsomedial, plantarolateral, or plantaromedial). The earliest radiographic sign is flattening of the trochlear ridge and apparent widening of the tibiotarsal joint space (Fig. 8–17) as a result of thickening of the articular cartilage and deviation of the subchondral bone line. Soft tissue swelling often is visible as a result of synovial effusion and the proliferation of periarticular fibrous tissue. If the flap is calcified, it may be visible in situ. If the flap has detached from the underlying bone, it may be visible within the joint. Osteophytes may be seen as well.

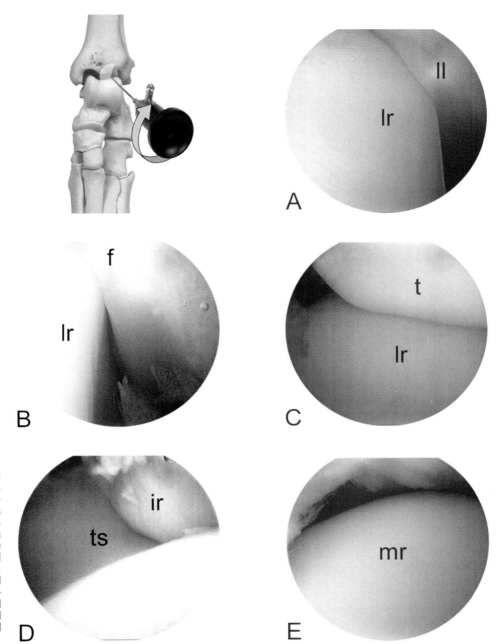

FIGURE 8–14 Positioning and normal joint findings for arthroscopic evaluation of the left tibiotarsal joint using a dorsolateral arthroscope portal. The images are obtained by rotating the light post in a clockwise direction from its starting position. *A,* Lateral collateral ligament (*ll*) and lateral trochlear ridge (*lr*). *B,* Distal fibula (*f*) and lateral trochlear ridge (*lr*). *C,* Lateral trochlear ridge (*lr*) and lateral aspect of the distal tibia (*t*). *D,* Intermediate ridge of the distal tibia (*ir*) and trochlear sulcus (*ts*) between the medial and lateral trochlear ridges. *E,* Medial trochlear ridge (*mr*).

Diagnosis. A complete orthopedic examination is essential because other conditions may occur in association with tarsal OCD. These conditions include shoulder OCD, elbow dysplasia [fragmented medial coronoid process (FCP), ununited anconeal process (USP)], panosteitis, and hip dysplasia. The diagnosis of OCD is based on signalment and history and physical findings, and confirmed radiographically. Radiographic evaluation often requires oblique and skyline views in addition to traditional survey views.

Treatment. OCD is usually treated with a combination of medical and surgical approaches. Most orthopedic specialists perform early surgical removal of osteochondral flaps, followed by symptomatic treatment of osteoarthritis as needed with NSAIDs and chondroprotectant therapy (oral and injectable). Whether treated medically or surgically, these patients also require controlled exercise to maintain function of the joint.

Anesthetic Considerations and Perioperative Pain Management. Young, healthy patients require minimal preoperative laboratory evaluation. Table 3–1 shows a standard anesthetic protocol, including preemptive pain medication. Postoperative pain is controlled with cold therapy, opioids, and NSAIDs.

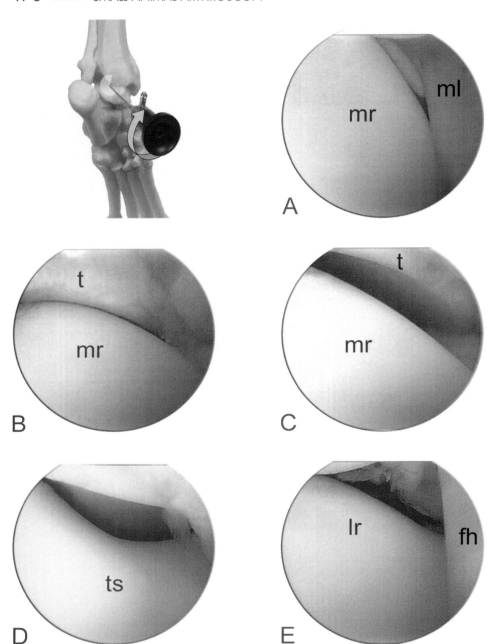

FIGURE 8-15 Positioning and normal joint findings for arthroscopic evaluation of the left tibiotarsal joint using a plantaromedial arthroscope portal. The images are obtained by rotating the light post in a clockwise direction from its starting position. *A,* Medial collateral ligament (*ml*) and medial trochlear ridge (*mr*). *B,* Distal tibia (*t*) and medial trochlear ridge (*mr*). *C,* Distal tibia (*t*) and medial trochlear ridge (*mr*) while the joint is fully flexed. *D,* Trochlear sulcus (*ts*) between the medial and lateral trochlear ridges. *E,* Lateral trochlear ridge (*lr*) and flexor hallucis longus tendon (*fh*).

Surgical Intervention. Surgery is performed to reduce pain and inflammation and slow the progress of osteoarthritis. Portal sites and surgical anatomy were discussed earlier. With the advent of arthroscopy and minimally invasive surgical approaches, both tarsi are treated at the same sitting if the condition is bilateral. The operative site is clipped and prepared according to the amount of limb maneuverability desired during surgery. A hanging limb preparation provides the greatest degree of freedom to manipulate the limb. Liberal clipping and thorough sterile preparation are necessary because an open arthrotomy may be required if arthroscopy is unsuccessful. In most cases, a 1.9-mm, 30-degree fore-oblique arthroscope is used. A 2.4- or 2.7-mm scope may be used in larger dogs. Basic instrumentation includes probes to inspect the cartilage surface or help raise a cartilage flap, graspers to remove the cartilage flap, and a hand curette or hand burr to prepare the lesion bed. Instrument cannulas are used in some larger patients, but the small tibiotarsal joint space present in most dogs often precludes their use. A motorized shaver can be helpful but is not essential. The shaver may be used for synovectomy to improve visualization, to débride the osteochondral flap, and to abrade the subchondral bed. The dog is positioned as described earlier, based on the anticipated location of the lesion.

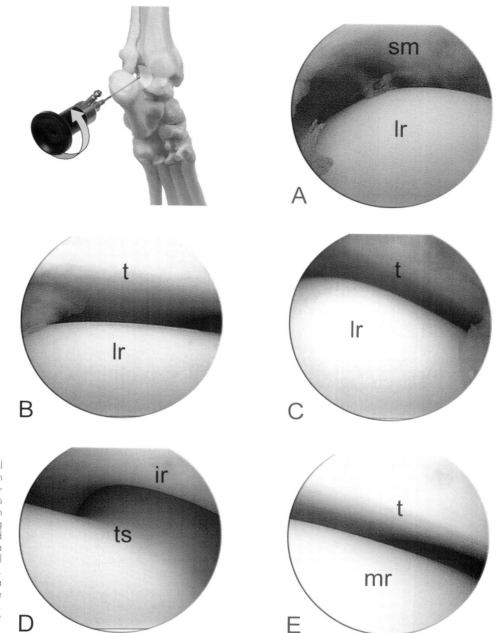

FIGURE 8–16 Positioning and normal joint findings for arthroscopic evaluation of the left tibiotarsal joint using a plantaro-lateral arthroscope portal. The images are obtained by rotating the light post in a clockwise direction from its starting position. *A,* Synovial membrane (*sm*) and lateral trochlear ridge (*lr*). *B,* Distal tibia (*t*) and lateral trochlear ridge (*lr*). *C,* Distal tibia (*t*) and lateral trochlear ridge (*lr*). *D,* Intermediate ridge of the distal tibia (*ir*) and trochlear sulcus (*ts*) between the medial and lateral trochlear ridges. *E,* Distal tibia (*t*) and medial trochlear ridge (*mr*).

Egress is established with a needle or cannula. The joint is distended with lactated Ringer's solution, and the arthroscope is inserted. Ingress flow is established through the arthroscope cannula. The medial and lateral joint compartments are inspected for evidence of inflammation and an osteochondral flap. The arthroscope is positioned to provide a clear view of the lesion, and a guide needle is used to triangulate the position for the instrument port. The most common reason for inability to visualize the guide needle in the joint is crossing the arthroscope. After the position for the instrument portal is established, the surgeon must decide whether to work through an open instrument portal, an instru-

ment cannula, or a combination. If the surgeon works through an open portal site, a no. 11 Bard-Parker scalpel blade is used to make a 0.5- to 1-cm soft tissue tunnel adjacent to the guide needle. If the cartilage flap is still attached, a probe or small elevator is inserted to partially free the edge of the flap. The cartilage flap is not freed completely but is left attached at one or more sites. Grasping forceps are inserted, used to hold the cartilage flap, and removed. To facilitate removal of the flap, the forceps are twisted to release the flap from the talus, fold the flap longitudinally, and ease its passage through the joint capsule. The cartilage flap may be removed as a single large fragment or in two or three smaller pieces

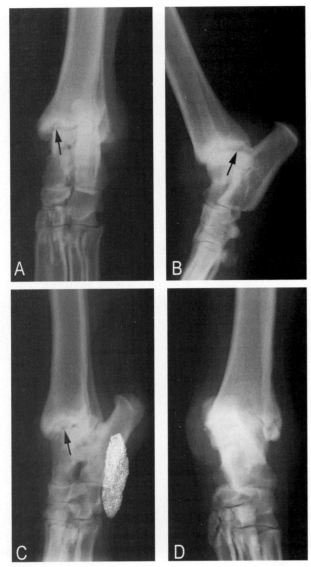

FIGURE 8-17 Radiographs of a canine tarsus with osteochondritis dissecans. *A*, Craniocaudal view showing flattening and a calcified fragment over the medial trochlear ridge (*arrow*). *B*, Lateral view showing flattening and irregularity on the ridge of the talus (*arrow*). *C*, Medial oblique view showing flattening and irregularity on the ridge of the talus (*arrow*). *D*, Lateral oblique view shows normal lateral trochlear ridge.

(Figs. 8-18 and 8-19). To ease removal of the flap, the tips of small Metzenbaum scissors can be used to enlarge the instrument portal. In patients with plantaromedial OCD, the joint can be hyperflexed to better separate the joint surfaces and improve access. If the surgeon works through an instrument cannula, a small cannula with a sharp trocar is inserted into the joint adjacent to the guide needle. Larger cannulas can be placed with switching sticks, but the smallest possible instrument cannula is used. A hand curette, hand burr, or motorized shaver is passed through the cannula and used to break the cartilage flap into small pieces. These pieces are usually small enough to flow out through the instrument cannula.

If a piece of cartilage is too large to pass freely through the cannula, small grasping forceps are inserted and used to capture the fragment. The fragment is pulled next to the instrument cannula, and the cannula and forceps are removed at the same time. The instrument port is reestablished by placing a switching stick into the joint, followed by the cannula. The cartilage flap is broken into small pieces until the surgeon sees that the cartilage that lines the periphery of the lesion bed is firmly attached to the underlying subchondral bone. Then the subchondral bed is treated by surface abrasion or microfracture. To optimize healing, a curette is used to débride the edges of the lesion to form a perpendicular edge of healthy articular cartilage at the periphery of the lesion. A handheld curette, handheld burr, or motorized shaver is used to abrade the subchondral bone surface of the lesion until the underlying bone bleeds freely. The surgeon stops the flow of ingress fluid frequently to observe the extent of bleeding bone, and abrasion arthroplasty is stopped after multifocal pinpoint bleeding is observed. Further abrasion may deepen the defect, inhibit recovery, and increase instability of the joint. After surface abrasion arthroplasty or microfracture is completed, fragments of bone or cartilage are flushed from the joint by increasing the ingress flow and allowing egress through a large instrument cannula. The joint is inspected for remaining bone or cartilage fragments, and the arthroscope and instrument cannula are removed. If necessary, the portals are sutured with nonreactive, nonabsorbable suture.

Postoperative Care. To relieve pain and reduce swelling during recovery, cold therapy is applied by alternating 15 minutes on and 10 minutes off for two applications. Commercial cold packs or a circulating cold water pack can be used. Alternatively, ice wrapped in a towel or packs of frozen vegetables can be used. If the dog is dismissed from the hospital on the day of surgery, NSAIDs and oral butorphanol (see Table 3-1) are dispensed for administration at home. If the dog remains in the hospital overnight, buprenorphine is administered in the evening. NSAIDs and butorphanol are dispensed for administration at home. NSAIDs are continued for 5 days, and butorphanol is discontinued after 48 hours. Cold therapy is continued at home for the first 2 days after surgery. After the surgical swelling is gone (48 to 72 hours), the owner should begin heat therapy and passive motion and stretch exercises. Moist heat is applied to the tarsus region with a commercial heat pack or a moistened warm towel. The owner should hold the warm pack against the inside of his own elbow for 30 seconds to ensure that it is not too hot. Then the owner holds the warm pack over the patient's tarsus area for 10 minutes. Afterward, the warm pack is removed and gentle flexion and extension movements of the tarsus joint are begun, starting with small movements and gradually increasing to the limit of comfort over 1 to 2 minutes. At the limit of comfort, the joint is held in position for 10 seconds. The motion and stretch exercise is repeated five times. The owner should examine the portal sites daily for signs of irritation or drainage.

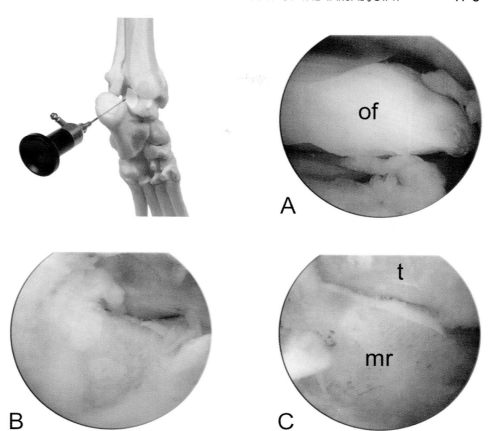

FIGURE 8-18 Positioning and abnormal joint findings for arthroscopic evaluation of the right tarsus using a plantarolateral arthroscope portal in a Labrador retriever with osteochondritis dissecans. *A,* Free-floating osteochondral fragment (*of*) originating from the plantar aspect of the medial trochlear ridge of the talus. *B,* Cartilaginous debris that is seen in addition to the main fragment is removed by lavage, with a minishaver, or with a grasping forceps. *C,* Subchondral defect of the medial trochlear ridge (*mr*) after fragment removal. Cartilage erosion is seen on the distal tibia (*t*) opposite the osteochondral fragment.

For the first 4 weeks, exercise is limited to controlled leash walking. Arthroscopically treated dogs usually use the affected leg immediately after surgery. To increase the weightbearing load, walking at a slow pace is recommended. As postoperative time increases, the pace is hastened. To increase the range of motion in the tarsus, the owner should walk the dog in high grass (e.g., weeds), shallow water, or sand, which forces the dog to pick up the feet and step high with the legs. After 4 weeks, a limited amount of free activity is added to the controlled walking, beginning with 5 minutes and increasing to 30 minutes over the next 2 weeks. After 6 to 8 weeks, free activity is gradually increased to normal levels. If, during any exercise period (controlled or free activity), the dog becomes sore or is sore the next day, the pace is decreased and the dog returns to controlled activity for 2 to 3 days.

Complications. Complications are unusual. Occasionally, excessive fluid extravasation occurs and results in swollen soft tissues around the tarsus in the immediate postoperative period. This fluid resorbs within the first 24 hours. Residual mild swelling adjacent to portal sites may be noticeable for the first 48 hours.

Prognosis. The prognosis for normal limb function is variable. Dogs that have small lesions and are treated early usually improve and do well. Large osteochondral defects and advanced osteoarthritis may be associated with long-term intermittent or persistent lameness. However, many dogs have adequate function if strenuous activity is avoided.

Fractures and Instability of the Tarsus

History and Signalment. Dogs have acute lameness of the hindlimb. Most exhibit non-weightbearing lameness that is associated with trauma and does not respond to anti-inflammatory medication. Any age or breed of dog may be affected.

Physical Examination Findings. Gait analysis shows visible lameness. Swelling is usually palpable in the tarsus region. Manipulation of the tarsus usually elicits discomfort and crepitus. Collateral instability is characterized by excessive valgus or varus deviation when the joint is stressed. To evaluate the function of the short and long components of the collateral ligament complex, collateral instability is assessed in flexion and extension, respectively. Injury to the plantar ligaments leads to hyperextension of the intertarsal and tarsometatarsal joints. Injury to multiple ligaments may cause subluxation or luxation at any level of the tarsus.

Differential Diagnosis. The differential diagnosis includes OCD, septic arthritis, and immune-mediated arthritis.

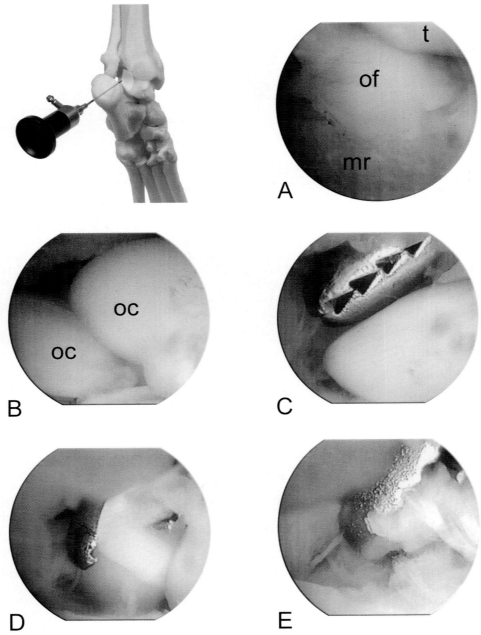

FIGURE 8–19 Positioning and abnormal joint findings for arthroscopic evaluation of the left tarsus using a plantarolateral arthroscope portal in a Labrador retriever with osteochondritis dissecans. *A,* Free-floating osteochondral fragment (*of*) originating from the plantar aspect of the medial trochlear ridge of the talus, subchondral defect of the medial trochlear ridge (*mr*), and distal tibia (*t*). *B,* Multiple large osteochondral fragments (*oc*) found after probing of the lesion and hyperflexion of the tibiotarsal joint. *C,* Insertion of a grasping forceps alongside the fragments. *D,* Grasping and removal of a fragment. *E,* Many lesions require multiple attempts with the grasper to completely remove free-floating fragments.

Radiographic Findings. Lateral and anteroposterior views may be insufficient to yield a definitive diagnosis. The collateral ligament may be injured if these views show soft tissue swelling or evidence of an avulsion fragment in the area of the collateral ligament. Stress radiographs often show instability of the collateral and plantar ligaments. To detect injury to the lateral and medial collateral ligaments, respectively, varus or valgus stress can be applied while an anteroposterior view is obtained. Injury to the plantar ligament is shown by a lateral view that is obtained while the tibiotarsal joint is hyperflexed. A skyline or oblique view also may be helpful in assessing tarsal fractures.

Diagnosis. The diagnosis of tarsal instability or fracture is based on the history and signalment, physical findings, and radiographic findings.

Treatment. Medical management relieves pain, but definitive therapy with coaptation or surgical stabilization, depending on the severity of the injury, is necessary. Arthroscopic intervention is performed to evaluate the collateral ligaments, remove small avulsion fragments, help to reduce an avulsed fragment, and examine the articular surfaces of the tibiotarsal joint. Articular fractures require anatomic reduction and rigid stabilization to reduce the chance of debilitating osteoarthritis.

Anesthetic Considerations and Perioperative Pain Management. Preoperative laboratory workup is based on the patient's physical status and surgical risk. Young, healthy patients with no underlying systemic problems require minimal laboratory evaluation. Older dogs should undergo a complete blood screen, chest radiographs, and an electrocardiogram. Table 3–1 shows a standard anesthetic protocol, including preemptive pain medication. Postoperative pain is controlled with cold therapy, opioids, and NSAIDs.

Surgical Intervention. Tarsal instability or fracture usually is treated with an open approach. Repair may include ligamentous reconstruction, fracture reduction and stabilization, or arthrodesis. Arthroscopy is used primarily for diagnostic and adjunctive purposes. Portal sites and surgical anatomy were discussed earlier. The operative site is clipped and prepared according to the amount of limb maneuverability desired during surgery. A hanging limb preparation provides the greatest degree of freedom to manipulate the limb and is recommended. Liberal clipping and thorough sterile preparation are necessary because an open arthrotomy may be required. In most cases, a 1.9-mm, 30-degree fore-oblique arthroscope is used. Basic instrumentation includes probes to inspect the joint capsule. If the surgeon works through an instrument cannula, different-sized cannulas and switching sticks facilitate the surgery. A motorized shaver is helpful to débride synovial proliferation but is not essential. The dog is positioned as described earlier, based on the anticipated site of the lesion.

The egress needle is established, and the joint is distended with saline. A guide needle is used to locate the joint line and the correct position for the arthroscope portal. The arthroscope is inserted, and ingress flow is established through the arthroscope cannula. The arthroscope and light post are positioned to allow the surgeon to visualize the trochlear ridges of the talus, the distal tibia, the fibula, the flexor hallucis longus tendon, the synovial membrane, and the collateral ligaments. The light post is rotated 360 degrees to allow thorough evaluation of the joint. The scope is tipped in different directions and retracted or advanced to enhance the view of the structures. The medial and lateral collateral ligaments are examined in extension and partial flexion. During this examination, the surgeon looks for avulsed fragments and assesses the practicality of stabilization versus fragment removal (Fig. 8–20). The condition of the articular cartilage is assessed, and fragments are examined to determine whether reduction or removal is needed.

If an instrument portal is needed, a guide needle is used to triangulate its position. The most common reason for inability to visualize the guide needle in the joint is crossing the arthroscope. To prevent crossing the arthroscope with the guide needle, the needle is inserted perpendicular to the skin surface. This orientation is maintained through the soft tissues. After the position for the instrument portal is established, a probe is inserted through a cannula or an open portal. If the articular surfaces of the tibiotarsal joint show excessive wear, arthrodesis rather than stabilization is considered.

In patients that require open reduction and stabilization, useful techniques include ligamentous reconstruction, transarticular external fixation, and arthrodesis. These techniques are described in detail in various veterinary surgical textbooks and journals.

Postoperative Care. Cold therapy is applied during recovery to relieve pain and reduce swelling. Cold therapy is applied by alternating 15 minutes on and 10 minutes off for two applications. Commercial cold packs or a commercial circulating cold water pack can be used. Alternatively, ice wrapped in a towel or frozen packs of vegetables can be used. If the dog is dismissed from the hospital on the day of surgery, NSAIDs and oral butorphanol (see Table 3–1) are dispensed for administration at home. If the dog remains in the hospital overnight, buprenorphine is administered in the evening. NSAIDs and butorphanol are dispensed for administration at home. NSAIDs are continued for 5 days, and butorphanol is discontinued after 48 hours. If adjunctive coaptation is not used, cold therapy can be continued by the owner at home for the first 2 days after surgery. In addition, the owner should examine the portal sites daily for signs of irritation or drainage. Leash walking is recommended for 4 to 8 weeks, followed by a progressive increase in activity. To increase the weightbearing load on the limb, walking at a slow pace is recommended. As postoperative time increases, the pace can be hastened. To increase the range of motion in the hip when walking, the owner should walk the dog in high grass, shallow water, or sand. Walking on this type of surface forces the dog to pick up the feet and step high with the legs. After

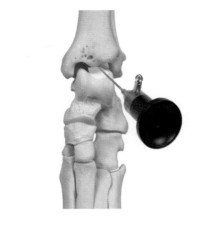
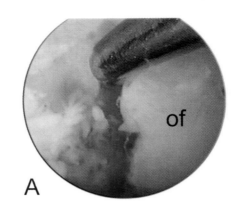
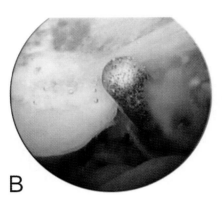
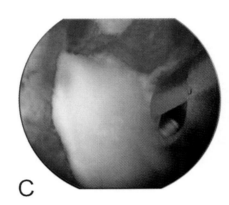

FIGURE 8-20 Positioning and abnormal joint findings for arthroscopic evaluation of the right tarsus using a dorsolateral arthroscope portal in a Labrador retriever that was injured while playing. *A,* Free-floating osteochondral fragment (*of*) originating from the insertion of a portion of the medial collateral ligament (avulsion fracture). The fragment is displaced with a probe. *B,* Fibers associated with the medial collateral ligament attached to the fragment and adjacent to the probe. *C,* Débridement and removal of the fragment with a mini-shaver.

6 weeks, a limited amount of free activity is introduced in combination with controlled walking. The owner should begin with 5 minutes of free activity and increase to 30 minutes over the next 2 weeks. After 8 weeks, free activity is gradually increased to normal levels. If the dog becomes sore during any exercise period (controlled or free activity) or is sore the next day, the owner should decrease the pace and return to controlled activity for 2 to 3 days. Adjunctive coaptation can be used for various lengths of time, depending on the severity of injury.

Complications. Complications are unusual. Occasionally, excessive fluid extravasation occurs and results in swollen soft tissues around the joint in the immediate postoperative period. This fluid resorbs within the first 24 hours. Residual mild swelling adjacent to the portal sites may be noticeable for the first 48 hours.

Prognosis. The prognosis for satisfactory limb function after treatment of ligamentous instability or fracture of the tarsus is fair to good, depending on the severity of injury and the surgical procedure required. Most dogs that undergo successful reconstruction of the collateral ligaments have a good outcome. If arthrodesis is necessary, functional outcome is usually fair because of the loss of range of motion in the tarsus. A good prognosis is typical if fractures can be reduced anatomically and rigidly stabilized.

Suggested Readings

Beale BS, Goring RL: Exposure of the medial and lateral trochlear ridges of the talus in the dog: Part 1. Dorsomedial and plantaromedial surgical approaches to the medial trochlear ridge. JAAHA 26:13–18, 1990.

Beale BS, Goring RL, Herrington J, et al: A prospective evaluation of four surgical approaches to the talus of the dog used in the treatment of osteochondritis dissecans. JAAHA 27:221–229, 1991.

Cook JL, Tomlinson JL, Stoll MR, et al: Arthroscopic removal and curettage of osteochondrosis lesions on the lateral and medial trochlear ridges of the talus in two dogs. JAAHA 37:75–80, 2001.

Goring RL, Beale BS: Exposure of the medial and lateral trochlear ridges of the talus in the dog: Part 2. Dorsolateral and plantarolateral surgical approaches to the lateral trochlear ridge. JAAHA 26:19–24, 1990.

van Ryssen B, van Bree HJ: Diagnostic and surgical arthroscopy in osteochondral lesions. Vet Clin North Am Small Anim Pract 28:161–189, 1998.

van Ryssen B, van Bree HJ, Vyt P: Arthroscopy of the canine hock joint. JAAHA 29:107–115, 1993.

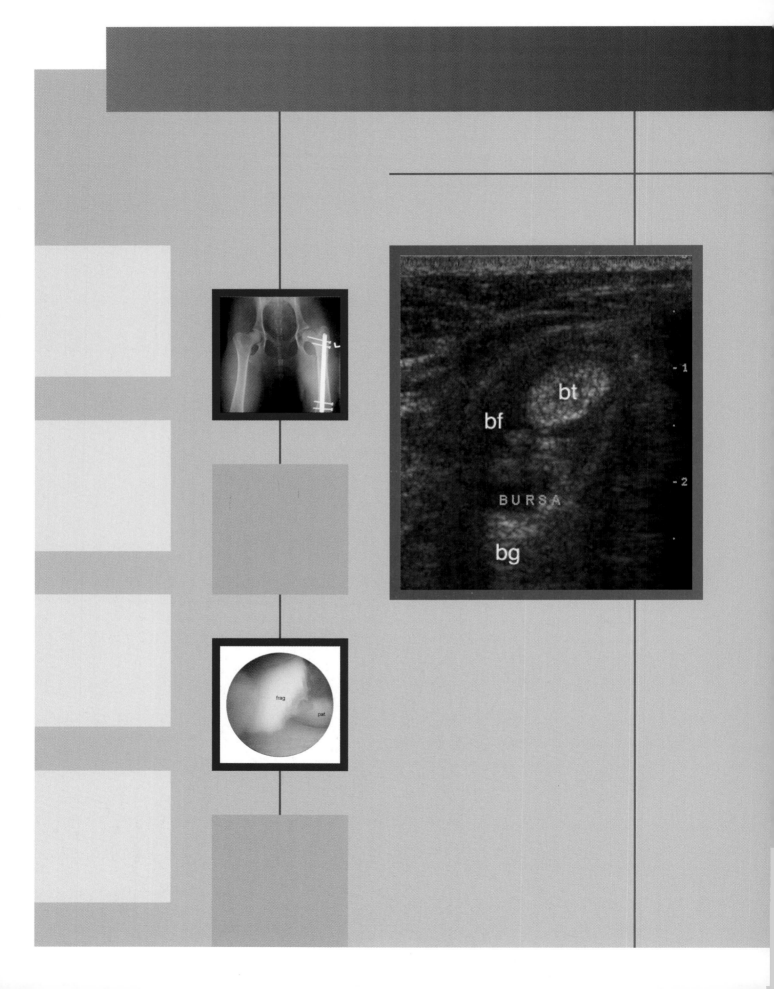

Case Studies

Clinical Case Study 1

Traumatic Displacement of an Osteochondritis Dissecans Fragment

Signalment. The patient is a 16-month-old, 30-kg female Gordon setter.

Chief Complaint. The chief complaint is acute-onset weightbearing lameness of the right forelimb.

History. One week before presentation, the dog returned from playing in the yard with non-weightbearing lameness of the right forelimb. The yard is an enclosed 2-acre area, and the dog plays vigorously with three other dogs. The dog was given carprofen (Rimadyl) for 5 days, which improved the patient's condition, but did not resolve the lameness.

Orthopedic Findings. The dog had a grade II of V lameness of the right forelimb. Flexion of the shoulder elicited a painful response. No other shoulder movements or palpation of the biceps tendon elicited discomfort. Three weeks before presentation, the dog underwent a thorough yearly physical examination that included shoulder manipulation. The findings were normal.

Diagnostic Findings. Radiographs of the right shoulder showed a lesion compatible with osteochondritis dissecans (OCD) (Fig. 9–1).

Arthroscopic Findings. Arthroscopic examination of the right shoulder showed an OCD lesion bed in the caudocentral region of the humeral head. A free cartilage flap characteristic of OCD was not present, and the surface of the lesion showed evidence of neovascularization (Fig. 9–2). Further examination showed that the cartilage flap was embedded in the caudal arm of the medial collateral ligament (Fig. 9–3).

Therapy. The embedded cartilage fragment was removed, and the lesion bed was treated with surface abrasion until bleeding cancellous bone was reached.

Postoperative Care. The dog was dismissed from the hospital the day of surgery with instructions for rehabilitation for 6 weeks. Rehabilitation included restricted leash walking, active and passive range of motion exercises, and flexion and extension stretch exercises.

Outcome. The dog had a grade III of V lameness for the first postoperative week. The lameness resolved gradually over the ensuing 4 weeks. Six months after surgery, the dog showed no lameness and had normal range of motion in the shoulder joint.

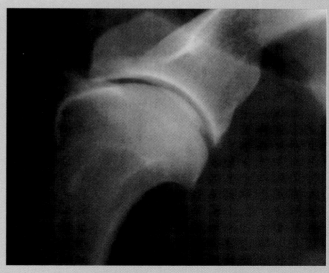

FIGURE 9–1 Lateral radiograph of the shoulder joint showing the typical appearance of caudocentral osteochondritis dissecans of the humeral head.

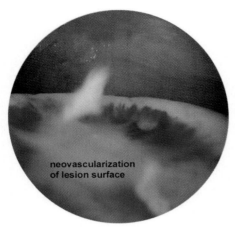

FIGURE 9–2 Arthroscopic view of the lesion bed. Neovascularization is consistent with acute traumatic displacement of the surface cartilage.

Comments. In this case, arthroscopy was used to confirm and treat an unusual case of developmental joint disease. Classically, clinical signs associated with shoulder OCD occur in dogs that are younger than 1 year of age. The lameness is slow in onset and initially improves with rest. This dog was clinically sound and had normal findings on physical examination 3 weeks before the onset of acute non-weightbearing lameness. Arthroscopically, the surface of the lesion showed signs of neovascularization and the cartilage fragment was embedded in the medial collateral ligament. The presumption is that this dog had traumatic displacement of a nonclinical OCD lesion. The advantage of arthroscopy in this case is the ability to examine the internal structures of the entire shoulder joint and locate and remove the fragment from an atypical location.

Clinical Case Study 2

Radial Tear of the Lateral Meniscus

Signalment. The patient is a 5-year-old, 35-kg male boxer.

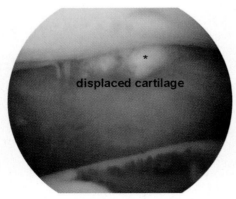

FIGURE 9–3 Arthroscopic view of the medial joint capsule and the caudal arm of the medial collateral ligament. Cartilage (*) is embedded in the medial collateral ligament.

Chief Complaint. The chief complaint is weight-bearing lameness of the left hindlimb.

History. Five months before evaluation, the dog showed weightbearing lameness associated with moderate activity. With rest, the dog returned to normal weight-bearing, but the lameness recurred with activity. As time passed, the lameness progressed and discomfort was noticeable even with decreased activity. The dog was given carprofen, which improved the condition but did not resolve the lameness.

Orthopedic Findings. All findings were normal except those that involved the left hindlimb. The dog had a grade II of V lameness and had moderate muscle atrophy of the left hindlimb. Palpable thickening of the joint capsule and medial restraints (medial buttress) was noted. When the dog was asked to sit, he sat with incomplete flexion of the stifle joint and rotated the stifle externally (negative sit test). No pain or crepitus was noted with manipulation of the stifle joint. The range of motion was normal, and no abnormal craniocaudal translation was present.

Diagnostic Findings. Radiographs of the left stifle joint showed joint effusion and mild osteophyte production (Fig. 9–4).

Arthroscopic Findings. Arthroscopic examination of the left stifle joint showed mild to moderate synovial inflammation, osteophytes adjacent to the medial and lateral trochlear ridges, and a proliferative fat pad. The cranial cruciate ligament was intact (Fig. 9–5). Further inspection of the lateral compartment showed a radial tear of the lateral meniscus (Fig. 9–6).

Therapy. The dog underwent radiofrequency ablation of the torn portion of the meniscus (Fig. 9–7).

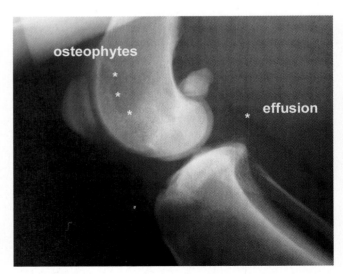

FIGURE 9–4 Lateral radiograph of a stifle joint showing the typical appearance of joint effusion (***) and osteophyte formation (*).

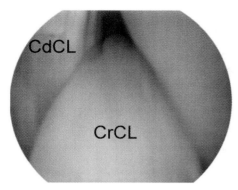

FIGURE 9–5 Arthroscopic view of the anterior cruciate ligament showing the normal appearance of the cranial cruciate ligament (*CrCL*) and the caudal cruciate ligament (*CdCL*).

Postoperative Care. The dog was dismissed from the hospital the day after surgery with instructions for rehabilitation for 6 weeks. Rehabilitation included restricted leash walking, active and passive range of motion exercises, and flexion and extension and stretch exercises.

Outcome. The dog had a grade III of V lameness for the first postoperative week. The lameness resolved gradually over the ensuing 4 weeks. Six months after surgery, the referring veterinarian reported normal function with the limb except for occasional soreness after strenuous exercise.

Comments. In this case, arthroscopy was used to explore the stifle joint thoroughly. This dog had clinical symptoms and diagnostic features that were characteristic of a partial cranial cruciate ligament tear. Although no side-to-side difference in joint stability was noted and the dog had a palpably stable joint, a partial tear of the cranial cruciate ligament was suspected. Arthroscopically assisted intervention allowed thorough inspection of the joint and led to the correct diagnosis and successful treatment.

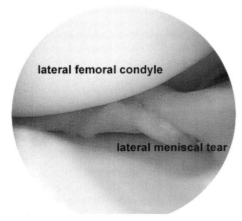

FIGURE 9–6 Arthroscopic view of the lateral compartment of the joint showing a radial tear of the lateral meniscus.

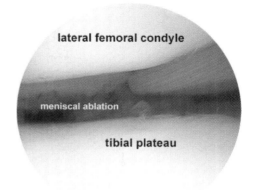

FIGURE 9–7 Arthroscopic view showing ablation of the torn portion of the posterior body of the lateral meniscus.

Clinical Case Study 3

Coxofemoral Osteoarthritis Caused by Femoral Malunion

Signalment. The patient is a 1-year-old, 22-kg spayed female German shepherd mix.

Chief Complaint. The chief complaint is intermittent weightbearing lameness of the left hindlimb.

History. The dog was adopted from a shelter approximately 2 months before the onset of lameness. The dog walked normally but collapsed intermittently on the left hindlimb when running. The gait abnormality did not improve with the administration of nonsteroidal anti-inflammatory drugs (NSAIDs).

Orthopedic Findings. All findings were normal except those that involved the left hindlimb. The dog had moderate internal rotation of the limb when standing or walking. A grade I of V lameness and moderate muscle atrophy of the left hindlimb were observed, and mild pain occurred on hyperextension of the left coxofemoral joint.

Diagnostic Findings. Radiographs of the left coxofemoral joint showed evidence of a previous fracture of the proximal femur, including malunion and mild osteoarthritis of the joint (Fig. 9–8). A skyline view of the left femur showed severe anteversion (104 degrees) (Fig. 9–9).

Arthroscopic Findings. Arthroscopic examination of the left coxofemoral joint showed mild synovial inflammation and grade I to II cartilage disease (mild to moderate fibrillation) (Fig. 9–10). The ligament of the head of the femur was intact.

Therapy. Because the ligament of the femoral head was intact and the cartilage did not show severe damage, corrective osteotomy of the proximal femur

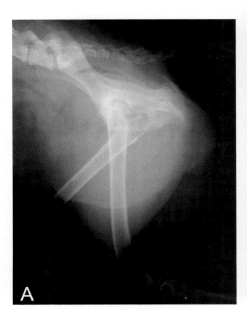

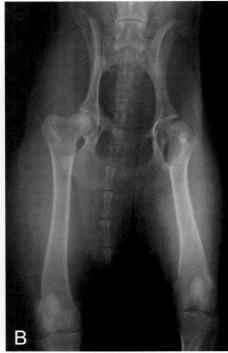

FIGURE 9–8 Preoperative lateral (A) and ventrodorsal (B) radiographs of a 1-year-old dog with femoral malunion and osteoarthritis of the left coxofemoral joint.

was performed with derotation and stabilization with an interlocking nail (Fig. 9–11).

Postoperative Care. The dog was dismissed from the hospital the day after surgery with instructions for strict exercise restriction for 6 weeks.

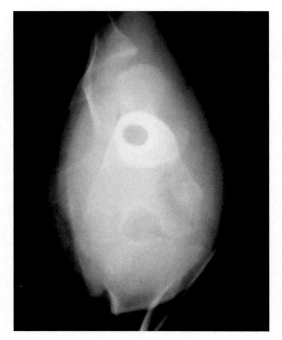

FIGURE 9–9 Coronal view of the left femur showing anteversion of 104 degrees.

Outcome. The dog had a grade III of V lameness for the first postoperative week.

Comments. In this case, arthroscopy was used to explore the coxofemoral joint thoroughly and determine the condition of the cartilage. Dogs that have hip dysplasia and are candidates for triple pelvic osteotomy (TPO) are evaluated similarly. When electing to perform corrective osteotomy, the surgeon must decide independently how much cartilage damage is permissible. No specific guidelines are in place. In this case, the surgeon decided to perform corrective osteotomy because the patient had no deep fissuring or full-thickness cartilage loss.

Clinical Case Study 4

Osteoarthritis of the Tarsus

Signalment. The patient is a 4-year-old, 32-kg male Border collie mix that is a working cattle dog.

Chief Complaint. The chief complaint is intermittent weightbearing lameness of the right hindlimb.

History. The dog had a 4-month history of a grade III of V lameness of the right hindlimb that was severe enough to limit the dog's ability to work cattle. An initial diagnosis of chronic partial tearing of the medial collateral ligament was made based on equivocal instability and radiographic evidence of osteophytosis in the region of the medial malleolus. The dog was discharged with

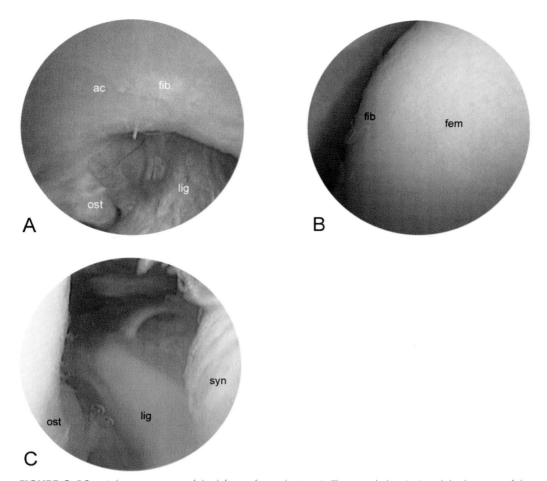

FIGURE 9–10 Arthroscopic view of the left coxofemoral joint. *A*, The acetabulum (*ac*) and the ligament of the head of the femur (*lig*). The ligament is intact, but the acetabulum shows mild fibrillation (*fib*) and osteophyte formation (*ost*). *B*, The femoral head (*fem*) shows mild fibrillation (*fib*). *C*, The transverse acetabular ligament (*lig*), moderate synovitis (*syn*) and early osteophytosis (*ost*) are seen at the base of the femoral head.

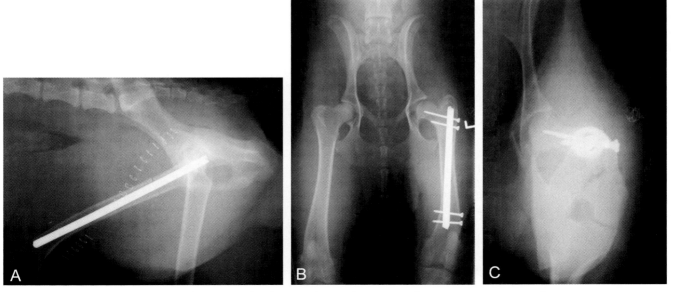

FIGURE 9–11 Lateral (*A*), ventrodorsal (*B*), and coronal (*C*) views after osteotomy, correction of excessive anteversion, and stabilization with an interlocking nail.

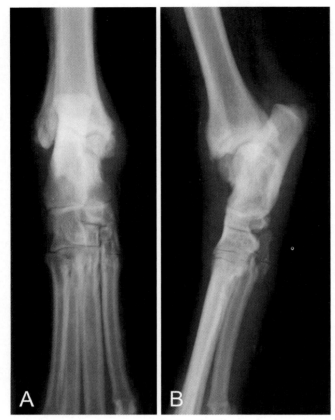

FIGURE 9–12 Craniocaudal (*A*) and lateral (*B*) radiographs of the right tarsus showing osteoarthritis of the tibiotarsal joint.

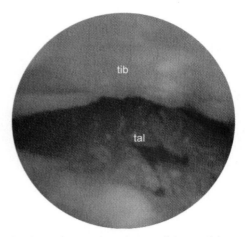

FIGURE 9–13 Arthroscopic evaluation of the caudal aspect of the tibiotarsal joint showing partial-thickness cartilage loss in the distal tibia (*tib*) and full-thickness cartilage loss in the talus (*tal*).

Therapy. Because damage to the cartilage was severe, pantarsal arthrodesis was performed (Fig. 9–14).

Postoperative Care. The dog was dismissed from the hospital the day after surgery with instructions for strict exercise restriction and maintenance of external

instructions for severe restriction of activity and administration of NSAIDs. The owner did not notice significant improvement, and the dog was presented for further evaluation.

Orthopedic Findings. All findings were normal except those that involved the right hindlimb. The dog had a grade I of V lameness and moderate muscle atrophy of the right hindlimb. Mild thickening and pain were noted on manipulation of the right tarsal joint.

Diagnostic Findings. Radiographs of the right tibiotarsal joint showed degenerative changes, including osteophyte formation along the medial malleolus and proliferative new bone along the cranial and caudal aspects of the distal tibia. Also apparent was irregular mineralization of the soft tissue along the plantaromedial aspect of the calcaneus (Fig. 9–12). On the craniocaudal projection, valgus stress caused the medial aspect of the tarsocrural joint to open slightly more than the lateral aspect. On the varus-stressed views, this area opened slightly more than on the contralateral limb.

Arthroscopic Findings. Arthroscopic examination of the tibiotarsal joint showed mild synovial inflammation and a grade IV of V cartilage disease (complete cartilage loss with early eburnation) (Fig. 9–13).

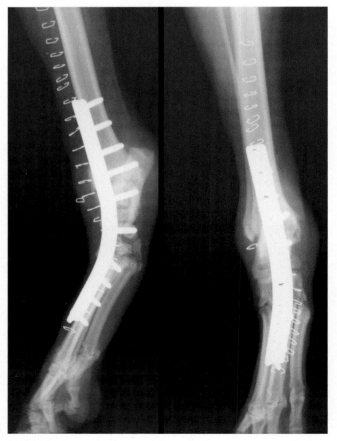

FIGURE 9–14 Postoperative radiographs showing pantarsal arthrodesis with a 3.5-mm dynamic compression plate.

coaptation for 6 weeks. After that, radiographic evaluation was performed to determine the adequacy of healing.

Outcome. Healing was evident after 8 weeks of exercise limitation. Over the following 4 months, the dog was progressively rehabilitated to return to working cattle.

Comments. In this case, arthroscopy was used to explore the tibiotarsal joint thoroughly and determine the condition of the cartilage. In this case, the surgeon needed to choose between ligament reconstruction and arthrodesis. Although the joint ultimately required an arthrotomy to perform arthrodesis, had the joint been salvageable, an arthrotomy would have been avoided. This case shows that arthroscopy can determine the severity of cartilage damage more accurately than radiography.

Clinical Case Study 5

Fracture of the Patella

Signalment. The patient is a 4-year old, 23-kg spayed female German shorthaired pointer.

Chief Complaint. The chief complaint is traumatic injury to the left stifle.

History. The dog has been non-weightbearing on the limb since she fell out of the back of a pickup truck 1 week earlier.

Orthopedic Findings. All findings were normal except those that involved the left hindlimb. The dog had non-weightbearing lameness of the left hindlimb. Moderate swelling and pain on manipulation of the left stifle joint, equivocal proximal displacement of the patella, and evidence of a small, healed wound on the lateral aspect of the stifle were noted.

Diagnostic Findings. Radiographs of the left stifle joint showed multiple bone fragments associated with a comminuted fracture of the distal aspect of the patella. The proximal fragment was displaced slightly proximally. No axial fracture lines were visualized. The patellar tendon was swollen, but intact (Fig. 9–15).

Arthroscopic Findings. Arthroscopic examination of the stifle joint showed synovial proliferation with multiple small fragments of the distal aspect of the patella. Most of the patella was intact, and numerous hairs were identified in the joint (Fig. 9–16).

Therapy. The comminuted fragments of the patella and the hairs contaminating the joint were removed arthroscopically. The patellar tendon was approached surgically and tenodesis was performed with a locking loop suture pattern. A box wire was placed proximal to the patella and then through the tibial crest (Fig. 9–17).

Postoperative Care. The dog was dismissed from the hospital the day after surgery with instructions for strict exercise restriction and maintenance of external coaptation for 6 weeks. Radiographic evaluation was performed to assess the adequacy of healing 6 weeks postoperatively.

Outcome. The wire was removed 6 weeks postoperatively, and the dog underwent physical therapy for rehabilitation. By 2 months postoperatively, the dog

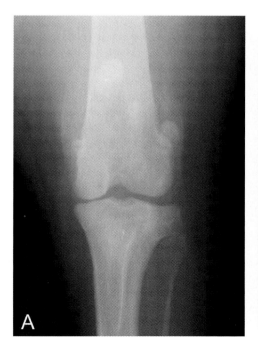 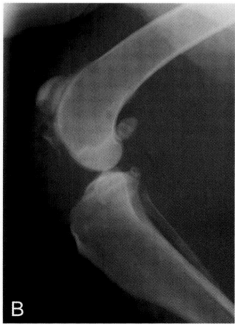

FIGURE 9–15 Craniocaudal (A) and lateral (B) radiographs of the left stifle of a dog with traumatic fracture of the patella.

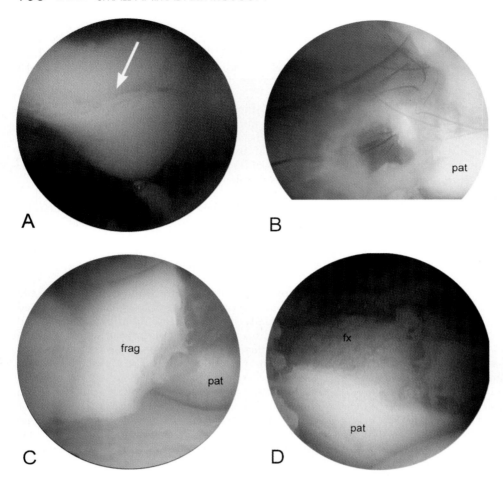

FIGURE 9-16 Arthroscopic evaluation of the left stifle. *A*, Articular surface of the patella showing a fissure line (*arrow*). *B*, Contamination of the stifle joint with hairs as a result of open trauma. The patella (*pat*) is visible. *C*, The distal fragment (*frag*) and the remaining body of the patella (*pat*). *D*, Patella (*pat*) and fracture surface (*fx*) after the visible fragments were removed.

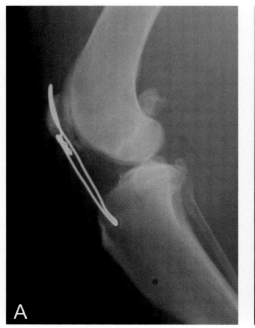
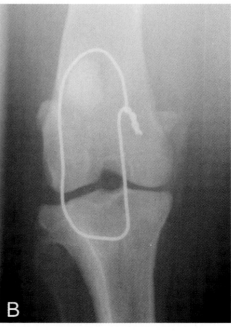

FIGURE 9-17 Postoperative lateral (*A*) and craniocaudal (*B*) radiographs after the visible fragments were removed arthroscopically and the patellar tendon was protected with a box wire. Several fragments remained postoperatively, but because of their position, they were not likely to cause additional damage to the cartilage surface.

resumed normal function without lameness or evidence of patella alta.

Comments. In this case, joint trauma was managed with arthroscopic assistance. Arthroscopy enabled complete débridement of the joint without disruption of the joint capsule. The patellar tendon had been partially torn, and arthrotomy would have contributed to the instability of the patella and the entire joint.

Clinical Case Study 6

Bilateral Biceps Tendonitis

Signalment. The patient is a 9-year-old, 36-kg castrated male Rottweiler mix.

Chief Complaint. The chief complaint is a 1-year history of progressive shifting forelimb lameness.

History. The referring veterinarian evaluated this dog 1 year before presentation for progressive shifting forelimb lameness. At that time, manipulation of both shoulder joints elicited pain. The dog was treated with strict rest and administration of NSAIDs. This treatment resulted in improvement, but not resolution, of the lameness. The dog was given intra-articular steroid injections that resulted in resolution of the lameness. After approximately 1 month, the lameness recurred, particularly in the left limb. The dog underwent arthrocentesis of the left shoulder, which showed hemarthrosis. Again treatment with strict rest was implemented. The left limb appeared to improve; however, the lameness in the right limb worsened significantly.

Orthopedic Findings. All parameters were normal except those that involved the forelimbs. The dog had a grade IV of V lameness and severe muscle atrophy of the right forelimb and moderate atrophy of the left forelimb. Manipulation of the right shoulder elicited severe pain. Manipulation of the left shoulder elicited mild pain.

Diagnostic Findings. Radiographs of the shoulders showed focal regions of increased opacity within the bicipital grooves and an angular osseous density associated with the supraglenoid tubercle (Fig. 9–18). Mild periarticular remodeling was seen at the caudal aspect of the humeral head and glenoid. Ultrasound scans showed a large volume of fluid within the bicipital bursa of the right shoulder (Fig. 9–19). The fiber pattern of the biceps tendon was disrupted near its origin at the supraglenoid tubercle, and a large spur of bone projected off the supraglenoid tubercle. On the left shoulder, the volume of fluid within the bicipital bursa was slightly increased. A large zone of fiber disruption was seen within the proximal aspect of the biceps tendon, and multiple sites of dystrophic mineralization were seen throughout the biceps tendon. In both shoulders, the bicipital groove showed significant sclerosis and bone reactivity.

Arthroscopic Findings. Arthroscopic examination of the right shoulder joint showed mild synovial inflammation and a partial tear of the biceps tendon (Fig. 9–20). Arthroscopic examination of the left shoulder joint showed a complete tear of the biceps tendon with adherence of the tendon to the bursal wall (see Fig. 9–20).

Therapy. On both sides, the tendons were completely transected below the level of disease and resection of the diseased portion of the tendons was attempted (Fig. 9–21).

Postoperative Care. The dog was dismissed from the hospital the day after surgery with instructions for strict exercise restriction for the first week followed by a gradual increase in controlled activity. Professional physical therapy was recommended but was not within the financial limitation of the owner.

Outcome. Lameness increased significantly during the first 48 hours after surgery, and the dog occasionally collapsed on the forelimbs. After approximately 3 weeks, the dog showed less lameness than he had shown preoperatively, and episodes of forelimb collapse were rare. Occasionally, the dog escaped from confinement and ran without lameness, although mild lameness was evident in the evening after these episodes.

Comments. In this case, arthroscopy was used to explore the shoulder joint and definitively diagnose and treat disease of the biceps tendon. Biceps tendonitis may be primary or secondary to other diseases of the shoulder joint and rotator cuff. Arthroscopy can be used to evaluate the joint for multiple problems within the shoulder. Transection of the biceps tendon is well accepted as treatment of biceps tenosynovitis in humans and also appears to have an excellent outcome in dogs.

Clinical Case Study 7

Occult Dysplasia of the Elbow

Signalment. The patient is a 10-year-old, 27-kg male vizsla.

Chief Complaint. The chief complaint is chronic recurrent lameness of the right forelimb.

History. The dog participated in agility training for 9 years. Two years before presentation, the dog showed vague signs of lameness, including crying out when landing from a jump and hunching of the back. The dog was treated with rest, acupuncture, and glucosamine administration. Approximately 1 year before presentation, the dog showed obvious lameness of the right forelimb. Biceps tendon disease was diagnosed based on the arthrographic finding of narrowing of the biceps tendon. Intra-articular corticosteroid injection was implemented and resulted in minimal improvement. Treatment with NSAIDs resulted in mild improvement.

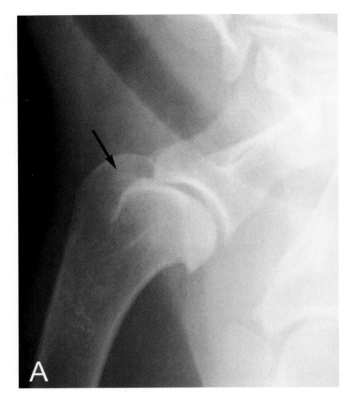

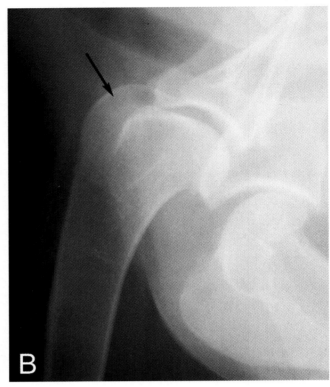

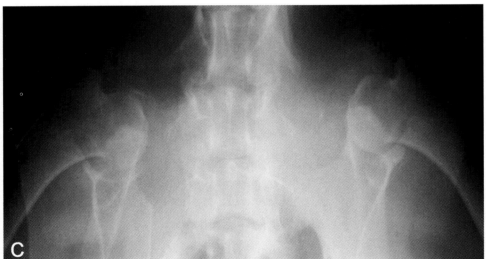

FIGURE 9–18 Left (A) and right (B) lateral radiographs and skyline view (C) of the shoulders of a dog with bilateral biceps tenosynovitis. Focal regions of increased opacity (arrow) are seen in the bicipetal groove.

Orthopedic Findings. All parameters were normal except those that involved the right forelimb. The dog had a grade I of V lameness and severe muscle atrophy of the right forelimb. The degree of atrophy did not coincide with the degree of lameness. Manipulation of the right shoulder and elbow elicited equivocal pain.

Diagnostic Findings. Radiographs of the right shoulder were within normal limits. Radiographs of the right elbow showed subtle changes that included mild lipping of the medial coronoid process and mild sclerosis in the ulnar notch (Fig. 9–22). Ultrasound scans of the shoulder were compatible with significant atrophy of the muscles. No other abnormalities were seen (Fig. 9–23).

Arthroscopic Findings. Arthroscopic examination of the shoulder joint showed no abnormalities. Arthroscopic examination of the elbow joint showed grade IV disease, or full-thickness cartilage loss, of the medial coronoid process (Fig. 9–24).

Therapy. Because the cartilage damage was severe, microfracture was performed until adequate bleeding of the subchondral bone was achieved.

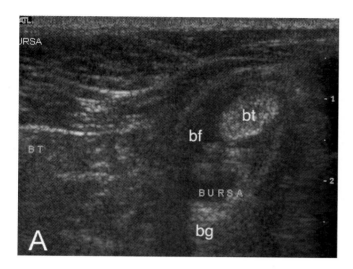
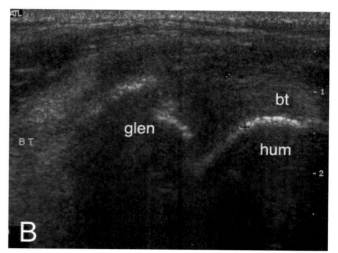
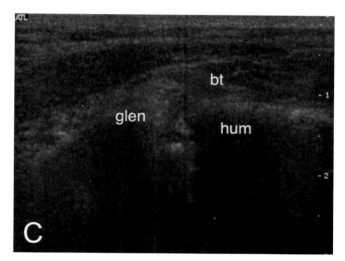

FIGURE 9-19 Transverse (*A*) and longitudinal (*B*) ultrasound scans of the right shoulder joint. A large volume of fluid (*bf*) is seen within the bicipital bursa of the right shoulder. The fiber pattern of the biceps tendon (*bt*) is disrupted near its origin. The bicipital groove (*bg*), supraglenoid tubercle (*glen*), and humerus (*hum*) also are visible. Longitudinal ultrasound scan (*C*) of the left shoulder showing a large zone of disruption of the biceps tendon fiber within the proximal aspect of the biceps tendon and multiple sites of dystrophic mineralization throughout the biceps tendon.

Postoperative Care. The dog was dismissed from the hospital the day after surgery with instructions for professional physical therapy beginning 5 to 7 days postoperatively. The dog was also treated with NSAIDs and glucosamine and chondroitin.

Outcome. Arthroscopic and medical management combined with intensive professional physical therapy resulted in significant improvement in lameness and restoration of function. As a result, the dog was able to resume agility work.

Comments. In this case, arthroscopy was used to perform a thorough workup of forelimb lameness. In many animals with forelimb lameness, the injury may be difficult to localize on physical examination. Shoulder ultrasound, full-limb radiographs, and joint taps are recommended, followed by arthroscopy of the shoulder and elbow. Bone scans also may be useful. This case also shows the value of shoulder joint ultrasound over arthrograms in thoroughly evaluating the joint. Finally, this case shows the possibility of severe cartilage disease in

the elbow joint even when radiographic changes are minimal. Arthroscopic inspection of the elbow joint is recommended in any dog that has forelimb lameness of unknown origin.

Clinical Case Study 8

Multiple Ligamentous and Tendinous Injury of the Right Shoulder

Signalment. The patient is an 8-year-old, 67-kg castrated male Rottweiler–German shepherd mix.

Chief Complaint. The chief complaint is a 4-month history of persistent weightbearing lameness of the left forelimb.

History. The patient underwent right-sided cemented total hip replacement 2 years earlier without complication. Lameness of the left forelimb has been present for 4 months and has not responded to carprofen

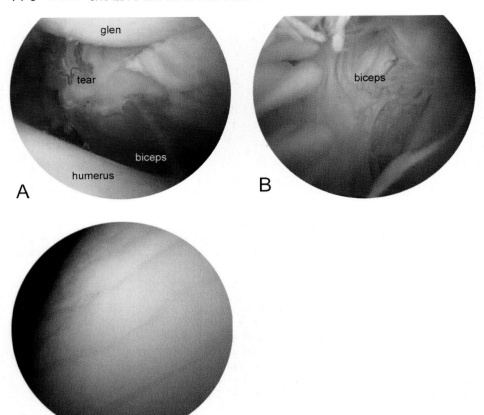

FIGURE 9–20 Arthroscopic views of the right and left shoulder joints. *A,* Right cranial region of the shoulder showing the supraglenoid tuberosity (*glen*), humerus, intact biceps tendon (*biceps*), and proximal tearing (*tear*). *B,* Left cranial region of the shoulder showing complete tearing of the biceps tendon from the supraglenoid tubercle and subsequent adherence of the biceps to the bursal wall (*biceps*). *C,* Caudal humeral head showing cartilage cracks associated with mild chronic osteoarthritis.

therapy. The owner reported possible right forelimb lameness this morning as well as previous intermittent lameness of the left hindlimb.

Orthopedic Findings. Palpation of the right shoulder elicited pain, especially when the shoulder was rotated internally or externally while flexed. The left hip was painful on extension. Severe weightbearing lameness (grade IV of V) of the right forelimb was evident. All findings were normal except those that involved the forelimbs. The left hindlimb showed mild muscle atrophy.

Diagnostic Findings. Radiographs of the shoulders showed bilateral focal regions of increased opacity in the region of the greater tubercle (Fig. 9–25). Radiographic examination of the left hip showed progressive remodeling and osteophyte proliferation, consistent with hip dysplasia. Radiographic evaluation of the right hip showed

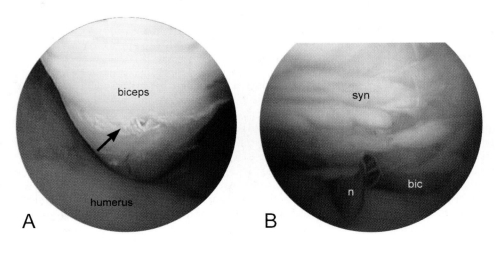

FIGURE 9–21 Arthroscopic views of the locations of biceps tenotomy. *A,* Proximal aspect of the right biceps tendon (*biceps*) showing the level where transection is performed (*arrow*). *B,* Proximal aspect of the left biceps tendon (*bic*). A needle (*n*) is visible through the proliferative synovium (*syn*) where transection is performed.

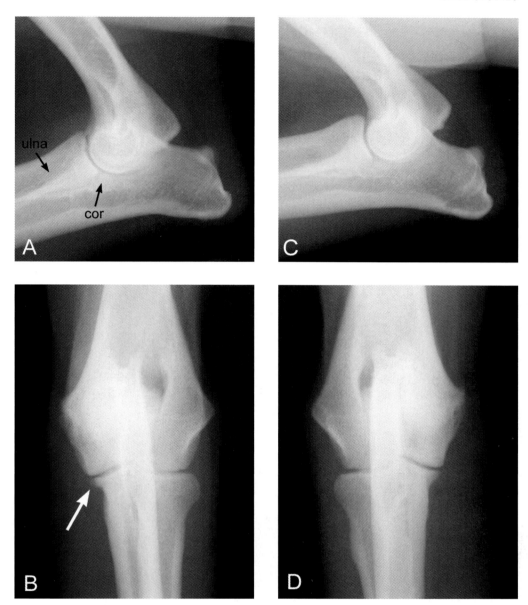

FIGURE 9–22 Lateral (*A*) and craniocaudal (*B*) radiographs of the right elbow joint. Lateral (*C*) and craniocaudal (*D*) radiographs of the left elbow joint showing subtle irregularity of the cranioproximal ulna (*ulna*) and mild sclerosis of the coronoid region (*cor*) of the right elbow compared with the left elbow. Note osteophyte formation (*arrow*) causing a "lipping" appearance at the medial coronoid process in Fig. 9–22*B*.

no problems with the previous total hip replacement. A force plate evaluation confirmed right forelimb lameness.

Arthroscopic and Surgical Findings. Bilateral arthroscopy of the shoulder with possible bilateral supraspinatus tenotomy was planned. Arthroscopic examination of the right shoulder joint showed mild synovial inflammation, partial tearing of the lateral glenohumeral ligament, mild fraying of the subscapularis tendon, and remodeling and full-thickness erosion of the cartilage of the humeral head (Fig. 9–26). A minimally invasive approach was made to the right supraspinatus tendon. Thickening of the tendon and proliferation of fibrous

tissue were noted. Arthroscopic examination of the left shoulder joint with supraspinatus tenotomy was postponed because multiple problems were detected in the right shoulder and the prognosis was uncertain.

Therapy. The insertion of the right supraspinatus tendon was transected. The abnormal portion of the tendon was resected and submitted for histopathologic diagnosis. The torn fibers of the lateral glenohumeral were débrided with a radiofrequency probe.

Histopathologic Diagnosis. Histologic changes in the right supraspinatus tendon included severe, chronic,

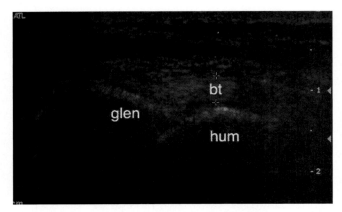

FIGURE 9-23 Ultrasound of the right shoulder showing no abnormalities. The supraglenoid tubercle (*glen*), biceps tendon (*bt*) and humerus (*hum*) are visible.

traumatic degeneration. Dystrophic mineralization and fibrocartilaginous metaplasia were noted among tendon fibers (Fig. 9–27).

Postoperative Care. The dog was dismissed from the hospital the day after surgery with instructions for strict exercise restriction for 2 months followed by a gradual increase in controlled activity.

Outcome. No change was seen during the first 48 hours after surgery. The right forelimb lameness improved slowly over the next 6 weeks and then suddenly became more severe after the dog returned from unsupervised activity in the yard. Four months following surgery,

the patient was much improved but still exhibited a grade II of V lameness.

Comments. In this case, arthroscopy was used to explore the shoulder joint and identify multiple pathologic findings. Without arthroscopic assistance, these intra-articular abnormalities may have been overlooked because the patient had an obvious supraspinatus tendon injury that was identified and treated with a minimally invasive surgical approach. Arthroscopy is recommended to evaluate the shoulder joint to detect multiple problems. Transection of the supraspinatus tendon is proposed as a treatment for supraspinatus tendon tears and mineralization. The long-term prognosis of this patient is unknown at the present time. Future reevaluation and treatment, including reconstruction of the lateral glenohumeral ligament and total replacement of the left hip, may be necessary.

Clinical Case Study 9

Bilateral Tearing of the Biceps Tendon and an Avulsion Fracture

Signalment. The patient is a 5-year-old, 31.2-kg castrated male Labrador retriever–chow chow mix.

Chief Complaint. The chief complaint is a 5-month history of right forelimb lameness.

History. Acute onset of right forelimb lameness occurred 5 months before presentation. The lameness

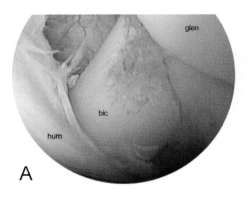

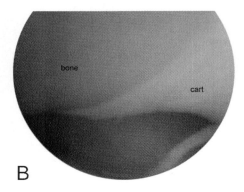

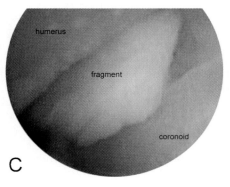

FIGURE 9-24 Arthroscopic views of the right elbow and shoulder. *A*, Arthroscopic view of the right shoulder showing a normal biceps tendon (*bic*) and supraglenoid tubercle (*glen*) and mild fibrillation of the bicipital groove (*hum*). *B*, Arthroscopic view of the right elbow. Severe medial compartmental osteoarthritis is seen as full-thickness cartilage loss (grade IV) of the medial aspect (*bone*) and mild cartilage damage (grade I) of the lateral aspect (*cart*). *C*, Arthroscopic view of the craniomedial region of the right elbow showing full-thickness cartilage loss of the humerus and coronoid as well as an osteochondral fragment between the joint surfaces.

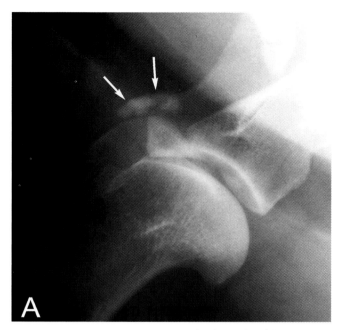
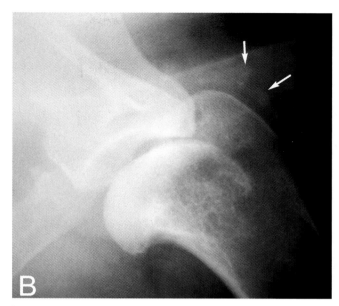

FIGURE 9–25 Lateral radiographs of the right (A) and left (B) shoulders of a dog with bilateral mineralization of the supraspinatus tendon. Focal regions of increased opacity (arrows) are visible adjacent to the greater tubercle.

usually was weightbearing but occasionally was nonweightbearing. Its severity was constant. NSAID therapy resulted in partial improvement.

Orthopedic Findings. All findings were normal except those that involved the forelimbs. The dog showed a grade IV of V lameness and muscle atrophy of the right forelimb. Extension, flexion, abduction, adduction, internal rotation and external rotation of the right shoulder elicited moderate pain.

Diagnostic Findings. Radiographs of the right shoulder showed a supraglenoid tuberosity avulsion fracture (Fig. 9–28).

Arthroscopic Findings. Arthroscopic examination of the right shoulder joint showed moderate synovial inflammation and a partial tear and hemorrhage of the biceps tendon. An avulsion fragment from the supraglenoid tuberosity was seen within the joint. Osteophytes were seen along the caudal aspect of the humeral head. The medial glenohumeral ligament and subscapularis tendon showed mild inflammation and fraying (Fig. 9–29).

Therapy. The avulsion fragment was removed, and complete transection of the biceps tendon was performed arthroscopically.

Postoperative Care. The dog was dismissed from the hospital the day after surgery with instructions for leash walking for 4 weeks.

Outcome. The dog had weightbearing right forelimb lameness equal to the preoperative status 24 hours after surgery. The lameness improved progressively and disappeared approximately 6 weeks after surgery.

Comments. In this case, arthroscopy was used to explore the shoulder joint and definitively diagnose and treat disease of the biceps tendon. Arthroscopy is recommended for thorough evaluation of the joint for multiple problems within the shoulder. Transection of the biceps tendon is well accepted as treatment of biceps tenosynovitis in humans and appears to have an excellent outcome in dogs as well.

Clinical Case Study 10

Incomplete Ossification of the Humeral Condyle

Signalment. The patient is a 5-year-old, 22-kg intact castrated male Brittany spaniel.

Chief Complaint. The chief complaint is chronic, intermittent lameness of the right forelimb that has lasted for several months.

History. Acute onset of weightbearing lameness of the right forelimb occurred 3 months before presentation. The lameness was intermittent, but persistent, and became more severe 2 weeks before presentation.

Orthopedic Findings. The dog had a grade III of V lameness and muscle atrophy of the right forelimb. Extension of the right elbow elicited moderate pain.

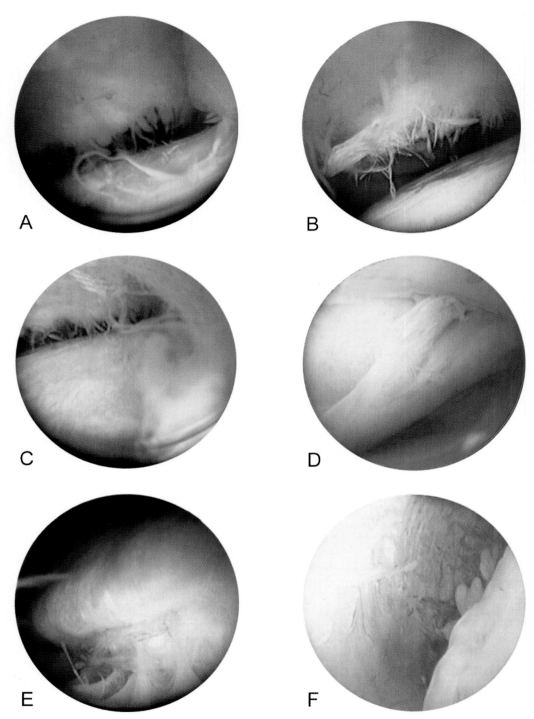

FIGURE 9–26 Arthroscopic views of the right shoulder joint. *A,* Torn fibers of the right lateral glenohumeral ligament and mild synovitis. *B,* Torn fibers of the right lateral glenohumeral ligament. *C,* Full-thickness erosion of the articular cartilage of the humeral head adjacent to the torn lateral glenohumeral ligament. *D,* Mild partial tearing of the subscapularis tendon. *E,* Remodeling of the caudal aspect of the humeral head associated with osteoarthritis. *F,* Remodeling of the glenoid fossa and humeral head associated with osteoarthritis.

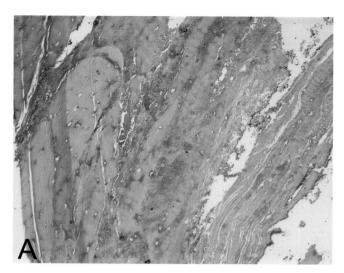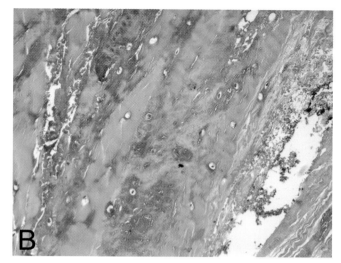

FIGURE 9–27 Histopathologic changes associated with the torn right supraspinatus tendon at 10× (A) and 20× (B) include degeneration of the tendon with dystrophic mineralization and fibrocartilaginous metaplasia replacing tendon fibers.

Diagnostic Findings. Radiographs of the right elbow showed a probable radiolucent line within the humeral condyles, consistent with incomplete ossification of the humeral condyle (IOHC) (Fig. 9–30).

Arthroscopic Findings. A caudomedial arthroscope portal was used for each elbow. Arthroscopic examination of the right elbow joint showed mild synovial inflammation and a fissure of the articular surface of the humeral condyle, just lateral to the central sulcus (Fig. 9–31A). No apparent displacement associated with a fracture was seen, and the remaining articular surfaces

appeared normal. No evidence of IOHC was seen on arthroscopic examination of the left elbow (see Fig. 9–31B).

Therapy. A 3.5-mm transcondylar lag screw was placed percutaneously from lateral to medial. Initially, a drill bit broke during attempted screw insertion and could not be retrieved. Typically, the bone of the humeral condyles is dense, especially in patients that have IOHC. A standard 3.5-mm cortical screw was placed in lag fashion by overdrilling the near cortex and redirecting the screw (Fig. 9–32).

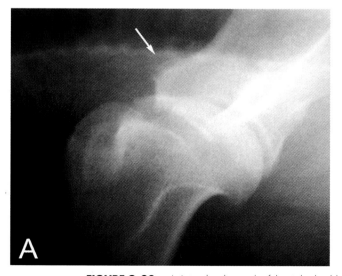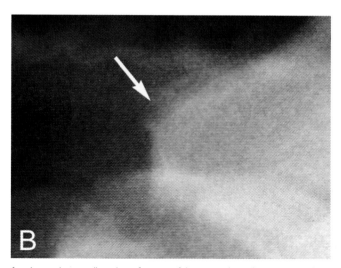

FIGURE 9–28 A, Lateral radiograph of the right shoulder of a dog with a small avulsion fracture of the supraglenoid tuberosity and partial tearing of the biceps tendon. A periosteal bone reaction is seen at the supraglenoid tuberosity (arrow). B, Magnified view of the supraglenoid tuberosity showing bony changes (arrow) associated with a minimally displaced, chronic avulsion fracture of the supraglenoid tuberosity.

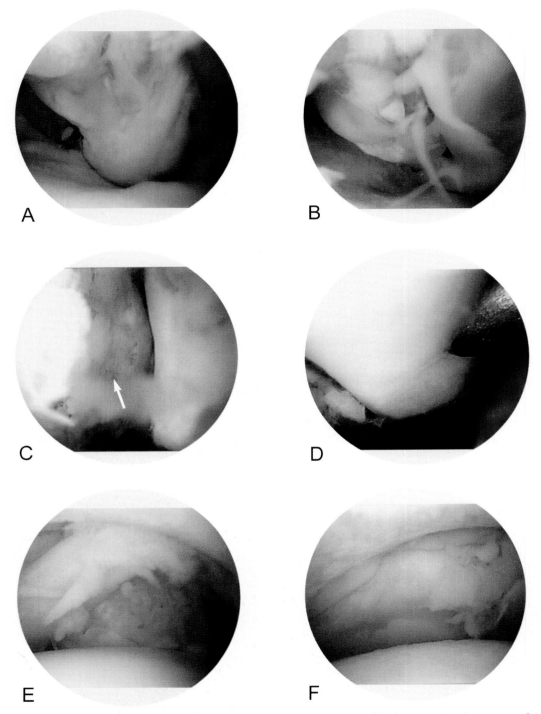

FIGURE 9–29   Arthroscopic views of the right shoulder joint. *A,* The origin of the biceps tendon shows areas of hemorrhage and tearing. *B,* The tip of the arthroscope is advanced to provide a better view of the partial tear of the biceps tendon. *C,* A fragment (*arrow*) arising from the supraglenoid tuberosity is seen adjacent to the biceps tendon. *D,* A grasping forceps is used to grasp and remove the fragment. *E,* Mild fraying and inflammation of the medial glenohumeral ligament and subscapularis tendon. *F,* Partial-thickness wear of the cartilage of the glenoid and humeral head (grade I) adjacent to the medial glenohumeral ligament.

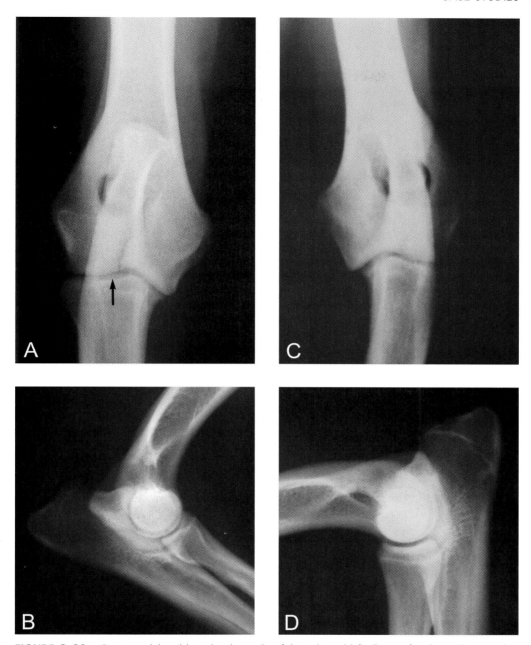

FIGURE 9–30 Craniocaudal and lateral radiographs of the right and left elbows of a dog with incomplete ossification of the right elbow. *A* and *B*, Anteroposterior view of the right elbow showing a radiolucent line (*arrow*) between the medial and lateral condyles. *C* and *D*, The normal left elbow.

Postoperative Care. The dog was dismissed from the hospital the day after surgery with instructions for leash walking for 8 weeks.

Outcome. The weightbearing right forelimb lameness was equal to the preoperative status 24 hours after surgery. The lameness improved progressively and disappeared approximately 4 weeks after surgery. The dog returned to running and jumping with no adverse effects. A radiolucent line between the humeral condyles of the right elbow was seen radiographically 12 months postoperatively (see Fig. 9–32). Despite compression with a transcondylar lag screw, the radiolucent line often persists indefinitely.

Comments. In this case, arthroscopy was used to explore the elbow joint and provide definitive diagnosis and treatment of incomplete ossification of the humeral condyle. This case is interesting because lameness attributable to IOHC was successfully diagnosed and treated before a potentially severe fracture of the elbow occurred. IOHC can be difficult to diagnose radiographically. Arthroscopic examination can confirm or exclude the condition.

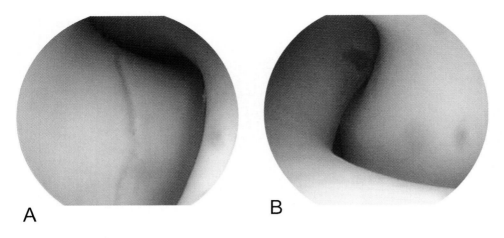

FIGURE 9–31 Arthroscopic views of the right and left elbow joints with a caudomedial scope portal. *A,* A fissure associated with incomplete ossification of the humeral condyle is seen just lateral to the central sulcus of the trochlea of the distal humerus and adjacent to the trochlear notch of the ulna. *B,* The normal articular surface of the left distal humerus.

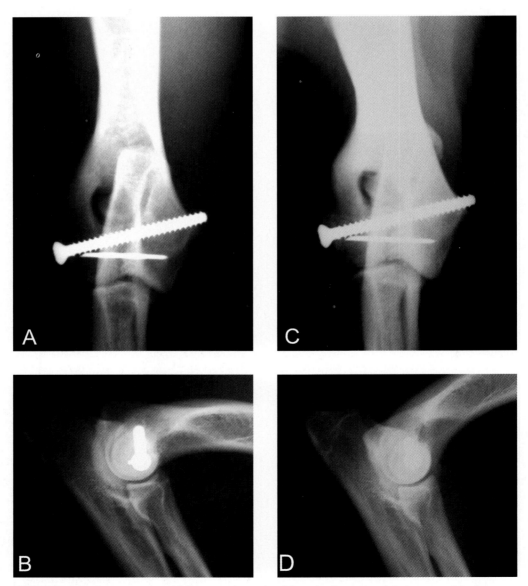

FIGURE 9–32 Postoperative and follow-up radiographs of the right elbow. *A* and *B,* A transcondylar lag screw was placed to treat incomplete ossification of the humeral condyle. A drill bit that broke and could not be retrieved during attempted insertion of the first cannulated screw into the dense cortical bone of the humeral condyle is seen. The screw was redirected on the second attempt at insertion. *C* and *D,* Follow-up radiographs 1 year after surgery show incomplete healing of the fissure after a lag screw was placed.

Clinical Case Study 11

Osteochondrosis of the Elbow

Signalment. The patient is an 11-month-old, 35-kg male black Labrador retriever.

Chief Complaint. The chief complaint is weightbearing lameness of the left forelimb.

History. Left forelimb lameness began 4 months before presentation. No evidence of trauma was observed, and the dog was restricted to a fenced yard. The lameness did not respond to NSAID and antibiotic therapy.

Orthopedic Findings. The dog had a grade III of V lameness of the left forelimb. Extension and flexion of both elbows elicited pain. Distension of the joint capsule was palpable in both elbows. The remaining orthopedic findings were normal.

Diagnostic Findings. Radiographs showed a subtle lesion compatible with OCD involving the medial humeral condyle of the left elbow and possibly the right elbow as well (Fig. 9–33).

Arthroscopic Findings. A caudomedial scope portal was used. Arthroscopic examination showed a loose OCD fragment on the weightbearing surface of the medial humeral condyle of each elbow (Fig. 9–34). Generalized moderate synovitis was seen. The remaining articular surfaces appeared normal.

Therapy. A craniomedial instrument portal was used. The loose cartilage fragment was elevated with a banana knife and removed with grasping forceps. A motorized mini-shaver and curette were used to treat the subchondral bed with surface abrasion until bleeding cancellous bone was achieved (Fig. 9–35).

Postoperative Care. The dog was dismissed from the hospital the day of surgery with instructions for rehabilitation for 6 weeks. Rehabilitation included restricted leash walking, active and passive range of motion exercises, and flexion and extension stretch exercises.

Outcome. The dog had a grade III of V lameness for the first postoperative week. The lameness gradually resolved over the ensuing 2 weeks. The dog presented 3 weeks postoperatively with bilateral hindlimb lameness and stiffness. The cause was suspected to be panosteitis, but the results of diagnostic tests were inconclusive. The lameness resolved spontaneously. One year after surgery, the dog showed no lameness and had normal range of motion in the elbow joints.

Comments. In this case, arthroscopy was used to confirm the diagnosis of elbow OCD and also to treat the condition. Arthroscopic removal of osteochondral fragments from the elbow can be performed completely and atraumatically. The subchondral bed can be treated

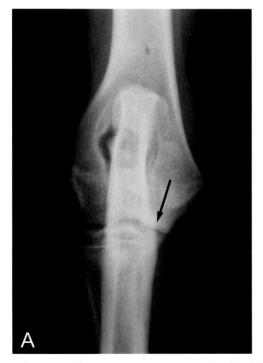 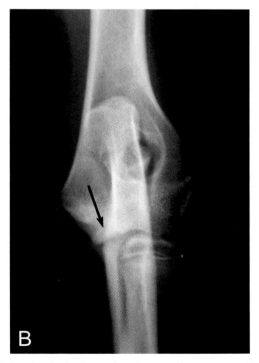

FIGURE 9–33 Anteroposterior radiographs of the left (A) and right (B) elbows show the typical appearance of subchondral defects due to osteochondritis dissecans of the medial humeral condyle (arrows).

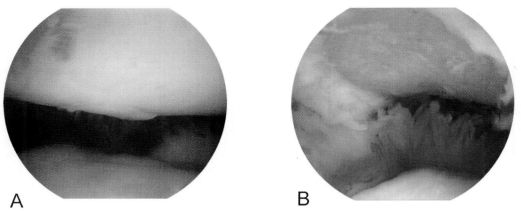

FIGURE 9–34   Arthroscopic views of the right elbow. *A,* A loose flap of cartilage is slightly elevated from the articular surface of the medial humeral condyle. *B,* Moderate synovitis is seen throughout the joint. Subchondral bone of the medial humeral condyle is seen after flap removal.

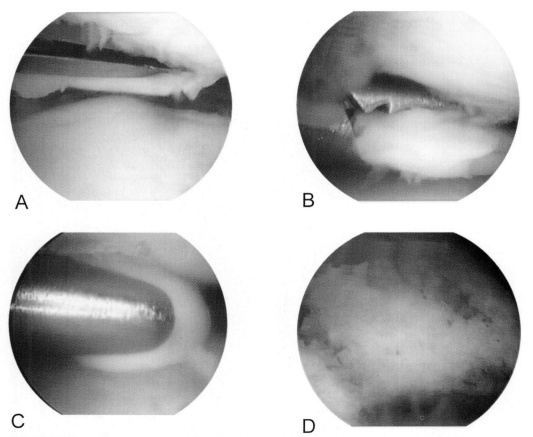

FIGURE 9–35   Arthroscopic views of the right elbow. *A,* A banana knife is used to elevate the flap, leaving it attached to the subchondral bed by a small amount of tissue. *B,* The flap is secured with grasping forceps. *C,* The flap is removed by twisting and retracting the forceps from the joint. *D,* The subchondral bed is treated with abrasion arthroplasty and curettage to provide a blood supply to the defect. This treatment is carried to a level at which bleeding is first recognized. Excessive removal of bone can be detrimental.

to encourage fibrocartilage repair of the defect. A good long-term clinical result can be achieved if the lesion is small or medium and if osteoarthritis is minimal at the time of treatment. Early arthroscopic intervention is recommended in patients with elbow OCD.

Clinical Case Study 12

Ligamentous Injury of the Carpus

Signalment. The patient is a 9-year-old, 43-kg neutered male English sheepdog.

Chief Complaint. The chief complaint is chronic weightbearing lameness of the right forelimb.

History. Right forelimb lameness began acutely 1 month before presentation. No evidence of trauma was observed, but the dog had free roam outside before the lameness occurred. Response to NSAID therapy and rest was poor.

Orthopedic Findings. The dog had a grade V of V right forelimb lameness. Extension and flexion of the right carpus elicited a painful response. When the dog stood, the right carpus appeared hyperextended. Bilateral hip dysplasia and secondary osteoarthritis also were also seen.

Diagnostic Findings. Radiographs of the right carpus showed osteoarthritis of the intercarpal and carpometacarpal joints. The joint spaces appeared decreased, and osteophytes were evident (Fig. 9–36). The radiocarpal joint showed minimal evidence of osteoarthritic changes. Stress views did not show obvious instability.

Arthroscopic Findings. Dorsomedial and dorsolateral scope portals were used. Arthroscopic examination of the right radiocarpal joint showed partial tearing of the palmar radiocarpal ligament and accessory carpal bone ligaments. Generalized synovitis was evident. A small area of articular cartilage erosion was present on the distal radius and ulnar carpal bone (Fig. 9–37).

Therapy. Because the radiocarpal joint was damaged, the surgeon elected to perform pancarpal arthrodesis rather than partial arthrodesis. Pancarpal arthrodesis was performed through a standard dorsal approach using a 10-hole, 3.5-mm broad plate and 10 screws (Fig. 9–38).

Postoperative Care. The dog was dismissed from the hospital the day after surgery with instructions for rehabilitation for 12 weeks. A fiberglass splint was placed on the palmar aspect of the carpus for 4 weeks. Rehabilitation included restricted leash walking, active and passive range of motion exercises, and flexion and extension stretch exercises. Activity was restricted to

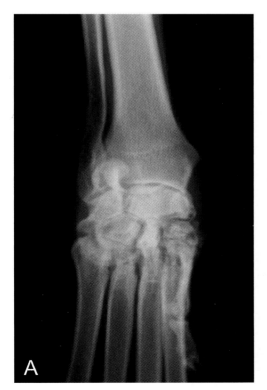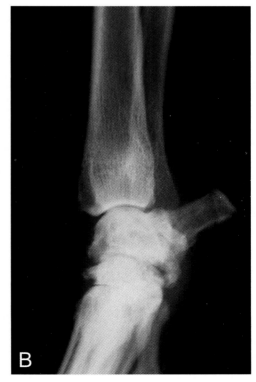

FIGURE 9–36 Anterior posterior (A) and lateral (B) radiographs of the right carpus showing osteoarthritis of the intercarpal and carpometacarpal joints. The joint spaces appear decreased, osteophytes are evident, and the radiocarpal joint shows minimal evidence of osteoarthritic changes.

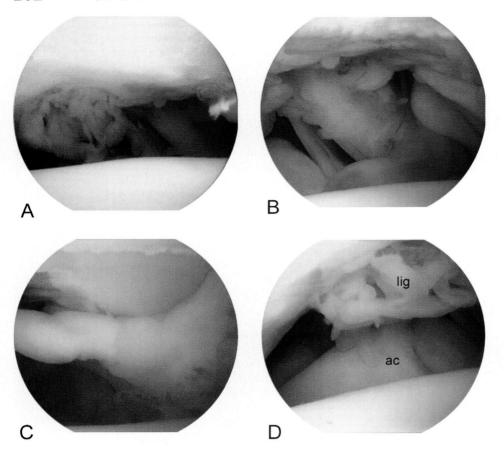

FIGURE 9-37 Arthroscopic views of the right carpus. *A,* Mild erosion of the distal radius and synovitis within the radiocarpal joint. *B,* Partial tearing of the palmar ulnocarpal ligament. *C,* Partial tearing of the palmar radiocarpal ligament. *D,* Partial tearing of the proximal ligament (*lig*) of the accessory carpal bone (*ac*).

short leash walks for 8 weeks, followed by a gradual increase to normal activity over a period of 4 weeks.

Outcome. The dog walked with a grade II of V lameness while the splint was in place. The lameness was increased for the first week after splint removal but improved to a grade I of V lameness by 3 months postoperatively. At that time, the dog was willing to run and jump on the affected leg.

Comments. In this case, arthroscopy was used to confirm the presence of intra-articular carpal ligament damage of the radiocarpal joint. Identification of damage to this joint was an important factor in the decision to perform pancarpal arthrodesis rather than partial arthrodesis. The use of both a dorsomedial and a dorsolateral scope portal allowed quick and thorough evaluation of the radiocarpal joint.

Clinical Case Study 13

Tear of the Subscapularis Tendon and Medial Glenohumeral Ligament in the Shoulder of a Rabbit

Signalment. The patient is a 5-year-old, 2.0-kg male rabbit.

Chief Complaint. The chief complaint is inability to walk on the front legs.

History. The patient was a rescue case; therefore, a complete history is not available. The owner reported an inability to walk and a splaying out of the front legs since the rabbit was adopted 1 week before presentation.

Orthopedic Findings. Palpation of the shoulders elicited mild pain that was more severe on the right. The rabbit was unable to walk on the front legs. Both front legs splayed out as a result of abduction of the shoulders. Severe medial instability and excessive abduction of the shoulders were palpable under anesthesia and were most severe on the right (Fig. 9–39).

Diagnostic Findings. Radiographs of the shoulders showed osteoarthritis of both shoulder joints. Instability of the shoulders was not seen radiographically (Fig. 9–40).

Arthroscopic and Surgical Findings. Arthroscopic examination of the right shoulder was performed with a standard lateral scope portal located just distal to the acromion process. A 1.9-mm arthroscope was used. Arthroscopic examination of the right shoulder joint showed moderate synovial inflammation, a complete tear of the subscapularis tendon, an advanced partial tear of the medial glenohumeral ligament, and wear of

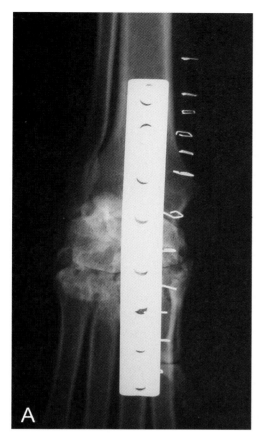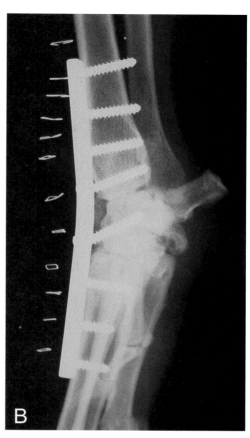

FIGURE 9–38 Postoperative anterior posterior (*A*) and lateral (*B*) radiographic views of the right carpus after pancarpal arthrodesis.

the cartilage of the humeral head and glenoid fossa (Fig. 9–41). Medial instability of the shoulder was noted arthroscopically while the medial side of the joint was stressed during surgery.

Therapy. The owner elected shoulder arthrodesis rather than ligamentous reconstruction because of the severity of the instability and a requirement for only one surgical procedure. Arthrodesis was initially attempted

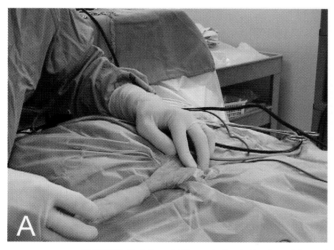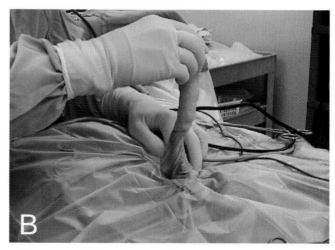

FIGURE 9–39 *A*, The right forelimb of a rabbit with medial shoulder instability in the normal lateral position. *B*, The right forelimb of the same rabbit placed in a stressed position, showing excessive abduction and medial instability of the shoulder.

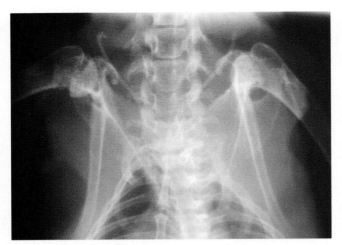

FIGURE 9–40 Radiograph of the shoulders of a rabbit with bilateral medial shoulder instability. Osteoarthritis is evident, but instability is difficult to confirm radiographically.

with a 2.0/2.7-mm veterinary cuttable plate, but complications occurred. Because of osteopenia, the quality of the cortical bone was insufficient to secure the screws. In addition, a proximal humeral fracture occurred during tightening of one screw. A transarticular tie-in external fixator combined with an intramedullary pin placed in the humerus was used to perform the arthrodesis and repair the humeral fracture. Cancellous bone graft was placed at the arthrodesis and fracture sites.

Postoperative Care. The rabbit was discharged from the hospital 5 days after surgery with instructions for cage rest for 2 months. The rabbit was placed on a balanced diet to improve bone quality.

Outcome. The rabbit was improved and using the leg 1 month postoperatively. Future arthroscopy with arthrodesis of the left shoulder is planned.

Comments. In this case, arthroscopy was used to explore the shoulder joint in a rabbit. An adequate joint space was present to allow visualization of all intra-articular structures that are normally visible arthroscopically in other species.

Clinical Case Study 14

Fracture of the Supraglenoid Tuberosity

Signalment. The patient is a 5-month-old, 11.0-kg female bullterrier.

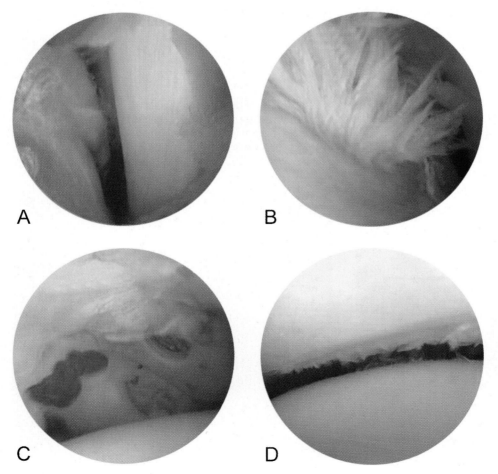

FIGURE 9–41 Arthroscopic views of the right shoulder joint of a rabbit with medial shoulder instability. A, Normal biceps tendons adjacent to the cranial edge of the torn subscapularis tendon. B, Torn fibers of the right subscapularis tendon. C, Torn fibers and hemorrhage associated with an advanced partial tear of the medial glenohumeral ligament. Cartilage wear also involves the medial lip of the glenoid cavity. D, Cartilage wear involves the lateral lip of the glenoid cavity. The articular cartilage of the humeral head appears normal in this region.

Chief Complaint. The chief complaint is acute onset of left forelimb lameness.

History. Acute onset of non-weightbearing lameness of the left forelimb occurred the day before presentation. No trauma was observed, and the dog was confined to the house.

Orthopedic Findings. Non-weightbearing lameness (grade V of V) of the left forelimb was observed. Marked pain was present on flexion and extension of the shoulder. Other findings of physical examination were normal.

Diagnostic Findings. Radiographs of the left shoulder showed an avulsion fracture of the supraglenoid tuberosity (Fig. 9–42).

Arthroscopic Findings. The supraglenoid tuberosity was easily visualized with a 1.9-mm arthroscope positioned in a standard lateral portal (Fig. 9–43). A fracture hematoma was present at the fracture line and

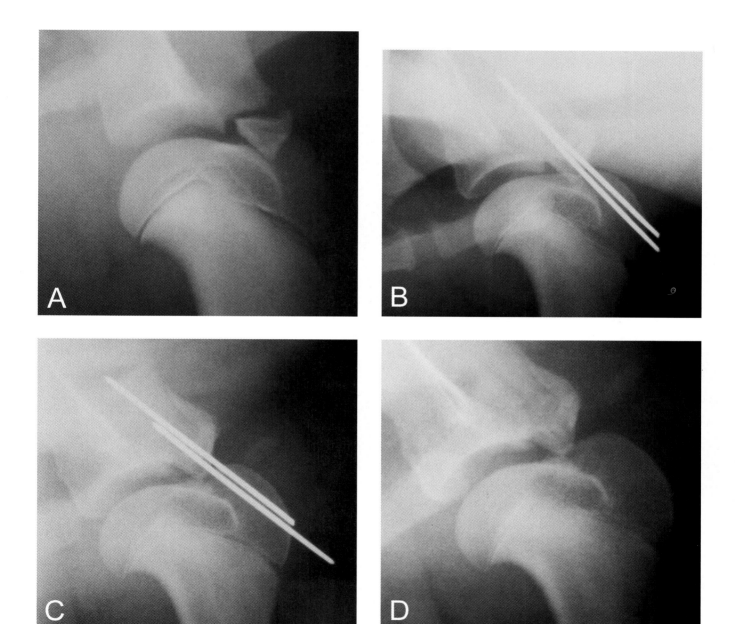

FIGURE 9–42 Lateral radiographs of the left shoulder of a dog with a fracture of the supraglenoid tuberosity. A, Fracture of the left supraglenoid tuberosity. B, Postoperative radiograph after percutaneous K-wire fixation of the fracture. C, Six-week follow-up radiograph showing healing of the fracture and migration of the implant. The fragment shifted slightly, compromising anatomic reduction, although reduction was adequate for good function. D, Radiographic appearance after removal of the implant.

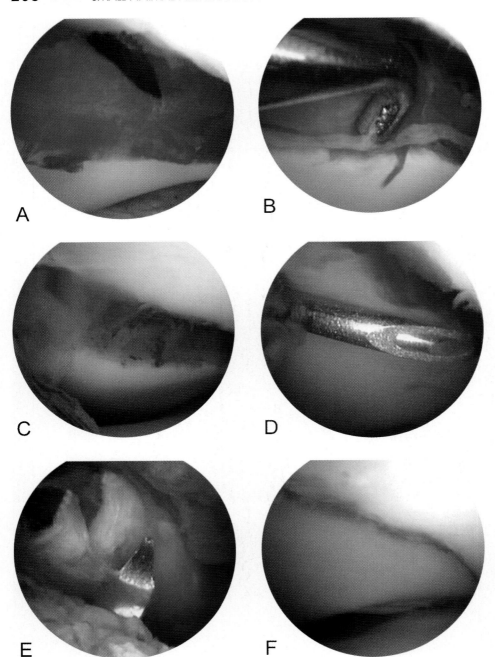

FIGURE 9–43 Arthroscopic views of the left shoulder joint. *A,* The fracture line associated with an articular fracture of the supraglenoid tuberosity. A fracture hematoma is seen. *B,* The fracture hematoma was removed with a blunt probe and graspers. *C,* The fracture after removal of the fracture hematoma. *D,* A guide needle is placed and viewed arthroscopically to assist in the orientation of the percutaneously placed K-wire in the fracture fragment. *E,* The position of the K-wire is assessed arthroscopically as it exits the fracture line. *F,* The fracture is reduced and the K-wire is driven into the bone of the distal scapula. Anatomic reduction at the level of the joint surface can be documented arthroscopically.

was removed with a blunt probe and graspers through a craniolateral instrument portal.

Therapy. A 22-gauge guide needle was placed alongside the fragment to use as a guide for positioning the K-wire. A 0.045-inch K-wire was placed in the fragment percutaneously. When viewed arthroscopically, the point of the wire could be seen exiting the fracture line. The fracture was reduced by digital pressure under arthroscopic visualization. After reduction of the fracture was confirmed, the wire was driven into the scapula. With the first wire used as a guide, a second 0.045-inch K-

wire was placed percutaneously (Figs. 9–42 to 9–44). A radiofrequency probe was used to transect the biceps tendon arthroscopically at its origin. The K-wires were left long to facilitate removal of the implant.

Postoperative Care. The dog was dismissed from the hospital the day after surgery with instructions for leash walking for 4 weeks.

Outcome. The dog had weightbearing left forelimb lameness equal to the preoperative status 24 hours after surgery. The lameness improved progressively, but mild

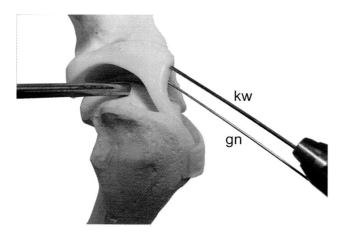

FIGURE 9–44 The fracture of the supraglenoid tuberosity is stabilized with arthroscopic assistance. A standard lateral arthroscope portal is used. A guide needle (*gn*) is placed alongside the fragment and used as a guide to insert the percutaneous K-wire (*kw*) that is used to stabilize the fracture. The guide needle is placed under arthroscopic visualization, and the K-wire is placed into the fragment in the same direction as the guide wire.

lameness persisted at follow-up radiographic examination 6 weeks postoperatively. Radiographic evaluation showed healing of the fracture and migration of one K-wire. Both K-wires were removed. Lameness resolved within 2 weeks, and no gait abnormalities were evident at walk, trot, or run 2 months later.

Comments. In this case, arthroscopy was used to evaluate, reduce, and stabilize an intra-articular fracture. Initially, a lag screw technique was planned, but this technique was abandoned because the fragment was small and an appropriately sized implant was not available. Divergent K-wire fixation provided adequate fixation and good postoperative function. The biceps tendon was transected to remove a potential distractive force from the stabilized fragment. Transection of the biceps tendon is used to treat fractures of the supraglenoid tuberosity in horses. Although this patient had a good outcome, stabilization with a lag screw is the preferred technique because of the benefits of interfragmentary compression on bone healing and fracture reduction.

Clinical Case Study 15

Lateral Condylar Fracture of the Distal Humerus

Signalment. The patient is a 3.5-month-old, 12.0-kg female Labrador retriever.

Chief Complaint. The chief complaint is acute onset of lameness of the right forelimb.

History. Acute onset of non-weightbearing lameness of the right forelimb occurred 4 days before presen-

tation. The lameness occurred while the dog was running unobserved in a fenced yard.

Orthopedic Findings. Non-weightbearing lameness (grade V of V) of the right forelimb was observed. Flexion and extension of the right elbow elicited marked pain and crepitus. Other findings were normal.

Diagnostic Findings. Radiographs of the right elbow showed a lateral condylar fracture of the humerus with minimal displacement (Fig. 9–45).

Arthroscopic Findings. The fracture line was visualized with a 1.9-mm arthroscope positioned in a standard caudomedial elbow portal (Fig. 9–46). A fracture hematoma was present at the fracture line but was difficult to remove completely because of the duration of the fracture.

Therapy. The fracture was reduced by digital pressure under arthroscopic visualization. Reduction was maintained and compression was applied across the fracture line with a vulsellum forceps (Fig. 9–47). A 4.0-mm partially threaded screw was placed percutaneously in routine fashion. A 0.062-inch K-wire was placed percutaneously across the lateral epicondylar crest to provide adjunctive stabilization. As the screw was tightened, compression of the fracture line was observed arthroscopically. As compression occurred, the fracture hematoma bulged from between the fragments.

Postoperative Care. The dog was dismissed from the hospital the day after surgery with instructions for leash walking for 6 weeks.

Outcome. Follow-up radiographs 6 weeks postoperatively showed healing of the fracture (see Fig. 9–45). The dog had mild weightbearing right forelimb lameness at this time. The lameness improved progressively over the subsequent month. Two years postoperatively, the dog occasionally favors the leg after hard exercise but does not show lameness with normal activity.

Comments. In this case, arthroscopy was used to evaluate, reduce, and stabilize an intra-articular fracture. Lateral condylar fractures with minimal displacement are candidates for this technique. Arthroscopic visualization of the fracture line at the level of the articular cartilage ensures anatomic reduction and helps to avoid step defects that may lead to osteoarthritis. Percutaneous fixation of lag screws can be performed if the lateral and medial epicondyles are readily palpable or if fluoroscopic imaging is available.

Clinical Case Study 16

Ununited Anconeal Process

Signalment. The patient is an 8-year-old, 42.0-kg male German shepherd.

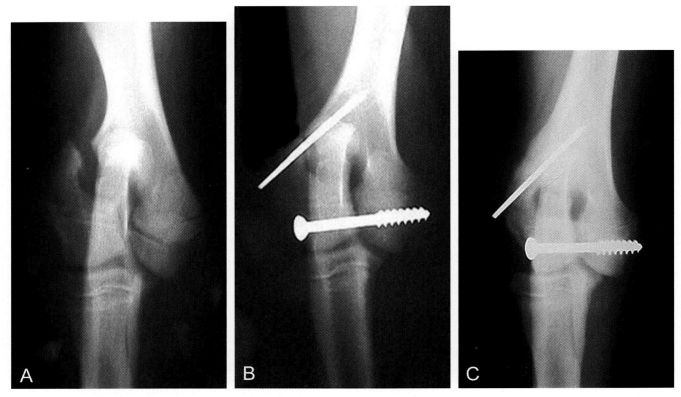

FIGURE 9–45 Radiographs of the right elbow of a dog with a fracture of the lateral condyle of the humerus. *A,* Minimally displaced fracture of the right lateral humeral condyle. *B,* Radiograph after arthroscopically assisted fixation of the fracture with a percutaneous lag screw and K-wire. *C,* Six-week follow-up radiograph showing healing of the fracture.

Chief Complaint. The chief complaint is acute onset of right forelimb lameness.

History. Acute onset of weightbearing lameness of the right forelimb occurred 1 week before presentation. The owner reported a history of chronic, mild, intermittent forelimb lameness. No trauma was observed, and the dog was confined to the house and a fenced yard.

Orthopedic Findings. Weightbearing lameness (grade III of V) of the right forelimb was observed.

Extension of the right elbow caused marked pain. The other findings were normal.

Diagnostic Findings. Radiographs of the right elbow showed a chronic ununited anconeal process and mild osteoarthritis (Fig. 9–48).

Arthroscopic Findings. The ununited anconeal process was visualized with a 1.9-mm arthroscope positioned in a standard caudomedial portal (Fig. 9–49). Full-thickness erosion of the articular cartilage on the caudal

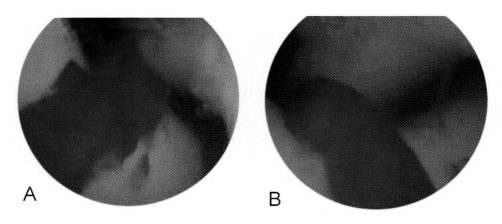

FIGURE 9–46 Arthroscopic views of the left elbow joint. *A,* The fracture line associated with an articular fracture of the lateral condyle of the elbow shows a fracture hematoma. *B,* The fracture hematoma bulges as compression is placed across the fracture. Fracture reduction can be assessed arthroscopically.

FIGURE 9–47 Arthroscopically assisted stabilization of a lateral condyle fracture of the elbow. *A,* A standard caudomedial arthroscope portal is used. The fracture is reduced with digital pressure while the articular surface is viewed arthroscopically. Anatomic reduction is maintained with vulsellum forceps. *B,* A lag screw is placed percutaneously, with the lateral and medial epicondyles used as landmarks. The screw is placed across the condyles cranial and distal to the epicondyles and can be placed from the medial or lateral side. A K-wire also is placed percutaneously across the lateral epicondylar crest (not shown) (see Fig. 9–45B).

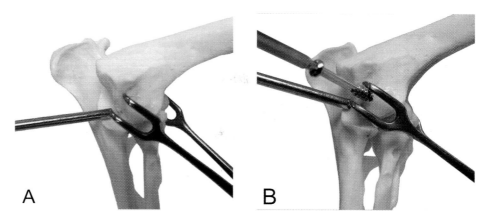

A B

aspect of the humeral trochlea was seen, and mild synovitis was present.

Therapy. A 22-gauge guide needle was placed alongside the medial aspect of the anconeal fragment to use as a guide for positioning a lag screw. A 0.045-inch threaded K-wire was placed percutaneously in the fragment. The point of the wire was seen exiting the anconeal process when viewed arthroscopically (see Fig. 9–49). The fragment was reduced under arthroscopic visualization by placing the elbow in extension and applying counterpressure with a Freer elevator that was placed into the joint through a caudal instrument portal. After the fragment was reduced, the wire was driven into the fragment. A self-tapping, self-drilling, cannulated 4.0-mm lag screw was threaded onto the guide wire and inserted into the fragment (see Fig. 9–49). As the screw was tightened, the gap narrowed and compression of

the fragment was observed (see Fig. 9–49). Anatomic reduction was confirmed arthroscopically. A proximal, dynamic ulnar osteotomy was preformed in routine fashion. The proximal ulna shifted a small distance proximally immediately after the osteotomy was completed. The osteotomy was not stabilized.

Postoperative Care. The dog was dismissed from the hospital the day after surgery with instructions for leash walking for 8 weeks. No bandage was used.

Outcome. The dog had weightbearing lameness of the left forelimb equal to the preoperative status 24 hours after surgery. The lameness improved progressively, but mild intermittent lameness was seen 2 months postoperatively. Radiographic evaluation 8 months postoperatively showed complete bony union of the anconeal process but incomplete union of the ulnar osteotomy.

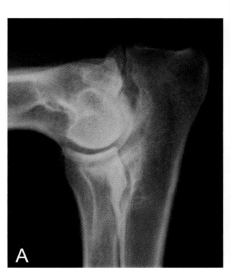 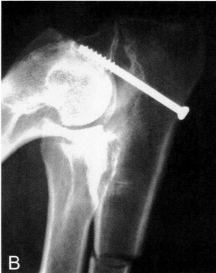 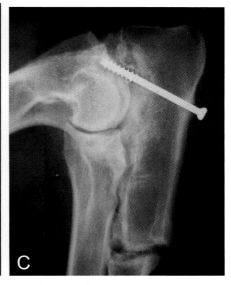

A B C

FIGURE 9–48 Lateral radiographs of the right elbow of a dog with an ununited anconeal process. *A,* Preoperative radiograph showing an ununited anconeal process and mild osteoarthritis. *B,* Radiograph after arthroscopically assisted percutaneous fixation of the anconeal process with a 4.0-mm cannulated lag screw and dynamic proximal ulnar osteotomy. *C,* Eight-month follow-up radiograph showing healing of the anconeal process, but incomplete healing of the ulnar osteotomy.

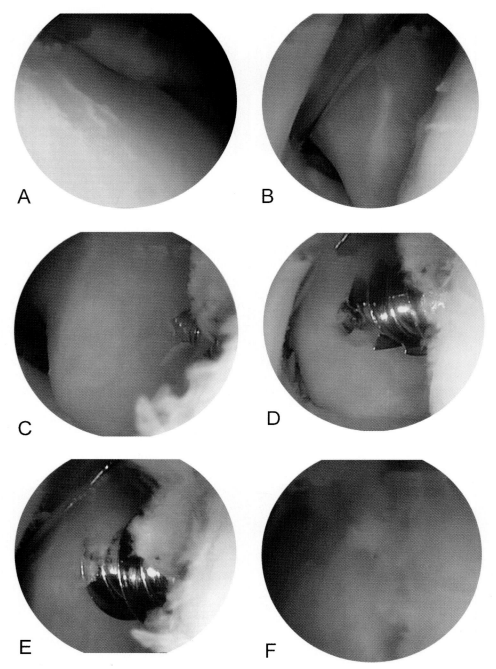

FIGURE 9–49 Arthroscopic views of the right elbow. *A,* Full-thickness erosion of the articular cartilage of the caudal and proximal aspects of the humeral trochlea adjacent to the anconeal fragment. *B,* A Freer elevator is inserted into the joint to apply counterpressure to the anconeal fragment during stabilization. *C,* A threaded K-wire protrudes from the anconeal process. The wire is advanced into the anconeal fragment after it is reduced to provide initial stability and guide placement of the screw. *D,* A 4.0-mm cannulated, self-drilling, self-tapping lag screw is inserted. *E,* The screw is partially engaged, and the fragment gap is beginning to close. *F,* The fragment gap is closed, and compression of the fragment line is seen arthroscopically as the screw is tightened. Anatomic reduction also is confirmed arthroscopically.

The dog was doing well clinically but continued to have mild lameness after exercising. Lameness was not present during normal daily activity. Pain was not evident when digital pressure was applied to the proximal ulna.

Comments. In this case, arthroscopy was used to evaluate, reduce, and stabilize a fragmented anconeal process. A cannulated lag screw was used to stabilize the process and provide compression, with good long-term results. The reason for the exacerbation of clinical lameness at 8 years of age is unknown, but the ununited fragment may have been dislodged by incidental trauma, causing acute pain. A dynamic ulnar osteotomy was performed to release tension on the stabilized anconeal process. The osteotomy was necessary because extensive articular erosion was present on the proximal and caudal aspect of the humeral trochlea. Follow-up radiographs 8 months later showed incomplete healing of the ulnar osteotomy. Placement of a small-diameter intramedullary pin in the ulna may have aided bony healing while allowing dynamic adjustment of the olecranon. The mild intermittent lameness noted after exercise may be caused by mild osteoarthritis or by incomplete healing of the ulnar osteotomy.

Acknowledgments

The authors thank Dr. Jeff Edwards, DVM, Diplomate ACVP with Antech Diagnostics for the histopathologic interpretation and histologic photomicrographs in Clinical Case Study 8.

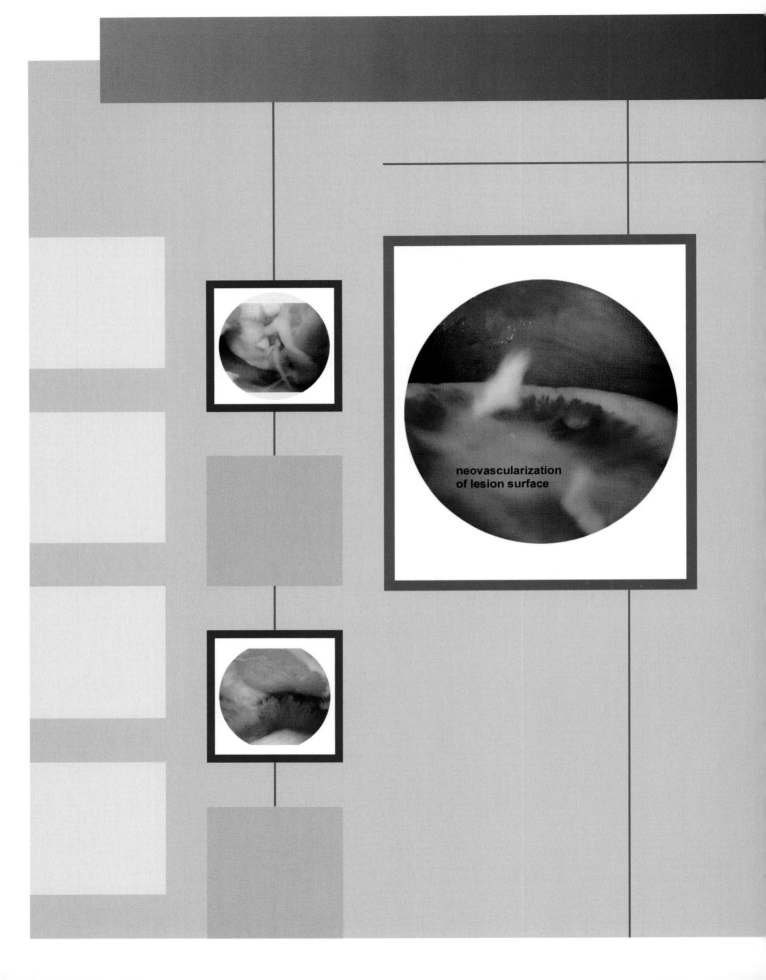

neovascularization
of lesion surface

Postoperative Management and Treatment After Arthroscopy

Introduction

Many patients that undergo arthroscopy have pre-existing osteoarthritis or will develop it in the future. Although arthroscopic treatment may be used as the sole method of managing a specific joint problem, a treatment plan that includes arthroscopy, medical therapy, proper nutrition, and physical rehabilitation usually leads to a higher level of performance. In addition, combining modalities may reduce the need for certain types of treatment. For example, attention to weight loss and proper nutrition may reduce the necessary dose or frequency of nonsteroidal anti-inflammatory drug (NSAID) therapy. In addition, adequate postoperative analgesia with NSAIDs and opiates may encourage the patient to participate in physical rehabilitation exercises. The use of chondroprotectant drugs and nutraceuticals may reduce the need for NSAIDs or enhance the response to medical therapy. Physical rehabilitation usually improves performance, decreases the need for medication, and encourages weight loss by increasing activity level. Arthroscopy enhances the surgeon's ability to evaluate the condition of the articular surface and synovium and formulate an appropriate postoperative plan. Patients with traumatic injury or osteoarthritis are best served by a management plan tailored to the individual. A cookbook approach toward treatment may lead to excessive, inadequate, or inappropriate treatment because of variations in patient signalment, severity of disease, duration of disease, and tissues involved (e.g., cartilage, synovium, bone). Patients with mild disease may need only short-term postoperative management, whereas severely affected patients may require lifelong management of osteoarthritis. This chapter provides an introduction to a variety of modalities that may improve clinical results. Veterinary textbooks and journal articles provide more detailed information.

Medical Therapy

NONSTEROIDAL ANTI-INFLAMMATORY DRUGS

NSAIDs have long been the gold standard for treating osteoarthritis in humans and domestic animals. These drugs reduce the synthesis of prostaglandin (primarily prostaglandin E2 [PGE2]) through inhibition of cyclooxygenase. Many types of NSAIDs are available. Aspirin and phenylbutazone were the first NSAIDs to be widely used in dogs. Recently, NSAIDs have been developed with greater specificity toward cyclooxygenase II (Cox II). In the past, most NSAIDs inhibited both cyclooxygenase I (Cox I) and Cox II. Inhibition of Cox I leads to widespread inhibition of PGE2, including prostaglandins that are found in the gastrointestinal tract, joints, and kidneys and provide homeostatic functions. Cox II inhibitors act predominantly on Cox II, an enzyme that produces inflammatory prostaglandins in the joint and other tissues. The use of NSAIDs that selectively inhibit Cox II should reduce side effects that involve the gastrointestinal tract, platelets, and kidneys.

Carprofen. Carprofen, a relatively new NSAID, relieves the clinical signs of osteoarthritis in dogs and causes fewer gastrointestinal side effects than NSAIDs that inhibit both Cox I and Cox II. Carprofen is rapidly replacing aspirin as the veterinarian's first choice of NSAID for the treatment of osteoarthritis. Carprofen is routinely used for preemptive and postoperative analgesia. In addition, it is administered after arthroscopy to reduce synovitis and swelling of periarticular tissues. Reducing postoperative inflammation encourages earlier use of the affected joint. Depending on the severity of the condition, some patients may require NSAID therapy for several weeks or months postoperatively. Gastro-duodenal protection occurs as a result of the enhanced Cox II activity offered by carprofen. In dogs, carprofen is administered at a dose of 2.2 mg/kg orally every 12 hours or 4.4 mg/kg orally every 24 hours. The flexibility to administer the drug once or twice a day is advantageous. Patients having clinical signs only at a particular time of the day may benefit from once daily dosing, whereas patients having persistent problems may do better with twice daily dosing. The flexibility in dosing also can be advantageous in meeting the scheduling needs of pet owners. Plasma and serum concentrations of carprofen are consistent throughout the treatment period. Serum concentrations peak at 2 hours, and synovial concentrations peak between 3 and 6 hours after administration. In both normal and osteoarthritic joints, the synovial concentration of carprofen reaches therapeutic levels during the treatment period. At therapeutic doses, carprofen significantly reduces the production of PGE2 from chondrocytes. A rare, idiosyncratic side effect of carprofen in dogs is hepatoxicity leading to icterus and elevation of alkaline phosphatase and hepatic transaminase levels. The incidence of this effect and other side effects is low (<1%), and many affected patients recover with symptomatic therapy and discontinuation of carprofen. In recent studies, carprofen had little effect on kidney and platelet function and was found to support cartilage metabolism and proteoglycan synthesis. The chondroprotective effects of carprofen are particularly important if long-term NSAID use is anticipated. In anecdotal reports, carprofen at a dose of 12.5 mg orally every 5 days was used successfully in the treatment of osteoarthritic and postoperative pain in cats. No severe adverse reactions were reported at this dose. However, this drug is not approved for use in cats, and no clinical research data are available to substantiate the anecdotally reported regimen. Cats are sensitive to NSAIDs because of differences in liver metabolism of this type of drug. NSAID toxicity in cats may be manifested in many ways, including gastrointestinal, hepatic, and renal dysfunction.

Etodolac. Etodolac is another relatively new NSAID that inhibits Cox II preferentially and ameliorates the clinical signs of osteoarthritis in dogs. It is administered at a dose of 10 to 15 mL/kg every 24 hours. Like carprofen, etodolac has a favorable Cox II:Cox I ratio. Side effects are uncommon but are typical of those seen with NSAIDs, with gastrointestinal ulceration the most common. Gastrointestinal ulceration can be severe at dosages well above the labeled dose. The effect of etodolac on proteoglycan synthesis and cartilage metabolism is not clear. The use of etodolac in cats has not been reported.

Aspirin. Aspirin is commonly used but is not approved for administration in dogs and cats. Aspirin does not inhibit Cox II preferentially. In dogs, aspirin is recommended to be administered with food at a dose of 25 mg/kg body weight every 12 hours. In cats, the dose is 10 to 20 mg/kg with food every 48 hours. Aspirin is available plain, buffered, or combined with various stomach protectants. Side effects include gastrointestinal irritation, platelet inhibition, and renal toxicity.

Phenylbutazone. Phenylbutazone is an older NSAID that does not preferentially inhibit Cox II. In dogs, it is given at a dosage of 10 to 22 mg/kg body weight divided three times a day. When the higher dose is used, after 48 hours, it is decreased to the lowest effective level, not to exceed a total daily dosage of 800 mg, regardless of patient body weight. The reported dose in cats is 6 to 8 mg/kg orally every 8 hours, but its use is not recommended in cats. Because of the potential for gastric ulceration, NSAIDs are used cautiously in dogs with orthopedic problems.

Other NSAIDs Used in Dogs

Other promising new Cox II NSAIDs, such as deracoxib and meloxicam, are anticipated to be available in the United States in the near future. These drugs are available for use outside of the United States.

Other NSAIDs Used in Humans

Although dosages have been suggested for naproxen, piroxicam, ketorolac tromethamine (Toradol), and ibuprofen in dogs, their use is discouraged because they appear to have greater ulcerogenic potential than aspirin.

STEROIDAL DRUGS

Steroidal drugs, such as prednisone, prednisolone, and dexamethasone, are not typically used after arthroscopic surgery unless immune-mediated polyarthritis is suspected. Steroid drugs can substantially inhibit the production of proteoglycan as a result of down-regulation of chondrocytes. Depletion of the extracellular matrix may increase the chance of cartilage erosion. If inflammation is severe and does not respond to NSAIDs, a short course of steroids can be considered to break the cycle of inflammation and osteoarthritis. A common dose for prednisone is 0.5 to 1.0 mg/kg orally divided twice a day. Intra-articular injections of steroids should be avoided, especially if long-term administration is anticipated. Intra-articular injection of steroids may increase the likelihood of septic arthritis or may inhibit the metabolic processes of the cartilage. If short term anti-inflammatory treatment is required, intra-articular steroid injections can be considered. Intra-articular steroids must be administered aseptically. Methyl prednisolone (SoluMedrol) and triamcinolone acetate (Vetalog) (0.5 to 2.0 ml depending on patient size) are options for steroid drugs suitable for intra-articular administration.

CHONDROPROTECTANTS

Optimal recovery from musculoskeletal disorders requires attention to mechanical, environmental, and biologic factors. Changes in one factor often affect other factors. For example, attention to mechanical and environmental factors improves the biologic environment of injured joints. Mechanical factors that enhance recovery may include an appropriate level of physical activity to build endurance, the use of special exercises to increase the range of motion in the joint, exercises to increase strength, and the use of aids to protect from or alleviate pain. Environmental factors that affect rehabilitation include patient compliance, owner compliance, weather conditions, terrain, and household environment. Biologic factors that affect the local environment of the joint include the quality and quantity of synovial fluid, the presence of degradative enzymes within the synovial fluid and articular cartilage, the condition of the extra-articular matrix of articular cartilage, and the metabolic state of the chondrocytes. Nutraceuticals and chondroprotectants may enhance joint health and promote healing by improving biologic factors.

Chondroprotectants and nutraceuticals can be an attractive adjunctive or alternative treatment for cats and dogs that undergo arthroscopy or that have osteoarthritis. Chondroprotectants are available as oral nutraceuticals and as oral and injectable pharmaceuticals. Because direct comparisons of these products have not been made, selection of the optimal chondroprotectant for a particular animal is not known. In addition, it is not known when different mediators of osteoarthritis play an important role. Different mediators of pain and cartilage degradation (e.g., prostaglandins, free radicals, metalloproteinases, serine proteases) may play a role at different points during the course of disease. Ideally, if the predominant mediators in an individual with osteoarthritis are known, the most appropriate product can be selected for treatment. The best recommendation is to use products that have undergone well-designed experimental and clinical research to evaluate their efficacy and safety as well as products that are manufactured under the high quality standards practiced by the pharmaceutical industry.

The term *chondroprotectant* is applied to various compounds that are proposed to promote the health and metabolism of chondrocytes and synoviocytes. This broad definition encompasses a wide variety of veterinary products that differ considerably in structure, function, and degree of purity. A number of other terms are used to describe these types of products, including *slow-acting, disease-modifying osteoarthritic agent* (SADMOA), *structure- and disease-modifying anti-osteoarthritis drug* (S/DMOAD), and *symptomatic slow-acting drug for osteoarthritis* (SYSADOA). Because of variations in the nomenclature and molecular structure of these compounds, care must be taken when one chondroprotectant agent is compared with another. When discussing the effects or comparing the merits of these agents, it is best to use generic compound names rather than trade names or broad descriptive terms (e.g., chondroprotectant, SADMOA). In this chapter, the term *chondroprotectant* is used to bridge the information presented here with that reported elsewhere. Chondroprotective agents have three primary effects:

1. Support or enhance the metabolism of chondrocytes and synoviocytes (anabolic)
2. Inhibit the degradative enzymes within the matrix of synovial fluid and cartilage (catabolic)
3. Inhibit the formation of thrombi in the small blood vessels that supply the joint (antithrombotic)

Many compounds are purported to have chondroprotective effects, including glycosaminoglycans, amino sugars, structural proteins, enzymes, minerals, preparations of whole tissue, and semisynthetic compounds. These compounds are available in oral and injectable forms. Most oral chondroprotectants are classified as dietary supplements. A subset of oral chondroprotectant agents is designated as *nutraceutical*. The North American Veterinary Nutraceutical Council defined a veterinary nutraceutical as "a nondrug substance that is produced in a purified or extracted form and administered orally to provide compounds that are required for normal body structure and function with the intent of improving health and well-being." Injectable chondroprotectants are drugs; these include glycosaminoglycan polysulfate ester, pentosan polysulphate, and hyaluronic acid.

Regulation

In the United States, dietary supplements for humans are regulated under the Dietary Supplements Health and Education Act (DSHEA). This law was enacted to assist consumers in making purchasing decisions about supplements. Although these products must be safe, no premarketing approval is required as is required for pharmaceuticals. The DSHEA does not apply to veterinary dietary supplements. Strict interpretation of the Food, Drug and Cosmetic Act classifies oral veterinary compounds as foods, food additives, or pharmaceuticals. Therefore, the same dietary supplements sold legally under DSHEA for human use are technically unapproved veterinary pharmaceuticals when sold for treatment in animals. However, to date, the Center for Veterinary Medicine has exercised regulatory discretion in allowing veterinary dietary supplements to be used to promote the health and well-being of animal patients. Veterinary dietary supplements have not been forced to withdraw from the market if they are safe, if they pose no risk to the human food supply, and if they do not claim to prevent, treat, cure, or mitigate a disease. Chondroprotective agents that are administered by routes other than the oral route (e.g., topical or injectable agents) are considered drugs and are regulated by the Food and Drug Administration.

Manufacturing and Quality Control

The manufacturing processes used to produce chondroprotectant products vary widely. Manufacturers of chondroprotectant products should follow high standards of quality similar to those practiced by the pharmaceutical industry. To ensure the label accuracy of the product that reaches the consumer, validated analytical methods should be used to test both the raw materials and the finished product for purity and consistency. Problems have been reported with truth-in-labeling and quality control of oral chondroprotectant products. Unfortunately, the consumer cannot always be certain that the ingredients listed on the container actually are present in the product at the claimed concentration or purity. The results of clinical and experimental research on one product cannot be extrapolated to another similar product because of inconsistencies in manufacturing and quality control standards. Until regulation of these products improves, it is probably best to heed the recommendation found in the Arthritis Foundation's Guide to Alternative Therapies: "When a supplement has been studied with good results, find out which brand was used in the study, and buy that brand."

Mechanism of Action

The mechanism of action of many of these products is unknown, whereas other products have been evaluated with experimental and clinical trials. Dietary supplements and nutraceuticals cannot be sold as a treatment for a medical condition. These products cannot be marketed with the intent to diagnose, treat, cure, or prevent disease. They must be marketed as nutrients that support or improve the normal structure and function of the joint.

Chondroprotective agents presumably influence the metabolism of cartilage by providing substrate and up-regulating chondrocytes. They also appear to inhibit degradative enzymes, including metalloproteinases, serine proteases, and free radicals. Finally, some of these products inhibit the formation of microthrombi in the periarticular vasculature, thus supporting a normal blood supply to the joint tissues. The mechanism of action of specific products is discussed later.

Nutraceutical

Glucosamine Hydrochloride, Chondroitin Sulfate, and Manganese Ascorbate. The combination of glucosamine hydrochloride, chondroitin sulfate, and manganese ascorbate is the most commonly used nutraceutical in companion animals that have osteoarthritis. A patented combination of high-purity glucosamine, low-molecular-weight chondroitin sulfate, and manganese ascorbate (Cosequin, Nutramax Laboratories, Edgewood, MD) is an important part of the management of osteoarthritis in dogs and cats.

Cosequin is marketed as a glycosaminoglycan enhancer that provides raw materials that are needed to synthesize endogenous synovial fluid and the extracellular matrix of cartilage. Cosequin contains glucosamine, which is described as the building block of the matrix of articular cartilage. It is a preferential substrate and stimulant of proteoglycan biosynthesis, including the synthesis of hyaluronic acid and chondroitin sulfate. Cosequin also contains chondroitin sulfate, mixed glycosaminoglycans, and manganese ascorbate to promote the production of glycosaminoglycan. Chondroitin sulfate appears to inhibit degradative enzymes associated with osteoarthritis, including metalloproteinases and collagenases. These degradative enzymes break down the cartilage and hyaluronan in synovial fluid. The combined action of glucosamine and chondroitin sulfate is synergistic. Manganese is a cofactor in the synthesis of glycosaminoglycans, and manganese supplementation may aid in the synthesis of the cartilage matrix. Manganese is also necessary for the synthesis of synovial fluid and may have antioxidant properties as well. Overdose safety studies have been conducted with Cosequin in the dog, cat, and horse. These studies found no persistent hematologic, serum chemistry, or hemostatic abnormalities. In addition, no clinically significant side effects were reported in cats or dogs.

Clinical and experimental studies support the use of glucosamine hydrochloride, chondroitin sulfate, and manganese ascorbate in combination or as individual components. Leeb et al. performed a meta-analysis of the clinical efficacy of chondroitin sulfate in humans. Sixteen published studies were examined, and seven trials of 372 patients were selected for the meta-analysis. All of the selected studies were randomized, double-blind designs in parallel groups; however, like human clinical studies, rescue medication (analgesics or NSAIDs) was permitted. According to the Lequesne index (a validated, subjective assessment of pain associated with osteoarthritis), chondroitin sulfate was significantly superior to placebo. Patients in the chondroitin sulfate group showed at least a 50% improvement in study variables compared with the placebo group. A double-blind clinical study in horses showed the efficacy of Cosequin for the treatment of OA associated with navicular disease. Cosequin was given to dogs with osteoarthritis that was induced experimentally through transection of the cranial cruciate ligament. In these dogs, the concentration of cartilage markers increased, indicating synthesis of the cartilage matrix. Glucosamine, chondroitin sulfate, and manganese ascorbate may act as signaling molecules for up-regulation of the genes for aggrecan and collagen II, not just as substrates for cartilage production. Cosequin also suppresses the inflammatory effects of chemically induced acute synovitis and experimental immune-mediated arthritis.

The fate of orally administered chondroitin sulfate appears to be affected by the molecular weight of the molecule. Low-molecular-weight chondroitin sulfate is absorbed in approximately 2 hours and accumulates in the serum over time. Its estimated bioavailability is 200%. Glucosamine hydrochloride is also absorbed in less than 2 hours, but does not accumulate over time. Orally administered glucosamine is readily absorbed and reaches the highest concentrations in the articular cartilage.

Mixed Glycosaminoglycan Products. Many other oral glycosaminoglycan or glucosamine products are available alone or as multiple-ingredient products. Most glycosaminoglycan products contain chondroitin sulfate or "mixed" glycosaminoglycans, and different glucosamine salts are available. There is controversy about the purity, concentration, and type of glycosaminoglycan or glucosamine product necessary to provide beneficial effects to cartilage.

The New Zealand green-lipped mussel (*Perna canaliculus*) contains glycosaminoglycans, omega-3 fatty acids, amino acids, vitamins, and minerals. This product is available as a sole dietary supplement or as an additive in canine diets. *P. canaliculus* may have mild anti-inflammatory and chondroprotective actions, but these effects have not been proven in humans and animals. One study showed beneficial effects in humans with rheumatoid arthritis and osteoarthritis. A recent study in dogs found improvement in joint pain and swelling in arthritic dogs that were fed a complete diet containing 0.3% *P. canaliculus*. No effect was seen on joint crepitus, range of motion, or mobility scores. Although the study concluded that a diet supplemented with *P. canaliculus* can alleviate symptoms of arthritis in dogs, several aspects of the study may be questioned. The dogs used in the study were not definitively diagnosed as having osteoarthritis. Joint swelling, which is not a consistent finding in osteoarthritic joints, was significantly improved. However, joint mobility, range of motion, and crepitus, which are commonly associated with osteoarthritis, showed no improvement. Additionally, control dogs showed marked worsening in joint pain and swelling over the 6-week study period, which is inconsistent with dogs selected for a chronic, slowly progressive condition such as osteoarthritis. This study also included a subjective scoring system, with scores for individual joints added to obtain a total score within the animal. However, certain scores, such as swelling of the hip and shoulder joints, would be difficult to obtain accurately or consistently. For this reason, the validity of the scoring system can be questioned. Further study is warranted before this substance can be recommended as a chondroprotective agent or nutraceutical for dogs with osteoarthritis.

Glucosamine. Glucosamine salt supplements are usually available as glucosamine hydrochloride or glucosamine sulfate. Although both forms are readily available, the hydrochloride form provides more glucosamine per unit weight than the sulfate form. Another form, *N*-acetylglucosamine, appears to have less activity than the hydrochloride and sulfate forms. Glucosamine is commonly found in combination products that include chondroitin sulfate and manganese ascorbate. Glucosamine is an amino sugar that is a precursor to glycosaminoglycans that are present in the extracellular matrix of articular cartilage. Normal chondrocytes synthesize glucosamine, but osteoarthritic cartilage appears to have a decreased ability to synthesize glucosamine. Exogenous glucosamine stimulates the production of proteoglycans and collagen by chondro-cytes in cell culture. Orally or parenterally administered glucosamine has good bioavailability and good distribution to all body tissues. It reaches the highest concentrations in the liver, kidney, and articular cartilage. Oral glucosamine has an intestinal absorption rate of 87%. In clinical and experimental studies in humans, orally administered glucosamine sulfate protected cartilage and relieved the clinical signs of osteoarthritis. Although glucosamine acts more slowly than ibuprofen in relieving the clinical signs of osteoarthritis, two clinical trials in humans found that the long-term efficacy was equal. Oral glucosamine improved clinical performance in humans with osteoarthritis. The use of this product as an individual agent in animals has been proposed, but adequately controlled clinical studies are needed to substantiate its efficacy.

Chondroitin Sulfate. Chondroitin sulfate is a predominant glycosaminoglycan that is found within the extracellular matrix of articular cartilage. Oral supplementation with exogenous chondroitin sulfate has been advocated anecdotally for many years as a treatment for osteoarthritis in humans and animals. This compound is often found in combination with other nutraceuticals, such as glucosamine and free radical scavengers. Chondroitin sulfate decreases the production of interleukin-1, blocks complement activation, inhibits metalloproteinases, inhibits histamine-mediated inflammation, and stimulates glycosaminoglycan and collagen synthesis. Oral absorption of chondroitin sulfate is reported with a variety of techniques. The fate of chondroitin sulfate after oral administration is not known. Various methods have been used to show that chondroitin sulfate is absorbed intestinally, but it is not known whether most of the chondroitin sulfate is absorbed intact or as a subunit of chondroitin sulfate. A highly pure, low-molecular-weight form of chondroitin sulfate has good absorption and bioavailability, and clinical studies showed that humans who received chondroitin sulfate supplementation had improvement in the clinical signs of osteoarthritis.

Free Radical Scavengers. Another class of nutraceutical that may reduce inflammation is free radical scavengers, such as superoxide dismutase, bioflavonoids, glutathione, and dimethyl sulfoxide (DMSO). Oxygen-derived free radicals (e.g., superoxide, hydrogen peroxide, hydroxyl radical) may play a role in the progression of osteoarthritis through their ability to damage cells by oxidative injury. Oxidative injury leads to depolymerization of hyaluronic acid, destruction of collagen, and decreased production of proteoglycans. Superoxide dismutase and glutathione are endogenous antioxidant enzymes that are present in mammalian cells and inhibit the production of oxygen free radicals. Those enzymes stabilize phagocyte cell membranes and lysosomes and reduce the level of superoxide radicals in tissues. The efficacy, bioavailability, and safety of many oral antioxidants are unknown. In addition, because of problems with manufacturing or storage, less active ingredient may be available than is indicated on the label. A recent study found discrepancies in the certificate of analysis and labeled contents in six superoxide dismutase products. Since this study was conducted, several new products have become available that may have resolved this problem.

DMSO, which is used as a topical agent to treat musculoskeletal disorders, penetrates most tissues, including skin. Topical application of 20 mL/day of a medical grade DMSO (70% to 90% solution) every 6 to 8 hours for as long as 14 days is recommended to treat local inflammation. Side effects with topical use are minimal but include a garlic odor to the breath.

Superoxide dismutase is an endogenous antioxidant that is present in mammalian cells and inhibits the production of oxygen free radicals. This enzyme stabilizes phagocyte cell membranes and lysosomes and reduces tissue levels of superoxide radicals, with a resultant decrease in the generation of free radicals. The efficacy of exogenous superoxide dismutase is unknown. One author recommends giving 5 mg subcutaneously for 6 days in the dog, followed by alternate-day therapy for 8 days. The manufacturer recommends giving 2.5 mg/kg subcutaneously five times a week for 2 weeks to treat spondylitis or disk disease. Oral superoxide dismutase products should be given based on manufacturer recommendations.

Bioflavonols are also reported to have strong antioxidant properties. They are believed to scavenge free radicals, alleviate inflammation caused by oxidative damage, and inhibit degradative enzymes released by oxidative cells. One double-blind, randomized study in dogs reported improvement in the clinical signs of hip osteoarthritis in dogs given a supplement containing bioflavonoids, superoxide dismutase, and glutathione. Other clinical studies reported improved function and decreased pain after 2 to 3 weeks of administration in dogs and horses with osteoarthritis. Grapeseed meal is a rich source of bioflavonols. Bioflavonols are available commercially, usually in combination with glucosamine and hydrolyzed collagen or an assortment of other antioxidants, including selenium, vitamin E, and superoxide dismutase.

Methylsulfonylmethane. Methylsulfonylmethane (MSM) is a white, crystalline, water-soluble, odorless, tasteless compound that is sold as a supplement. It is suggested for use in the management of pain and inflammation and as an antioxidant. According to the manufacturer and others, MSM can correct a dietary sulfur deficiency. MSM is a metabolite of industrial-grade DMSO. Although MSM is found naturally in certain foods, it is destroyed during processing. DMSO is a byproduct of the wood pulp processing industry and also is available in a medical grade. In the United States, it is approved only for the treatment of interstitial cystitis. After experimental oral administration of MSM in guinea pigs, radiolabeled sulfur was found in the amino acids (methionine and cysteine) of the animals' proteins. No controlled experimental or clinical studies support the use of MSM for the management of osteoarthritis in dogs. Manufacturers' claims that MSM relieves pain and inflammation are based on the results of studies conducted with DMSO, and little is known about the safety of the product. MSM is sold in capsules for human use and in powder form, tablets, and capsules for use in horses and small animals. Although manufacturer recommendations for dosage should be followed, the use of MSM cannot be unequivocally recommended because little is known about its safety and efficacy.

Omega-3 Fatty Acids. Omega-3 fatty acids recently gained popularity for their potential use in animals with osteoarthritis. These products are available naturally in fish and plant sources and commercially as nutraceutical supplements. Omega-3 fatty acids are desaturated in the body to produce eicosapentaenoic acid, which is an analog of arachidonic acid. Prostaglandins, thromboxanes, and leukotrienes are produced from both of these compounds through the action of cyclooxygenase and lipoxygenase. The products of arachidonic acid metabolism are proinflammatory, proaggregatory, and immunosuppressive. In contrast, the metabolic byproducts of eicosapentaenoic acid are less inflammatory, are vasodilatory, are antiaggregatory, and are not immunosuppressive. Theoretically, omega-3 fatty acids could benefit dogs and cats with osteoarthritis by decreasing inflammation and reducing the occurrence of microthrombi. However, objective data are lacking. The ideal ratio of N6:N3 fatty acids in the canine diet is controversial, but one current recommendation is between 10:1 and 5:1. A recent study reported a lower PGE2 level and reduced clinical and radiographic signs of osteoarthritis in experimental dogs that underwent transection of the cranial cruciate ligament while being fed a diet low in N6 fatty acids.

Chondroprotectant Drugs

Polysulfated Glycosaminoglycan. Adequan (Luitpold Pharmaceuticals, Shirley, NY) is a glycosaminoglycan polysulfate ester (GAGPS) that is available for use in dogs. It is reported to be both chondroprotective and chondrostimulatory. It provides chondroprotection by inhibiting various destructive enzymes and prostaglandins that are associated with synovitis and osteoarthritis. GAGPS inhibits neutral metalloproteinases (e.g., stromelysin, collagenase, elastase), serine proteases, hyaluronidase, and a variety of lysosomal enzymes. It also inhibits the synthesis of PGE_2, the generation of oxygen-derived free radicals, and the complement cascade. In numerous studies, gross and histologic examination also showed protection of articular cartilage. GAGPS stimulates anabolic activity in synoviocytes and chondrocytes. Chondrostimulatory effects are characterized by increased secretion of hyaluronate by synoviocytes and enhanced production of proteoglycan, hyaluronate, and collagen by articular chondrocytes. GAGPS also has anticoagulant and fibrinolytic properties that facilitate the clearing of thrombotic emboli that are deposited in the subchondral and synovial blood vessels. Although most experimental and clinical studies support the premise that GAGPS promotes chondro-protection and chondrostimulation, some studies show either no benefit or a detrimental effect on cartilage metabolism.

A clinical study in dogs with hip dysplasia found the greatest improvement in orthopedic scores at a dose of 4.4 mg/kg (2 mg/lb) given intramuscularly every 3 to 5 days for eight injections. The use of GAGPS in cats also has been reported at the same dose. Another study reported less coxofemoral subluxation in growing pups that were susceptible to hip dysplasia and were given GAGPS 5.0 mg/kg intramuscularly twice weekly from 6 weeks to 8 months of age. The duration of relief provided by GAGPS is unknown. Most studies have evaluated only its short-term effect. In anecdotal reports, the duration of amelioration of the clinical signs ranged from days to months. In addition, it is not known whether the complete series of injections is needed once the clinical signs return or whether a shorter regimen would suffice.

Side effects of GAGPS in dogs include short-term inhibition of the intrinsic coagulation cascade and inhibition of platelet aggregation when given at a dose of 5 mg/kg or 25 mg/kg intramuscularly. Also, GAGPS inhibits neutrophils and complement, which may predispose the patient to infections, especially when the drug is injected intra-articularly under contaminated conditions. GAGPS causes sensitization reactions in humans, but this effect has not been reported in dogs.

Pentosan Polysulphate. Pentosan polysulphate (Cartrophen-Vet, Biopharm Australia, Sydney, Australia) is a polysaccharide sulfate ester with a mean molecular weight of 6000 daltons that is prepared semisynthetically from beech hemicellulose. The drug is approved in Australia for use in dogs and horses. Like Adequan, it is used to relieve the clinical symptoms of DJD. Pentosan polysulphate is administered intra-articularly, intramuscularly, subcutaneously, or orally. The recommended intra-articular dose is 5 to 10 mg per joint weekly, as necessary. The intramuscular or subcutaneous dose in dogs is 3 mg/kg once weekly for 4 weeks. This regimen is repeated as necessary. A double-blind study that evaluated the efficacy of this drug in the treatment of osteoarthritis in dogs found this dose to be ideal. This dose also has been used anecdotally in cats. Oral calcium pentosan polysulphate at a dose of 10 mg/kg weekly for 4 weeks, repeated every 3 months, reduced the presence of cartilage breakdown products in osteoarthritic cartilage.

Sodium hyaluronate is reported to promote joint lubrication, increase the endogenous production of hyaluronate, decrease prostaglandin production, scavenge free radicals, inhibit the migration of inflammatory cells, decrease the permeability of the synovial membrane, protect and promote healing of the articular cartilage, and reduce joint stiffness and the formation of adhesions between tendons and tendon sheaths. The molecule lines the synovial membrane and acts like a sieve that prevents bacteria and inflammatory cells from reaching the synovial compartment by steric hindrance.

The actions of exogenous and endogenous hyaluronan appear to be similar. Sodium hyaluronate is recommended for mild to moderate synovitis and capsulitis rather than osteoarthritis. It appears to have a chondroprotective effect, but it is unclear whether this effect is direct or is a byproduct of the effect of the drug on the articular soft tissues. Sodium hyaluronate is administered intra-articularly or intravenously. When hyaluronate was administered intra-articularly in experimental dogs at a dose of 7 mg per joint once weekly, the progress of osteoarthritis was slowed.

Postoperative Physical Rehabilitation and Chondroprotectant Use

The goal of rehabilitation programs is to improve function and decrease pain in dogs and cats that have musculoskeletal compromise or have undergone orthopedic surgery. Rehabilitation includes a variety of physical modalities that are designed to improve strength, flexibility, and coordination. Chondroprotectants can be used concurrently. These drugs accelerate and enhance recovery by the following mechanisms:

1. They relieve pain to increase the patient's willingness to perform rehabilitation exercises.
2. They reduce the levels of degradative and inflammatory enzymes to help protect the cartilage.
3. They stimulate the production of synovial fluid, proteoglycan, and collagen to promote repair of the cartilage matrix.

Agents that reduce the expression of inflammatory mediators or up-regulate the normal expression of chondrocytes may provide a microenvironment that is favorable for optimal homeostasis of cartilage and connective tissue. A recent study evaluated the effect of a nutraceutical on intra-articular graft ligamentization in dogs that underwent unilateral transection of the cranial cruciate ligament. Cosequin appeared to have two primary effects in this study. It returned the joint capsule or reconstructed cranial cruciate ligament complex to a more physiologic state, and it reduced the severity of osteoarthritis in the treated joints. After transection of the reconstructed cranial cruciate ligaments, translation was similar in the Cosequin group and the control group, suggesting preservation of a more normal, physiologic joint capsule. Dogs that did not receive Cosequin had less translation after transection of the reconstructed cranial cruciate ligament, suggesting thickening and fibrosis of the joint capsule. Dogs that received Cosequin had less severe osteoarthritis, both subjectively as judged by morphologic observation and according to mean modified Mankin scores.

The treated limb may be immobilized postoperatively to provide adjunctive support, restrict use, reduce pain, treat open wounds, or control swelling. Whatever the indication, immobilization can adversely affect joint health. Joint immobilization reduces the production of synovial fluid and leads to depletion of proteoglycan as a result of decreased loading. The changes seen are similar to those observed in osteoarthritic cartilage. Chondroprotectant treatment may reduce damage to the joint during periods of immobilization. To improve and speed joint recovery, immobilization should be limited to the shortest possible time.

Nutrition and Body Condition

Obesity increases the progression of osteoarthritis in humans and likely in animals as well. After weight loss of 5 kg or more, humans who have arthritis experience decreased pain, improved function, and reduced need for medical therapy. Similar improvement is seen in obese, osteoarthritic dogs that undergo weight loss. Body conditioning scores for dogs and cats are available to help assess, document, and monitor the patient's initial body condition as well as changes in body condition over time. On a scale of 1 to 5, a score of 3 is considered ideal. The ideal conformation is as follows: the ribs are palpable but not visible; a waistline is seen behind the ribs when viewed from above; and the abdomen is tucked up when viewed from the side. An important component of a successful weight loss program is careful counseling of the owner. The owner needs to understand the importance of the program and must be committed to adhering to its guidelines. Proper body condition should be maintained in dogs with joint disorders. Overweight dogs are more susceptible to osteoarthritis and exhibit pain and lameness more readily.

Dogs and cats should be fed a fresh, high-quality food. Many good choices are available from reputable pet food manufacturers. Foods can be selected to match the animal's phase of growth, age, physical condition, and general health. Dogs and cats that have joint disorders may benefit from low-calorie foods. Some foods also contain supplements (nutraceuticals, such as N-3 fatty acids, chondroitin sulfate, and glucosamine) that are purported to improve joint health, although the effectiveness of these diets is unknown.

Owners should be assisted when developing and implementing a weight management plan for a pet. The management plan should include dietary modifications and recommendations for exercise. Realistic goals should be set, and regular follow-up visits should be scheduled to assess the animal's progress.

Physical Rehabilitation

Dogs and cats are often affected by conditions that compromise joint function. Osteoarthritis alone likely affects more than 20% of dogs. Osteoarthritis in cats appears to occur much more commonly than previously thought. Regardless of the etiology, chronic joint disease or inflammation often leads to decreased range of motion, chronic pain, and secondary muscle atrophy. Stiff, painful joints and loss of muscle mass dramatically affect a dog's quality of life and athletic performance.

Some dogs have a restricted, stiff gait rather than obvious lameness. Many dogs have trouble rising or posturing to eliminate. Some dogs have a history of joint trauma (e.g., intra-articular fracture, ligamentous injury, dislocation), osteochondral disease (e.g., osteochondrosis, ununited anconeal process, fragmented coronoid process), or congenital deformity (e.g., patellar luxation, hip dysplasia). Cat owners may report that the animal seems to be getting old or frequently seems tired. Traditional methods of minimizing functional loss secondary to joint disease include eliminating underlying causes of disease (e.g., stabilizing the joint, removing an osteochondral flap, improving joint congruity), optimizing body weight (e.g., weight loss), and administering drug therapy (e.g., NSAIDs, chondroprotectants). Physical therapy is an important adjunctive therapy for the treatment of orthopedic disorders in humans. Recently, the importance of incorporating exercise and physical modalities into the treatment of musculoskeletal disorders in dogs has been recognized.

Physical rehabilitation can take many forms. Rehabilitation may require loss of excess body weight, improved cardiovascular conditioning, a supervised exercise program, concomitant medical therapy, and a variety of topically applied physical modalities (e.g., cold therapy, heat therapy, ultrasound therapy, and magnet therapy). When used in reference to animals, the term *physical rehabilitation* is preferred to *physical therapy* because, unlike in humans, no formal licensure is available. The term *rehabilitation* also conveys a broader scope of management than the term *therapy*. To obtain the best results, each patient must be assessed independently and a program designed to meet the patient's specific needs. The use of a cookbook approach that is the same for every patient leads to suboptimal results.

Exercise. Although once contraindicated in patients with osteoarthritis, exercise is now believed to be beneficial. Frequent, low-impact exercise is preferable to high-impact or prolonged exercise. Moderate exercise is believed to diminish the likelihood that osteoarthritis will develop. Exercise offers several benefits. Moderate activity enhances chondrocyte metabolism, leading to increased production of proteoglycans. In contrast, proteoglycan content is decreased in the articular cartilage of immobilized joints. Joint motion is also important for optimal cartilage nutrition. Nutrients diffuse from the synovial fluid into the cartilage. This action is enhanced by a pumping motion that is created during joint motion. Exercise benefits the joint and improves muscle strength and flexibility. Because muscles and ligaments work together to support the joint, it is important to encourage good muscle tone and resiliency.

The goals of therapeutic exercise are to reduce body weight, increase joint mobility, improve cardiovascular condition, and reduce joint pain through the use of non-weightbearing or low-impact weightbearing exercises that are designed to strengthen supporting muscles. However, before an exercise program is initiated, underlying inflammation or predisposing problems must be treated.

If necessary, joint stability and congruity should be corrected surgically. Initially, anti-inflammatory drugs should not be administered before exercise because it is important to determine whether the exercise program is too strenuous and causes pain. After the appropriate level of exercise is determined, oral anti-inflammatory drugs are administered about 1 hour before exercise as necessary. Acceptable forms of exercise include walking on a flat surface, walking in high grass or sand to increase the range of motion in the joint, walking in a pool, swimming, slowly climbing a ramp or stairs, sitting and standing repeatedly, holding up the opposite limb, performing passive range of motion exercises, and wheelbarrow walking. Exercise sessions should be short initially, usually 5 to 10 minutes. The length and intensity of the session can be increased slowly as tolerated. A 5- to 10-minute cooldown period is recommended after each exercise session is completed.

External devices are used topically to encourage joint and muscle health. The use of most of these devices requires appropriate education and proper training. Modalities that have been proposed for rehabilitation include superficial heat therapy, superficial cold therapy, massage, hydrotherapy, ultrasound therapy, and electrotherapy. Most of these techniques are unproven in dogs, and their use is extrapolated from their application in humans.

Topical Treatment

Superficial Application of Heat. Application of superficial heat is recommended after inflammation and edema subside. Because heat is soothing and increases blood flow to the affected region, it decreases pain, increases the range of motion in the joint, and improves muscle flexibility. Superficial heating agents typically heat the skin and subcutaneous tissue to a depth of 1 to 2 cm, although deeper tissues may be heated through conduction, especially with long application times. Usually, the tissue is heated to 40° to 45°C for 15 to 20 minutes one to two times daily to promote hyperemia. Heat may be applied with hot water packs; moist, heated towels; heated, rice-filled stockings; or circulating water blankets. To prevent accidental burns, the temperature of the heating instrument should be tested by holding it against the therapist's skin for 30 seconds. Electric blankets are not recommended because of the increased chance of burns.

Superficial Application of Cold. Application of superficial cold is useful if inflammation or edema is present. This therapy is especially valuable for the first 2 to 3 days after surgery. Cooling the affected tissue causes vasoconstriction and reduces vascular permeability. As a result, swelling and inflammation are decreased. Cold therapy is applied with commercial cold packs, towels soaked in cold water, or plastic bags filled with water and ice. The affected area also can be immersed in a cold water bath. To increase comfort, a thin cloth towel can be placed on the skin before the cold pack is applied. Cold therapy is applied for 15 to 20 minutes two to three times daily until inflammation and edema resolve.

Other Modalities

Massage, hydrotherapy, shock wave, ultrasound, and electrotherapy also can help to rehabilitate patients with musculoskeletal compromise. The use of these modalities requires special training. This training can be obtained through the University of Tennessee College of Veterinary Medicine (Dr. Darryl Millis) or at various national veterinary meetings. Indications and methods are described elsewhere.

Suggested Readings

Adebowale A, Cox D, Liang Z, et al: Analysis of glucosamine and chondroitin sulfate content in marketed products and the Caco-2 permeability of chondroitin sulfate raw materials. JANA 3:37–44, 2000.

Altman RD, Dean DD, Muniz OE, et al: Prophylactic treatment of canine osteoarthritis with glycosaminoglycan polysulfuric acid ester. Arthritis Rheum 32:759–766, 1989.

Altman RD, Dean DD, Muniz OE, et al: Therapeutic treatment of canine osteoarthritis with glycosaminoglycan polysulfuric acid ester. Arthritis Rheum 32:1300–1307, 1989.

Anderson MA: Oral chondroprotectant agents: Part 1. Compend Contin Educ Pract Vet 21:601–609, 1999.

Auer DE, Ng JC, Seawright AA: Effect of palosein (superoxide dismutase) and catalase upon oxygen derived free radical induced degradation of equine synovial fluid. Equine Vet J 22:13–17, 1990.

Basleer C: Stimulation of proteoglycan production by glucosamine sulfate in chondrocytes isolated from human osteoarthritic articular cartilage in vitro. Osteoarthritis Cartil 6:427–434, 1998.

Beale BS: Evaluation of active enzyme in six oral superoxide dismutase products. Veterin Comparative Orthopaedics and Traumatology 11(4):A68, 1998.

Beale BS: The role of chondroprotectants and nutraceuticals in osteoarthritic dogs and cats. In Millis D, Taylor R (eds): Physical Rehabilitation in Dogs and Cats. Philadelphia, WB Saunders (in press).

Beale BS, Clemmons RM, Goring RL: The effect of a semi-synthetic polysulfated glycosaminoglycan on coagulation and primary hemostasis in the dog. Vet Surg 19:57, 1990.

Beale BS, Goring RL: Degenerative joint disease. In Bojrab MJ (ed): Disease Mechanisms in Small Animal Surgery. Philadelphia, Lea and Febiger, 1993, pp 727–736.

Beren J, Hill SL, Diener-West M, et al: The effect of pre-loading oral glucosamine/chondroitin sulfate/manganese ascorbate combination on experimental arthritis in rats. Exp Biol Med 226:144–152, 2001.

Boothe DM: Nutraceuticals in veterinary medicine: Part 1. Compend Contin Educ Pract Vet 19:1248–1255, 1997.

Bourgeois P, Charles G, Dehais J, et al: Efficacy and tolerability of chondroitin sulfate 1200 mg/day vs 3 × 400 mg/day vs placebo. Osteoarthritis Cartil 6(Suppl A):25–30, 1998.

Bucsi L, Poor G: Efficacy and tolerability of oral chondroitin sulfate as a symptomatic slow-acting drug for osteoarthritis (SYSADOA) in the treatment of knee osteoarthritis. Osteoarthritis Cartil 6 (Suppl A):31–36, 1998.

Budsberg S, Barteges J, Schoenherr W, et al: Effects of different N6:N3 fatty acid diets on canine stifle osteoarthritis. Proceedings of the 28th Annual Veterinary Orthopedic Society Meeting, Feb. 24–Mar. 3, 2001, Lake Louise, Canada, p 40.

Bui LM, Pawlowski K, Bierer TL: Influence of green lipped mussels (Perna canaliculus) in alleviating signs of arthritis in dogs. Poster at Experimental Biology 2000 (meeting), April 15–18, 2000, San Diego, CA, program 160.9.

Burkholder W, Taylor L, Hulse D: Weight loss to optimal body condition increases ground reactive force in dogs with OA.

Proceedings of the Purina Nutrition Symposium, St. Louis, MO, August 2000.

Canapp SO, McLaughlin RM, Hoskinson JJ, et al: Scintigraphic evaluation of glucosamine HCL and chondroitin sulfate as treatment for acute synovitis in dogs. AJVR 60:1552–1557, 1999.

Carreno MR, Muniz OE, Howell DS: The effect of glycosaminoglycan polysulfuric acid ester on articular cartilage in experimental osteoarthritis: effects on morphological variables of disease severity. J Rheumatol 13:490–497, 1986.

D'Ambrosio E, Casa B, Bompani R, et al: Glucosamine sulfate: a controlled clinical investigation in arthrosis. Pharmacotherapeutica 2:504–508, 1981.

Das AK, Hammad TA: Efficacy of a combination of FCHG49™ glucosamine hydrochloride, TRH122™ low molecular weight sodium chondroitin sulfate and manganese ascorbate in the management of knee osteoarthritis. Osteoarthritis Cartil 8:343–350, 2000.

Davidson G: Glucosamine and chondroitin sulfate. Compend Contin Educ Pract Vet 36:454–458, 2000.

de Haan JJ, Goring RL, Beale BS: Evaluation of polysulfated glycosaminoglycan for the treatment of hip dysplasia in dogs. Vet Surg 23:177–181, 1994.

Dettmer N, Nowack H, Raake W: Platelet aggregation by heparin and arteparon. Munch Med Wochenschr 125:540–542, 1983.

Edington ND, Du J, Liang Z, et al: Bioavailability and disposition of the dietary supplements TRH 122 Glucosamine and FCHG 49 Chondroitin sulfate in dogs after single and multiple dosing. Amer Assoc of Pharmaceutical Scientists 3(3):W417, 2001.

Egg D: Effects of glycosaminoglycan polysulfate and two nonsteroidal anti-inflammatory drugs on prostaglandin E$_2$ synthesis in Chinese hamster ovary cell cultures. Pharmacol Res 15:709–717, 1983.

Felson DT, Zhang Y, Anthony JM, et al: Weight loss reduces the risk for symptomatic knee osteoarthritis in women. Ann Intern Med 116:535, 1992.

Ghosh P, Smith M, Wells C: Second-line agents in osteoarthritis. In Dixon JS, Furst DE (eds): Second-Line Agents in the Treatment of Rheumatic Diseases. New York, Marcel Dekker, 1993, pp 363–427.

Hannen N, Ghosh P, Bellenger C, et al: Systemic administration of glycosaminoglycan polysulphate provides partial protection of articular cartilage from damage produced by meniscectomy in the canine. Orthop Res 5:47–59, 1987.

Hansen RR, Smalley LR, Huff GK, et al: Oral treatment with a glucosamine-chondroitin sulfate compound for degenerative joint disease in horses: 25 cases. Equine Pract 19:16–22, 1997.

Hellio MP, Vigron E, Annefeld M: The effects of glucosamine on the human osteoarthritic chondrocyte: In vitro investigations. Proceedings of the 9th Eular Symposium, Basel, Switzerland, 1996, pp 11–12.

Hill's Pet Nutrition, Inc. Body Condition Scoring System Poster, Topeka, KS, 1996.

Howard RD, McIlwraith CW: Sodium hyaluronate in the treatment of equine joint disease. Compend Cont Educ Pract Vet 15:473–481, 1993.

Hulse DA, Hart RC, Slatter M, et al: The effect of Cosequin in cranial cruciate deficient and reconstructed stifle joints in dogs. Veterinary Comparative Orthopedics and Traumatology 11(4):A68, 1998.

Hulse DS: Treatment methods for pain in the osteoarthritic patient. Vet Clin North Am Small Anim Pract 28:361, 1998.

Hungerford D, Navarro J, Hammad T: Use of nutraceuticals in the management of osteoarthritis. JANA 3:23–27, 2000.

Impellizeri JA, Lau RE, Azzara FA: A 14 week clinical evaluation of an oral antioxidant as a treatment for osteoarthritis secondary to canine hip dysplasia. Vet Q 20(Suppl 1): S107–108, 1998.

Innes JF, Barr AR, Sharif M: Efficacy of oral calcium pentosan polysulphate for the treatment of osteoarthritis of the canine stifle joint secondary to cranial cruciate ligament deficiency. Vet Rec 146:433–437, 2000.

Jimenez SA, Dodge GR: The effects of glucosamine on human chondrocyte gene expression. Proceedings of the 9th Eular Symposium, Basel, Switzerland, 1996, pp 8–10.

Johnson KA, Hulse DA, Hart RC, et al: Effects of an orally administered mixture of chondroitin sulfate, glucosamine hydrochloride and manganese ascorbate on synovial fluid chondroitin sulfate 3B3 and 7D4 epitope in a canine cranial cruciate transection model of osteoarthritis. Osteoarthritis Cartil 9:14–21, 2001.

Karzel K, Domenjoz R: Effect of hexosamine derivatives and uronic acid derivatives on glycosaminoglycan metabolism on fibroblast cultures. Pharmacology 5:337–345, 1971.

Kirker-Head RP: Safety of an oral chondroprotective agent in horses. Vet Ther 2:345–353, 2001.

Kuck JC, Mulnix JA: Clinical evaluation of an antioxidant joint nutrient and relief of the signs of pain associated with osteoarthritis and gait irregularities in the horse. Proprietary data. Animal Health Options, Golden, CO, 2001.

Kuck JC, Mulnix JA: Clinical evaluation of an antioxidant joint nutrient and relief of the signs of pain associated with osteoarthritis in the dog. Proprietary data. Animal Health Options, Golden, CO, 2001.

Leeb BF, Schweitzer H, Montag K, Smolen J: A metaanalysis of chondroitin sulfate in the treatment of osteoarthritis. J Rheumatol 27:205–211, 2000.

Leffler CT, Philippi AF, Leffler SG, et al: Glucosamine, chondroitin and manganese ascorbate for degenerative joint disease of the knee or low back: a randomized, double-blind, placebo-controlled pilot study. Mil Med 164:85–91, 1999.

Li Hirondel JL: Double-blind clinical study with oral administration of chondroitin sulfate versus placebo in tibiofemoral gonarthrosis. Litera Rheumatol 14:77–82, 1992.

Lippiello L, Woodward J, Karpman R, et al: Chondroprotection and metabolic synergy of glucosamine and chondroitin sulfate. Clin Orthop 381:229–240, 2000.

Lust G, Williams AJ, Burton-Wurster N, et al: Effects of intramuscular administration of glycosaminoglycan polysulfates on signs of incipient hip dysplasia in growing pups. Am J Vet Res 53:1836–1843, 1992.

McGoey BV, Deitel M, Saplys RJ, et al: Effect of weight loss on musculoskeletal pain in the morbidly obese. J Bone Joint Surg Br 72:323, 1990.

McNamara PS, Barr SC, Erb HN: Hematologic, hemostatic and biochemical effects in dogs receiving an oral chondroprotective agent for thirty days. AJVR 57:1390–1394, 1996.

McNamara PS, Barr SC, Erb HN, et al: Hematologic, hemostatic and biochemical effects in cats receiving an oral chondroprotective agent for thirty days. Vet Ther 1:108–117, 2000.

McNamara PS, Johnston SA, Todhunter RJ: Slow-acting, disease-modifying osteoarthritic agents. Vet Clin North Am Small Anim Pract 27:863–867, 951–952, 1997.

Millis DL, Levine D: The role of exercise and physical modalities in the treatment of osteoarthritis. Vet Clin North Am Small Anim Pract 27:913–930, 1997.

Mulnix JA: Promotion study, canine formula. Proprietary data. Animal Health Options, Golden, CO, 2001.

Nishikawa H, Mori I, Umemoto J: Influences of sulfated glycosaminoglycans on hyaluronic acid in rabbit knee synovia. Arch Biochem Biophys 240:146–148, 1985.

O'Grady CP, Marwin SE, Grande DA: Effects of glucosamine hydrochloride, chondroitin sulfate, and manganese-ascorbate on cartilage metabolism. Proceedings of the 68th Annual Meeting of the American Academy of Orthopedic Surgeons, San Francisco, CA, 2001, p 157.

Rashmir-Raven AM, Coyne CP, Fenwick BW, et al: Inhibition of equine complement activity by polysulfated glycosaminoglycans. Am J Vet Res 53: 87–90, 1992.

Read R, Cullis-Hill D: The systemic use of the chondroprotective agent pentosan polysulfate in the treatment of osteoarthritis: Results of a double-blind clinical trial in dogs. J Small Anim Pract 37:108–114, 1996.

Schiavinato A, Lini E, Guidolin D, et al: Intraarticular sodium hyaluronate injections in the pond-nuki experimental model of osteoarthritis in dogs: II. Morphological findings. Clin Orthop 241:286–299, 1989.

Setnikar I, Giacchetti C, Zanolo G: Pharmacokinetics of glucosamine in dog and in man. Arzneimittelforschung Drug Res 36:703–705, 1986.

Setniker I, Giaccheti C, Zanolo G: Pharmacokinetics of glucosamine in the dog and in man. Arzneimittelforschung 36:729, 1991.

Smith G: Influence of diet and age on subjective hip score and hip OA: a life long study in Labrador retrievers. Proceedings of the 29th Annual Meeting of the Veterinary Orthopedic Society, The Canyons, Utah, March 3–8, 2002, p 41.

Smith MM, Ghosh P: The effect of polysulfated polysaccharides on hyaluronate (HA) synthesis by human synovial fibroblasts. Agents Actions 18:55–62, 1986.

Tsuboi I, Matsuura T, Shichijo T, et al: Effects of glycosaminoglycan polysulfate on human neutrophil function. Jpn J Inflamm 8:131–135, 1988.

Vaz AL: Double-blind clinical evaluation of the relative efficacy of ibuprofen and glucosamine sulphate in the management of osteoarthrosis of the knee in outpatients. Curr Med Res Opin 8:145–149, 1982.

Verbruggen G, Goemaere S, Veys EM: Chondroitin sulfate: S/DMOAD (structure/disease modifying anti-osteoarthrosis drug) in the treatment of finger joint OA. Osteoarthritis Cartil 6 (Suppl A):39–46, 1998.

Verbruggen G, Veys EM: The effect of sulfated glycosaminoglycan on the proteoglycan metabolism of synovial lining cells. Acta Rheumatol Belg 1:75–92, 1971.

Verbruggen G, Veys EM: Treatment of chronic degenerative joint disorders with a glycosaminoglycan polysulfate. In Proceedings of the Euler IX European Congress on Rheumatology. Basel, Switzerland, 1980, pp 51–69.

von der Mark K: Collagen synthesis in cultures of chondrocytes as effected by arteparon. In Proceedings of the Euler IX European Congress on Rheumatology. Basel, Switzerland, 1980, pp 39–50.

Appendix: Manufacturers of Arthroscopic Equipment

Arthrex
2885 South Horseshoe Drive
Naples, FL 34104
Phone: 800-934-4404
Fax: 800-643-9310
http://www.arthrex.com/

ArthroCare Corporation
680 Vaqueros Avenue
Sunnyvale, CA 94085-3523
Phone: 800-348-8929 or 408-736-0224
Fax: 408-736-0226
http://www.arthrocare.com/

Instrument Makar, Inc.
2950 East Mount Hope
Okemos, MI 48864
PO Box 885
Okemos, MI 48805
Phone: 517-332-3593
Fax: 517-332-2043
http://www.instmak.com/

Karl Storz Veterinary Endoscopy
175 Cremona Drive
Goleta, CA 93117
Phone: 800-955-7832 or 805-968-7776
Fax: 805-685-2588
E-mail: info@karlstorzvet.com
http://www.ksvea.com/

Linvatec Customer Service
Phone: 800-237-0169
Fax: 727-399-5256
E-mail: cust_serv@linvatec.com
http://www.linvatec.com/

ORATEC Interventions, Inc.
3700 Haven Court
Menlo Park, CA 94025
Phone: 888-996-1996 or 650-369-9904
Fax: 650-369-9913
http://www.oratec.com/

Richard Wolf Medical Instruments Corporation
353 Corporate Woods Parkway
Vernon Hills, IL 60061
Phone: 847-913-1113
Fax: 847-913-1488
http://www.richard-wolf.com/

Smith-Nephew, Inc.
150 Minuteman Road
Andover, MD 01810
Phone: 800-343-5717
Fax: 978-748-1599
http://www.smith-nephew.com/

Spectrum Instruments (Dr. Fritz distributor)
4575 Hudson Drive
Stow, OH 44224
Phone: 800-444-5644 or 330-686-4550
Fax: 330-686-4555
E-mail: sales@spectrumsurgical.com
http://www.spectrumsurgical.com/

Stryker Endoscopy
2590 Walsh Avenue
Santa Clara, CA 95051
Phone: 800-624-4422 or 408-567-9100
Fax: 800-729-2917 or 408-567-2503
http://www.strykerendo.com/

3M Corporation
Phone: 888-364-3577
http://www.3m.com/US/

Index

Note: Page numbers followed by f indicate an illustration; page numbers followed by t indicate a table.